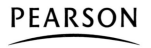

ALLYN & BACON AND MERRILL EDUCATION
RELATED TITLES OF INTEREST FOR CLASSROOM
USE AND PROFESSIONAL DEVELOPMENT

Articulatory and Phonological Impairments: A Clinical Focus, 3/e, Jacqueline Bauman-Waengler, © 2008, ISBN: 020554925X

Introduction to Phonetics and Phonology: From Concepts to Transcription, Jacqueline Bauman-Waengler, © 2009, ISBN: 0205402879

Audiologic Interpretation Across the Lifespan, Debra Busacco, © 2010, ISBN: 0205463983

The Development of Language, 7/e, Jean Berko Gleason and Nan Bernstein Ratner, © 2009, ISBN: 0205593038

Language and Communication Disorders in Children, 6/e, Deena K. Bernstein and Ellenmorris Tiegerman-Farber, © 2008, ISBN: 0205584616

Articulation and Phonological Disorders, 6/e, John E. Bernthal, Nicholas W. Bankson, and Peter Flipsen Jr., © 2008, ISBN: 0205569269

The Voice and Voice Therapy, 8/e, Daniel R. Boone, Stephen C. McFarlane, Shelley L. Von Berg, Richard I. Zraick, © 2010, ISBN: 0205609538

Language Development: Monolingual and Bilingual Acquisition, Alejandro E. Brice and Roanne Brice, © 2008, ISBN: 0131700510

Survey of Audiology: Fundamentals for Audiologists and Health Professionals, 2/e, David A. DeBonis and Constance L. Donohue, © 2008, ISBN: 0205531954

Diagnosis and Evaluation in Speech Pathology, 7/e, William O. Haynes and Rebekah H. Pindzola, © 2008, ISBN: 020552432X

Understanding Research and Evidence-Based Practice in Communication Disorders: A Primer for Students and Practitioners, William O. Haynes and Carole E. Johnson, © 2008, ISBN: 0205453635

Aural Rehabilitation: A Transdisciplinary Approach, Carole E. Johnson, © 2010, ISBN: 0205424171

Communication Sciences and Disorders: An Introduction, 2/e, Laura M. Justice, © 2010, ISBN: 0135022800

Teaching Students with Language and Communication Disabilities, 3/e, S. Jay Kuder, © 2008, ISBN: 0205531059

Introduction to Audiology (with CD-ROM), 10/e, Frederick N. Martin and John Greer Clark, © 2008, ISBN: 0205593119

Childhood Language and Literacy Disorders in Context: Infancy Through Adolescence, Nickola W. Nelson, © 2010, ISBN: 0205501788

Language Development: An Introduction, 7/e, Robert E. Owens Jr., © 2008, ISBN: 0205525563

Language Disorders: A Functional Approach to Assessment and Intervention, 5/e, Robert E. Owens, Jr., © 2010, ISBN: 0205607640

Linguistics for Non-Linguists: A Primer with Exercises, 5/e, Frank Parker and Kathryn Riley, © 2010, ISBN: 0137152043

Language Development: From Theory to Practice, Khara L. Pence and Laura M. Justice, © 2008, ISBN: 0131708139

Foundations of Audiology: A Practical Approach, Miles E. Peterson and Theodore S. Bell, © 2008, ISBN: 0131185683

Communication and Communication Disorders: A Clinical Introduction, 3/e, Elena M. Plante and Pélagie M. Beeson, © 2008, ISBN: 0205532098

Building ASL Interpreting and Translation Skills: Narratives for Practice (with DVD), Nanci A. Scheetz, © 2008, ISBN: 0205470254

Language Disorders in Children: Real Families, Real Issues, and Real Interventions, Ellenmorris Tiegerman-Farber and Christine Radziewicz, © 2008, ISBN: 0130915769

FOR A FULL LISTING OF THE LATEST RESOURCES OF INTEREST, BROWSE OUR ONLINE CATALOG AT

www.pearsonhighered.com

EIGHTH EDITION

The Voice and Voice Therapy

Daniel R. Boone
University of Arizona

Stephen C. McFarlane
University of Nevada Medical School

Shelley L. Von Berg
California State University, Chico

Richard I. Zraick
University of Arkansas for Medical Sciences
University of Arkansas at Little Rock

Allyn & Bacon

Boston   New York   San Francisco
Mexico City   Montreal   Toronto   London   Madrid   Munich   Paris
Hong Kong   Singapore   Tokyo   Cape Town   Sydney

Executive Editor and Publisher: Stephen D. Dragin
Editorial Assistant: Anne Whittaker
Marketing Manager: Jared Brueckner
Production Editor: Gregory Erb
Editorial Production Service: Omegatype Typography, Inc.
Composition Buyer: Linda Cox
Manufacturing Buyer: Megan Cochran
Electronic Composition: Omegatype Typography, Inc.
Interior Design: Omegatype Typography, Inc.
Cover Designer: Linda Knowles

For related titles and support materials, visit our online catalog at www.pearsonhighered.com.

Between the time website information is gathered and then published, it is not unusual for some sites to have closed. Also, the transcription of URLs can result in unintended typographical errors. The publisher would appreciate notification where these errors occur so that they may be corrected in subsequent editions.

Library of Congress Cataloging-in-Publication Data

The voice and voice therapy / Daniel R. Boone . . . [et al.].—8th ed.
   p. cm.
  Includes bibliographical references and index.
  ISBN-13: 978-0-205-60953-6 (hardcover)
  ISBN-10: 0-205-60953-8 (hardcover)
 1. Voice disorders—Textbooks.   I. Boone, Daniel R.
  RF540.B66   2010
  616.85'506—dc22

                     2008043476

Printed in the United States of America

10   9   8   7   6   5   4   HAM   13   12   11

Allyn & Bacon
is an imprint of

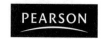

www.pearsonhighered.com

ISBN-10: 0-205-60953-8
ISBN-13: 978-0-205-60953-6

ABOUT THE AUTHORS

Daniel R. Boone celebrates his 55th year as a speech-language pathologist with the publishing of this eighth edition of *The Voice and Voice Therapy*. Dr. Boone has held professorships over the years at Case Western Reserve University, University of Kansas Medical Center, University of Denver, and the University of Arizona (where he is now a professor emeritus).

Dr. Boone is a former president of the American Speech-Language-Hearing Association and holds both a fellowship and the honors of that organization. He is the author of over 100 publications and is well known nationally and internationally for his many lecture and workshop presentations. Perhaps Dr. Boone is best known for his love of his students and turning them on to the excitement of clinical voice practice.

Stephen C. McFarlane is a professor emeritus at the School of Medicine at the University of Nevada, Reno. He received ASHA honors in 1999. He received both his B.S. and M.S. from Portland State University and his Ph.D. from the University of Washington. Dr. McFarlane has a long history of research interests in the area of voice disorders. Study of the outcomes from voice therapy and the development of new treatment techniques is of particular interest. He has been published in dozens of books and journals, among them *Seminars in Speech and Language, American Journal of Speech Language Pathology, Phonoscope*, and *Current Opinion in Otolaryngology & Head and Neck Surgery*.

Shelley L. Von Berg teaches, practices, and researches in the areas of voice, dysphagia, and motor speech disorders in adults and children at the department of communication sciences and disorders at California State University, Chico. She earned her M.S. and Ph.D. from the School of Medicine at the University of Nevada, Reno. She has presented on the assessment and intervention of neurogenic speech-language disorders nationally and abroad. Dr. Von Berg has been published in the ASHA *Leader* Series; *Unmasking Voice Disorders; Language, Speech, and Hearing Services in Schools; Current Opinion in Otolaryngology & Head and Neck Surgery;* and *Cleft Palate-Craniofacial Journal*.

Richard I. Zraick is an associate professor in the department of audiology and speech pathology at the University of Arkansas for Medical Sciences and the University of Arkansas at Little Rock. He was awarded his doctorate in 1998 by Arizona State University. Dr. Zraick is a clinician and scholar with over 20 years of experience in private practice and academia. His research grants, journal articles, and book chapters are in the areas of voice disorders, neurogenic speech-language disorders, speech and voice perception, and clinical skills training. He has been invited to speak about these topics at state, regional, and national scientific and professional conventions. In 2003 he was honored with a Faculty Excellence in Research Award by UALR, and in 2004 he was honored with a Faculty Excellence in Teaching Award by UAMS.

CONTENTS

5 Functional Voice Disorders   113

8 Management and Therapy for Special Problems 247

Therapy for Resonance Disorders   276

8 Management and Therapy for Special Problems   247

Therapy for Resonance Disorders   276

CONTENTS TO THE DVD

Case Studies

Facilitating Approaches (See Table 7.1 in text)

Laryngeal Images Photo Gallery

PREFACE

The original edition of *The Voice and Voice Therapy* was written in the late 1960s and first published in 1971. The preface to this first edition concluded with a statement that has as much relevance today as it did some forty years ago:

> *The Voice and Voice Therapy* is an attempt to take some of the magic out of voice therapy. I hope there is something here not only for the student of voice therapy, but also for the clinical speech pathologist and the practicing laryngologist. I think there is.

The "magic" in voice therapy is still there and it always will be. This magic is related to the art of applying science and clinical knowledge to the people receiving voice therapy.

The reader will see that our present knowledge of airway and laryngeal structures remains similar to the anatomical knowledge base of yesteryear; however, vast differences are quickly apparent in our early chapters describing our present understanding of the physiology of respiration, phonation, and resonance. Also, huge advances in equipment and instrumentation permit us to actually portray laryngeal physiology as it is happening. Our new voice assessment in Chapter 6 encourages the speech–language pathologist (SLP) to measure aspects of airway/laryngeal physiology, such as measuring various air volumes and pressures or recording the nuances of vocal frequency, intensity, and perturbation, or determining structural/physiologic variances contributing to faulty oral or nasal resonance. The four authors of this eighth edition have collected an extensive literature representing the latest scientific and clinical publications developed by an expanding collection of national and international investigators.

Despite our expanded science base, clinical voice writers are always faced with the question: "In voice therapy, does known science support the art?" Paul Moore posed this question in his seminal article, "Have the Major Issues in Voice Disorders Been Answered by Research in Speech Science? A 50-Year Retrospective," in the *Journal of Speech Hearing Disorders* (1977). In many personal (D.R.B.) discussions with Moore over the years at professional meetings and a few workshops we did together, Moore thoughtfully answered his question with a big "NO." He realized that when we apply our scientific knowledge to the person in the voice clinic, the "art of application" becomes the prominent factor. For example, the physician or SLP working with patients having voice disorders primarily uses an individual knowledge base; when and where the professional was trained can be a limiting or enhancing factor. Another example is the laboratory that may answer every voice question through a particular research bias or causative "filter." Or the clinical setting's time and cost constraints will have an obvious impact on application. Moreover, the quality of the clinician–client relationship will play a direct role in the outcome of therapy.

In Chapters 7, 8, and 9, we present management and therapy suggestions for children and adults. We recognize that the typical voice client has very little background specific to the anatomy and physiology of the larynx and vocal mechanisms. Therefore, what we present to the clients must be in language they can understand. You will see that in our beginning voice therapy sessions, we employ some therapy techniques as "diagnostic probes" to see whether the probes are effective in positively changing the voice. In Chapter 7, we present the view that voice therapy is highly individualized. The client's response dictates the order and the approaches to be used. We recommend that, in this therapy management chapter, the SLP should develop a number of management and therapy techniques beyond the minimal 25 presented in the chapter.

Today, in all of the healing arts there are growing concerns about evidence-based practice. Medical, social, and psychological clinical services are placing more emphasis on outcome data. Voice therapy is similarly challenged. Throughout this text, in discussing evaluation and therapy, we have attempted to present literature citations that support SLP intervention and management of voice disorders. Under the umbrella name "voice therapy," there are perhaps hundreds of literature studies reporting particular outcome benefits from particular therapy regimens. These positive outcome data are usually generated from pre- and posttherapy comparison measurements, and, while lacking a comparison no-therapy control group, they can offer high construct validity. There are a few voice clinical studies that offer one therapy technique for a population with a particular clinical problem, comparing it with a control group of similar patients who did not receive the particular intervention. Besides being ethically questionable (such as denying a voice patient therapy because he or she is in a control group), such studies may well lack clinical validity for generalized application. As this eighth edition of this text comes to print, there appears fortunately to be an emerging literature specific to the value of voice therapy in children and adults. The query for evidence-based practice is a welcoming stimulus for the SLP community to develop studies that look at therapy effectiveness.

As *The Voice and Voice Therapy* evolved over the years, the senior author needed to enlarge his knowledge base. Accordingly, the fourth edition (1988) added a co-author, Stephen C. McFarlane (former department head, dean of the Medical School, and finally the president of the University of Nevada at Reno). Dr. McFarlane has played an active and vital role in the last four editions, particularly in the use of instrumentation for both voice diagnosis and therapy with emphasis given to acoustic analyses and videostroboscopy. While on many visits to Reno working in collaboration with McFarlane, I became aware of the clinical genius of Shelley L. Von Berg. My direct observation of Dr. Von Berg and her students showed a continuous array of positive therapy outcomes for children with muscle tension dysphonia and adults with various neurogenic problems. With Dr. McFarlane's blessings, we added Dr. Von Berg as a seventh edition co-author.

Dr. Richard I. Zraick has been a very active clinical investigator in the past decade looking at the science/art dimensions of voice therapy, developing a literature on patient self-perceptions of voice quality and improvement and executing critical examinations of evidence-based practice. I know the intensive work ethic of Dr. Zraick firsthand as he earned both undergraduate and master's of science degrees at the University of Arizona. He later went on for doctoral study in voice with Dr. James Case at Arizona State University, where he was awarded his Ph.D. in 1998. Our profession's increasing demand for evidence-based practice and Dr. Zraick's long interest in this area made him a strong selection as a new co-author of the eighth edition of *The Voice and Voice Therapy.* When Dr. Zraick accepted our invitation to author parts of the book, he readily accepted the invitation, with the request of dedicating his part of the book to one of his mentors, the late Dr. James L. Case.

In this eighth edition, we have replaced much of the old text, placed increased focus on the book's pedagogy value, increased its clinical practicality, and expanded our DVD portrayals of both voice evaluation and therapy.

CHAPTER OVERVIEWS

Chapter 1, The Voice and Voice Therapy, introduces the reader to the biological, emotional, and linguistic role of the larynx. New to this chapter are prevalence data on voice disorders among populations at risk, such as teachers and children. Also, we have introduced four distinct categories to allow for easy identification of voice disordered populations. These categories are expanded on throughout the text.

Chapter 2, The Normal Voice, retains its strong foundation of the normal aspects of laryngeal and voice functions; however, this edition features new illustrations and expanded text to give the reader an increased appreciation of the anatomy and physiology of the vocal tract structures. In addition, a new section on changes of the larynx across the lifespan is intended to help the SLP work effectively with clients of all ages. This chapter continues to serve as a functional review of the readers' studies in speech and voice science as well as anatomy and physiology for speech and voice.

Chapter 3, Organic Voice Disorders, has been revised to feature the etiology and various behavioral, surgical, and pharmacological approaches to voice disorders of an organic nature. The latest research on congenital abnormalities has been added, along with new approaches to contact granulomas, laryngopharyngeal reflux, and sulcus vocalis. Many of the conditions described in this chapter can be seen in still images included on the DVD.

Chapter 4, Neurogenic Voice Disorders, continues to offer a solid foundation in the neurological bases of human laryngeal function while introducing new evidence-based data on approaches to unilateral vocal fold paralysis and spasmodic dysphonia, among other disorders.

Chapter 5, Functional Voice Disorders, is a new chapter devoted to the assessment and treatment of those voice disorders that are psychogenic or hyperfunctional in origin. Because functional voice disorders are the most common voice disorders encountered by the SLP, and because functional voice disorders are best addressed behaviorally, it was imperative that these disorders be operationally defined and addressed so that the most appropriate facilitation techniques from Chapter 7 could be considered.

Chapter 6, Voice Evaluation, continues to guide the reader through instrumental and noninstrumental assessment of voice. Ever mindful of the clinician with limited access to instrumental devices for measurement of voice, we illustrate how we approach the quantification and description of respiratory function, pitch, and resonance with light technology using low-cost approaches. New to this chapter are sections on the medical evaluation for voice disorders and the American Speech-Language-Hearing Association's preferred practice patterns for voice assessment. Other new additions are the ever-important quality-of-life scales and a section on auditory–perceptual measurement of voice.

Chapter 7, Voice Therapy, remains the bedrock of the text. The 25 *facilitating approaches* are described in detail, along with case histories showing the utilization of each approach. The DVD has been updated to illustrate a sample of each approach with one or more voice clients.

Chapter 8, Management and Therapy for Special Problems, considers special voice problems, focusing on management strategies, potential therapy approaches, and psychosocial management, when applicable. There are updated sections on the aging voice, pediatric voice, and the transsexual voice. This section also addresses current management approaches to the laryngectomee.

Chapter 9, Therapy for Resonance Disorders, focuses on assessment and intervention for resonance disturbances. The reader will appreciate updated references and approaches to hypernasality, hyponasality, assimilative nasality, and cul-de-sac resonance.

We have updated and expanded the Thought Questions at the end of each chapter so that the reader—whether student, practitioner or instructor—is compelled to engage in substantive dialogue with his or her colleagues on the material in the chapters. We have avoided "cookbook case studies," preferring to challenge the reader to investigate the questions further, using the expanded references in the eighth edition.

To increase the currency of the text with respect to evidence-based research and intervention, we have completely overhauled the reference section. Approximately 130 older references have been removed and replaced by more than 250 current references.

In accordance with the practice of the American Speech-Language-Hearing Association, we have added Learning Objectives to each chapter so that the reader appreciates the skills and knowledge to be demonstrated after reading each chapter. As always, we invite the reader to let us know your thoughts about the questions, learning objectives, and facilitation approaches, as well as the updated DVD.

ACKNOWLEDGMENTS

We would like to thank our reviewers: Raymond J. Dalfonso, Kutztown University; R. Kevin Manning, Texas State University, San Marcos; and Peter Watson, University of Minnesota. Deep gratitude is also extended to Teaching and Learning Technologies at the University of Nevada, Reno. The DVD would not have been possible without the expertise of Mark Gandolfo, manager of Media Design and Production, and camera and production specialists Shawn Sariti, Theresa Danna-Douglas, Maryan Tooker, Ted Cook, and Matt Blagen. Manuscript scrutiny was made possible by Douglas Kucera.

Daniel R. Boone
Stephen C. McFarlane
Shelley L. Von Berg
Richard I. Zraick

The Voice and Voice Therapy

Learning Objectives

- Describe the biological and emotional functions of the larynx
- List the kinds of voice disorders
- Describe voice disorders in the normal population
- Identify the types of intervention for voice disorders
- Recognize those populations at risk for voice disorders

When we hear the long-awaited birth cry of the newborn infant, we are hearing the infant's first coordination of the outgoing use of the breath stream passing between the vocal folds. More importantly, we are hearing the confirming evidence that a new life has been born. From that moment on, the mother and those nearby listen closely to the baby's vocalizations. The mood states of anger, loving, and hunger can be heard in the baby's vocal shadings. Similarly, for a lifetime, the sound of the voice often carries the message more than the words that we say.

The act of using voice while speaking is a distinctive way of using the vocal mechanism. The act of singing is even more so. Both speaking and singing demand a combination and interaction of respiration, phonation, resonance, and speech articulation. The best speakers and singers are often those persons who by natural gift or training, or by a studied blend of both, have mastered the art of optimally using these vocal mechanisms. For most of the population, however, we count on our voices being there when we speak, sing, cry, or laugh with very little conscious effort required.

Sitting at the top of the airway, it appears that the primary function of the larynx in mammals (including humans) is protecting the airway from any kind of obstruction. Production of the human voice is a secondary function. While the focus of this book is on voice habilitation and rehabilitation, whatever we do in therapy must be consistent with the primary demands of the respiratory system. We will also see that beyond breathing problems, voicing difficulties can be the result of anatomic deviation and disease, or by emotions overriding normal vocal function, or by a change of vocal function resulting from misuse and overuse of vocal mechanisms. The voice evaluation by both the physician and the speech–language pathologist (SLP) attempts to identify the causal factors of a particular voice disorder. The dual evaluation of voice documents and quantifies the elements for possible vocal change, recommending management of the voice problem by medical treatment and/or voice therapy.

The focus of this book is on voice therapy by the SLP, regardless of the setting (school, clinic, hospital) in which he or she works with the patient with a voice disorder.

THE BIOLOGICAL FUNCTION OF THE LARYNX

A description of the biological aspects of laryngeal function provides us an early hint of how the biological demands of the airway and the larynx will always take precedence over artistic or communicative vocal production. When the brain signals the body's need for renewal of oxygen in the breath cycle, we automatically take in a breath. Oxygen-laden air flows through the passages of the upper airway into the lungs, followed by the outgoing carbon dioxide–loaded air flowing out of the body through the airway. This transportation of air into and out of the lungs is the primary function of the airway. Protecting the airway for an unobstructed passage of the air supply is the larynx. The primary biological function of the larynx is to keep fluids and foods from going into the airway (aspiration).

The larynx sits in a vital site at the front, bottom of the throat (pharynx), and at the top of the windpipe (trachea). As fluids and chewed food (bolus) come down the posterior throat, they are diverted from the lower throat (hypopharynx) into the open esophagus, where they continue their journey through the esophagus down into the stomach. As part of the swallowing act, the laryngeal mechanism rises high (elevating the esophagus and trachea with it) in the neck. As the swallow progresses, the tongue comes back, and the epiglottis cartilage of the larynx, which acts as a partial cover, closes over the open larynx.

Whenever the larynx plays this sphincteral role of closing off the airway to permit the posterior passage of liquids or food, the entire laryngeal body rises. Also, in fear situations, the larynx may reflexively elevate as part of its primary role in protecting the airway. Some voice patients, sometimes those with excessive fears, will attempt voice with the larynx in its elevated "protector" posture. Such excessive laryngeal elevation is not a good posture for producing a normal voice.

Besides the elevating capability of the larynx, which helps prevent aspiration, airway closure is aided by three laryngeal muscle valves, described in Chapter 2 as the aryepiglottic folds, the ventricular folds (false folds), and the thyroarytenoid muscles (the true vocal folds). The most vertical of these valve pairs in the larynx are the aryepiglottic folds, which are considered part of the supralarynx. Under vigorous valving conditions, such as severe coughing, they begin to approximate (adduct). Below them are the ventricular folds; only during vigorous adductory activities, like the cough, do they approach each other. The lowest and most medial of the three laryngeal valves are the thyroarytenoid muscles, the true vocal folds. During swallow, they always adduct to prevent possible aspiration. Also, the individual has fine control of the true vocal folds, with some capability of altering their shape, length, and tension, producing various voicing changes.

When one breathes naturally, all three valve sites are open. The vocal folds separate further on inspiration, allowing a greater volume of air to pass through quickly; on expiration, they move slightly toward (adduct) one another. As further described in Chapter 2, voice is produced when the vocal folds adduct slightly together, allowing expired air to pass between them, setting the folds into vibration. This vibration produces voice (phonation). This phonation is then resonated through various sites of the vocal tract. The resonance of the voice begins with this vibratory sound in the larynx, traveling up through the pharynx and the oral and nasal cavities above. The voice we hear, then, is produced by a combination of respiratory activation, phonation, and amplifying resonance. Although the primary role of the larynx is to protect the airway, the larynx and voice in the human plays an important role in emotional and linguistic expression.

THE EMOTIONAL FUNCTION OF THE LARYNX

The infant seems to express emotions by making laryngeal sounds. Certainly, the caregiver can soon detect differences in the emotional state of the baby by changes in the sound of the baby's vocalizations: A cry from hunger may sound different from a cry of discomfort or the vocalization of anger. Contentment (after a full stomach or being held) can be heard in the cooing responses of the baby. From early infancy throughout the life span, the sound of one's vocalization often mirrors one's internal emotional state.

Our voice can sound happy or sad, contented or angry, secure or unsafe, placid or passionate. How one feels affectively may be heard in the sound of the voice as well as in changes of the prosodic rhythm patterns of vocalization. Our emotional status plays a primary role in the control of respiration; for example, nervousness may be heard in one's shortness of breath. Our emotional state seems to dictate the vertical positioning of the larynx, the relative relaxation of the vocal folds, the posturing and relaxation of the muscles of the pharynx and tongue.

One's emotionality can be heard in the voice, a fact that can be threatening to the professional singer, or harmful to sales for the nervous salesperson, or embarrassing to someone who sounds like he or she is crying when actually happy. Our mood state can be harmful to voice. Many voice disorders are the result of various affective excesses; for example, a young professional woman attempts to use normal conversational voice when her larynx is postured in a high, sphincterly closed position, resulting in a tight, tense voice. Her problem may be more related to unchecked and unrealistic fear than it is to faulty use of the vocal mechanisms per se.

Because emotionality and vocal function are so closely entwined, effective voice therapy often requires the treatment of the total person and not just fixating on the remediation of voice symptoms. Therefore, as we will see in ensuing chapters, getting to know the patient is an important prerequisite to taking a case history or making an instrumental–perceptual voice evaluation. Voice clinicians have long recognized that the patient in the office may not resemble the same person in play or stress settings; the patient's voice will change according to his or her mood state. To assess voice realistically, we have to observe and listen to the patient in various life settings.

THE LINGUISTIC FUNCTION OF THE VOICE

Voice seems to hold spoken language together. From the primitive emotional vocalization that may color what we say to the skilled use of voice stress to emphasize a particular utterance, the voicing component of spoken language plays a primary role. It is not always what we say that carries the message, but how we say it.

New interest in infant vocalization is producing a fascinating literature. By the time typical one-year-old babies utter their first word, they have already used their voices in highly elaborate jargon communication. While human babies all seem to babble about the same way from four to six months of age, babbling becomes more language differentiated beyond that age. That is, babies no longer sound alike after six months; rather, they begin to sound like the primary language they have been hearing. The melody of the parent language, or its prosody, begins to color the vocalizations of the baby. The jargon of Chinese babies begins to sound like the sweeping tonal patterns of the Chinese Mandarin language; the pharyngeal sounds of an Arab language begin to be heard in the jargon of Arab babies.

These prosodic vocal patterns exist far beyond the individual word or segment. Such voicing is known as *suprasegmental phonation*. In young babies, suprasegmental vocalization far exceeds the voicing of actual word segments. As infants acquire new words, they often place them in the proper place of their ongoing voicing rhythm. If they want to say *milk*, rather than say the word in isolation, they are far more likely to say the word at the end of a jargon phrase, such as "gawa na ta milk." The jargon leading up to the word is suprasegmental voicing. The jargon voice carries an uncoded message with no specific meaning but seems to convey some general meaning by the overall sound of it. The mood and need state of the baby influence the sound of the vocalization.

Although jargon speech appears to diminish after the first 18 months of life, we continue to use suprasegmental vocalization in all aspects of spoken communication. We may add vocal stress patterns to augment the meaning of what we say. The actual words we say are only part of the communication. The "how we say it" is conveyed by various vocal stress strategies, such as changing loudness, grouping words together on one breath, changing pitch level, changing vocal quality and resonance to match our mood. These stress changes of the suprasegmentals can be produced with or without intent. That is, if it serves our purpose, we can sound angry by talking louder, or we may sound angry despite our best efforts to hide our anger from our listener. Once again, the voice carries much of the message. The same words spoken or written may convey different messages (as any lawyer taking depositions will tell you) depending on the stress patterns given the words by the speaker, with or without intent.

Considering the role of the voice in both emotional and linguistic expression, it is no wonder that people with voice disorders may find themselves handicapped in their communication. A young girl with vocal nodules, for example, may have developed them in part from excessive emotional vocalization (such as constantly yelling). Once the nodules were developed, however, she may be unable to use the vocal suprasegmentals and stress patterns she had previously used with ease in communication. As one knows who has ever suffered a complete loss of voice from severe laryngitis, the lack of voice prevents you from being you. Somehow whisper and gesture do not carry the communication effectiveness that normal voice allows you to add to the words you say.

While a primary role of the human larynx appears to be biological (guarding the airway), laryngeal voicing plays a vital role in the expression of both emotional and linguistic communication. When we add the voicing dimensions of acting and singing as laryngeal functions, we can truly appreciate the amazing artistic capabilities of the vocal tract (that a few people are fortunate to have and sometimes use). The role of the human larynx is obviously more complex and more subtle than the way the larynx functions as an airway protector in most other mammals.

VOICE DISORDERS IN THE NORMAL POPULATION

It is difficult to establish normative incidence data on voice disorders for several reasons. For example, voice can become temporarily disordered from a common cold that changes laryngeal tissue vibration and may fill resonating sinuses with infected mucus; almost everyone at some time of life has experienced some voice change (phonation or resonance) as a result of a cold. Or some people experience allergies. Therefore, if we were to take a large segment of the population and determine the present and past incidence of a voice disorder, our incidence reporting would be near 100%. Such incidence data would be meaningless. Rather, if we took a segment of a population, such as airline pilots, and looked back at the occurrences of hoarseness (dysphonia) in a certain time period, we would determine some prevalence data for that particular group. Even this data would have far more meaning if the pilots' voices were compared with the voices of matched controls (matched, for example, by gender and age). Let us look at a few recent voice prevalence–incidence studies.

Teachers as a group have been studied specific to voice disorders more than any other population group, providing some interesting prevalence data. A study (Munier and Kinsella, 2008) of 550 primary school teachers found that "27% suffered from a voice problem" with 53% having voice problems at some time in their teaching careers. Similar prevalence data (Roy et al., 2004) found that over 70% of more than 1,200 teachers experienced voice problems over their teaching careers compared with less than 10% of 1,200 adults in other occupations.

In summarizing prevalence studies, Verdolini and Ramig (2001) suggest the prevalence of voice disorders is 3 to 9% in the normal adult population. A much higher prevalence for voice problems was found among 117 normal senior adults (Roy, Stemple, Merrill, and Thomas, 2007); over their lifetime, 47% of the seniors experienced a voice problem, with 29.1% of them reporting a current voice disorder. At the other end of the adult spectrum, of young adult college cheerleaders examined by Case (2002) over time, 75% experienced a voice disorder after a season of cheerleading. It appears that the prevalence of voice disorders is highest in adults who experience high vocal demands.

It was estimated by the National Institute on Deafness and Other Communication Disorders (NIDCD, 2007) that over 7.5 million American children have some "trouble using their voices." Duff and colleagues (2004) looked at 2,445 American preschool children and found that 95 (3.9%) of them had hoarse voices. At any one time, the actual incidence of voice disorders in children is difficult to determine because of temporary voice interference from allergies and chest/head infections. Faust (2003) found among populations of schoolchildren that, over time, "6%–23% displayed hoarseness." In summarizing incidence studies in primary school children, Andrews and Summers (2002) found that 6 to 9% of them displayed voice problems, with approximately only 1% receiving voice therapy intervention. This is consistent with school SLPs who report a much higher incidence of children with voice disorders than they are able to accommodate in their caseloads. Few data are available on the incidence of voice disorders among students in middle school (where among students most normal voice changes occur) or in high school.

If one were to generalize from existing literature on the incidence of voice disorders, it would appear that about 7% of school-age children experience continuing voice problems compared with 3% of the adult population.

KINDS OF VOICE DISORDERS

When we talk about *kinds of voice disorders,* we are usually talking about classifying the causes of voice disorders, which over time has led to the historic causal simplification, the organic and functional dichotomy. In most classification systems, there is a mixture of etiologic causations and descriptive names of conditions, such as *cancer* as a causative form of an organic disorder and *aphonia* as the name of a condition that may have organic or functional origins.

Let us look at a few literature presentations of voice disorder classifications. The *Classification Manual for Voice Disorders-I* (Verdolini, Rosen, and Branski, 2006) describes seven distinct causal classifications: laryngeal problems—related to structural pathologies, inflammatory conditions, and trauma or injury—and systemic conditions—nonlaryngeal aerodigestive disorders, psychiatric/psychological disorders, and neurological disorders. The *Manual* also offers two other categories—other disorders and undiagnosed. Each causative category lists specific information about etiology, behavioral description of the voice disorder, severity criteria, and so on, all of which can be most helpful to the SLP. Such diversity of nomenclature, however, generates many categories of voice patient groups, complicating the task for generating evidence-based data.

The need for developing useful outcome data led to an Australian effort (Baker et al., 2007) to present a diagnostic classification system as part of an inter-rater reliability study that basically modifies the historic two broad categories of voice disorders, organic and functional. The organic classification of voice disorder causation combines structural changes of the vocal folds or cartilages with "interruption of neurological innervations of the laryngeal mechanism." Such a combination of organic problems under one heading may present a real hindrance in evaluating treatment outcome effectiveness. Study of clinical effectiveness would probably be simpler if the organic causations and neurogenic categories were separated out. Similarly, the functional voice disorder categories might be separated into two separate classifications: psychogenic voice disorders (PVD) and muscle tension voice disorder (MTVD, otherwise known as muscle tension dysphonia). While both PVD and MTVD are functional voice disorders, they have distinctly different origins.

A different etiologic classification for causes of voice disorders was introduced by Stemple (2007), who presented these four pathology classifications: congenital laryngeal pathologies, pathologies of the vocal fold cover, neurogenic laryngeal pathologies, and pathologies of muscular dysfunction. The first category, congenital, includes only five relatively rare congenital conditions, such as congenital web or congenital cyst. The vocal cover category lists 15 various laryngeal conditions from nodules to papilloma to sulcus vocalis. The neurogenic category does not include degenerative diseases and their possible influence on vocal fold function.

In this edition of *The Voice and Voice Therapy*, we have made an effort to include the organization of the kinds of voice disorders to allow easy identification of a voice disorder population that will promote valid and reliable clinical research. There appear to be four distinct categories of voice problems, two of them *organic* in origin and two of them *functional* in causation. The first category retains the name **organic voice disorders** and includes any laryngeal structural deviation that affects vocal fold vibration. The second kind of voice disorder is titled **neurogenic voice disorders**, related to neurological conditions that cause faulty vocal fold closure from either paralysis (or weakness) or from neurological disease. There also appears to be two distinct kinds of functional voice problems under the traditional label of functional voice disorders: psychogenic voice disorders, which are caused by psychosocial factors, and muscle tension voice disorders (muscle tension dysphonia), which can develop from excessive muscle usage. In summary, these four categories of the causative classification system clearly appear not to overlap one another: organic voice disorders, neurogenic voice disorders, psychogenic voice disorders, and muscle tension voice disorders, which will be referred to as muscle tension dysphonia throughout the text.

Organic Voice Disorders

Organic voice disorders are related to structural deviations of the vocal tract (lungs, muscles of respiration, larynx, pharynx, and oral cavity) or to diseases of specific structures of the vocal tract. An example of a structural deviation is cleft palate, where there is abnormal coupling of the oral and nasal cavities, producing hypernasality during voicing attempts. An example of a vocal tract disease is viral papilloma of the larynx, where the child or adult experiences additive growths in the larynx, which might compromise the airway and interfere with vocal fold vibration. In Chapters 3 through 9 we will consider various organic diseases that may affect voice. Although the speech–language pathologist (SLP) may play an active role in the identification and evaluation of the patient with an organic voice disorder, the primary treatment of the disorder is often medical, dental, or surgical. Treatment by the SLP may have several goals, such as helping to improve the physiologic function of a damaged larynx. When the structural problem is controlled or stablized, the SLP will work with the patient to develop the best voice possible using various therapy methods.

Neurogenic Voice Disorders

The muscle control and innervation of the muscles of respiration, phonation, resonance, and articulation may be impaired from birth or from injury or disease of the peripheral or central nervous systems occurring at any age. For example, the SLP may work closely with the young child with cerebral palsy, perhaps working on both respiratory–voice control and helping the child to develop language. Or the SLP may work with the adult patient with a motor speech disorder acquired after a stroke, not only to improve respiration, voice, and articulation, but also to address concomitant swallowing problems. The tight, spasmodic voices of patients diagnosed with adductor spasmodic dysphonia appear to have unspecified neurogenic origins. Most of the neurological diseases presented in Chapter 4 alter normal voice in some way. The SLP plays a vital role in the assessment and management of the patient with a neurological voice disorder, such as assessing the patient's respiratory volumes and expiratory control, or visualizing through endoscopy a paralyzed vocal fold, or applying diagnostic probes to the Parkinson's disease patient to determine which therapy approaches produce a better voice.

While the majority of neurological impairments and diseases that impair swallowing, breathing, voice, and resonance cannot be cured or eradicated, the SLP frequently plays a vital role in maximizing function to as near normal levels as possible. For many neurologically impaired patients, there is a functional margin of disability that can be minimized by improved patient management and direct therapy intervention.

Psychogenic Voice Disorders

Some children and adults experience severe emotional trauma or conflict that shows itself in some kind of physical alteration. In this case, reaction to the trauma may manifest itself in a complete loss of voice, often labeled as a conversion aphonia. Or more commonly, the emotional reaction may show itself in a functional dysphonia, a hoarseness that has no physical cause. Excessive emotionality may cause an alteration of voice pitch or speaking style that has no physical cause. In aphonia, the patient usually continues to whisper when making conversational attempts to speak. The complete lack of voice prevents the patient from having normal conversational interactions and may have devastating effects vocationally. Clinically, we have seen aphonic teachers unable to teach, an airline pilot unable to fly, a politician unable to continue a political campaign. Similarly, patients with a psychogenic dysphonia may suffer severe social and vocational limitations. Conversion-type voice problems vary dramatically, perhaps only showing in particular emotional or physical situations. For example, a Jesuit priest could interact with a normal voice with his Jesuit-order teaching peers, but lose his voice completely when he entered the classroom. In psychogenic aphonia or dysphonia, the patients are not willfully experiencing voice limitation. Rather, their vocal symptoms are often the result of long-term or recent psychologically damaging circumstances, such as loss of a loved one or from continued sexual abuse. Although the patient with a psychogenic voice disorder may experience some voice improvement from direct voice therapy, in most cases, the voice disorder will not resolve unless there is some concomitant counseling or psychotherapy to address the underlying emotional problem.

Muscle Tension Dysphonia

Muscle tension dysphonia (MTD), the most prevalent voice disorder of both children and adults, is commonly a manifestation of vocal hypertension, using too extensive an effort in phonation. This overuse of respiratory, phonation, pharyngeal, and tongue functions when voicing usually begins gradually. After talking awhile, the individual begins to experience some pain and discomfort in the throat area. Before any dysphonia can be heard in the voice, the patient may experience fatigue and effort that increases with voice use. Children's loud voices and yelling over time seems to produce some hoarseness of voice. Also, adults may experience more hoarseness after prolonged voice use, indicating the problem is voice use itself. Physical examination of voicing structures shows no organic pathologies, and the voice problem is considered "functional" in origin. Baker and colleagues (2007) classify the patient's discomfort coupled with hoarseness (and normal laryngeal structures) as representing "primary" muscle tension dysphonia. With continued misuse of voice over time, however, children and adults may develop "secondary" organic changes related to this vocal hyperfunction, resulting in vocal fold tissue changes such as swelling, nodules, polyps, and so on. Both primary and secondary forms of MTD can usually be minimized with voice therapy, designed to restore the normal balance between respiratory, phonatory, and resonance systems.

MANAGEMENT AND THERAPY FOR VOICE DISORDERS

There are probably no client/patient groups seen by the SLP that are more responsive to management and therapy than children and adults with voice disorders. Successful intervention for a voice disorder first requires the identification of cause. We have grouped causal factors of voice disorders into four etiologic categories: organic, neurogenic, psychogenic, and inappropriate muscle tension disorders. The typical history shows the patient experiencing some problem in respiration, voice, and/or resonance. Breathing and resonance problems are often long-standing. Voice or phonation problems, such as hoarseness, are likelier to be more recently developed. The SLP often counsels patients that unless they are experiencing hoarseness (dysphonia) as part of an allergy or upper respiratory infection (URI), they should wait no more than seven days to have a medical evaluation of the hoarseness. The SLP and otolaryngologist (ear–nose–throat physician, ENT) have a close working relationship (Thibeault, 2007); an SLP will refer the hoarse patient to an ENT for identification of the problem and possible medical treatment.

Conversely, an ear–nose–throat physician often refers the patient to the SLP, who by training is able to evaluate and diagnose the voice problem and its respiration-phonation-resonance components. The SLP takes a detailed history, observes the patient closely, and uses instrumental and noninstrumental assessment approaches. The SLP collects measurement values related to respiratory volumes and performance, performs acoustic measurement of vocal function, visualizes the larynx, and determines resonance function, particularly as related to velopharyngeal closure. Added to these observations and measurements of structure and function, the SLP determines how the patient feels about his or her voice problem, its effect on personality and interaction with others, and the influence of the voice problem on vocational performance. For many voice problems at the time of the evaluation, the SLP tests voice stimulability by trying a few voice therapy approaches with the patient, often called *diagnostic probes*. The SLP determines the outcome from using a particular technique, such as opening one's mouth more or speaking in a louder voice. If such an approach is facilitative in producing a target voice, it might well be among the first techniques used in therapy.

There are many forms of voice therapy available for the SLP to use with different kinds of voice problems. The client's response to the diagnostic probe may indicate the general direction of the therapy to be provided. For example, changing the loudness of the patient's voice may be an option. Perhaps for a young boy with vocal nodules, we would recommend using a softer voice, "Change of Loudness, Voice 2" as the procedure (Boone, McFarlane, and Von Berg, 2005)—"the voice to use when not wanting to awaken a sleeping person, a quiet voice" (p. 188). Such a quiet voice is also presented by Casper (2000) as the "confidential voice." Or increasing loudness with an aging Parkinson patient may improve both articulation and voice, achieved by employing the loudness regimen of a specified program such as the Lee Silverman voice treatment program (Ramig et al., 2001) or following the steps of "Voice 4," using a voice loud enough to be heard "20 or 30 feet away" (Boone and Wiley, 2000). Working on loudness changes may go either way, developing a softer voice or a louder voice.

Despite our professional need to develop scientific evidence to support different therapies, group data are difficult to gather because voice therapy is so individualized. Two patients with the same causative voice problem may require a distinctively different combination of therapy procedures. It is possible, however, to look at therapy effectiveness using different levels of evidence, as suggested by Butler and Darrah (2001) in their determination of treatment outcomes for patients with cerebral palsy. Their five levels of evidence range from "Type I" (clinic vs. control group study) to "Type V" (descriptive case series/case reports). The construct validity of each level of typing may have to be questioned. The effectiveness of voice therapy facilitating techniques presented in Chapter 7 can probably best be determined by comparing pretherapy evaluation measurements with posttherapy evaluation of the same measurements. As we shall discuss in evaluating outcomes of therapy techniques in Chapter 7, validity of outcome data is often compromised by the limited number of voice patients available, SLP fiscal requirements, patient fee difficulties, and the need for rapid progress.

For organic voice problems, the SLP may work closely with other specialists, such as physical medicine or respiratory therapy, depending on the particular problem. For example, a preschool youngster with a growth in the airway called papilloma (caused by a virus) may require the clinical services of a surgeon, a respiratory therapist, extra nursing care, and close observation by an SLP, who may need to work with the child to address breath support and voice. The voice therapy goal with such a child may be solely to develop the best voice possible using a vocal mechanism heavily laden with multiple papilloma growths. When such papillomas become large enough to impinge on the airway, the surgeon excises or reduces them, as needed, to improve breathing function.

Neurogenic voice problems come in many varied forms as we will see in Chapter 4. The SLP may be the first health care professional to see a patient just beginning to experience voice symptoms. For example, a recent patient seen in our clinics felt he was experiencing a new problem pronouncing occasional words. A subsequent evaluation by the SLP found evidence of tongue fasciculations and a problem in tongue diadochokinesis (he could not move his tongue rapidly when making alternating movements, such as saying "ta-ka" in a rapid series). A subsequent referral by the SLP to a neurologist confirmed that the patient was showing beginning signs of amyotrophic lateral sclerosis. Or the neurologist may be the first professional to see a patient with a neurogenic disorder, referring the patient to the SLP for detailed assessment of breathing, phonation, and speech. The SLP sends his or her evaluation back to the neurologist, and together they may develop a management plan for the patient. Such a plan frequently includes medications for improving the patient's motor functions, with specific goals for the patient to achieve with the SLP in voice resonance and articulation therapy.

The SLP will often work with actors, singers, and teachers who want to improve their speaking voices. The role of the SLP working to improve the speaking voice of the professional user of voice was defined in a joint statement by the American Speech-Language-Hearing Association, the National Association of Teachers, and the Voice and Speech Trainers Association (ASHA/NATS/VASTA, 2005), which defines how the SLP would work collaboratively with members of NATS and VASTA. Since the establishment of roles for each voice specialist, there has been an increase in cross-referrals among the three voice specialties. For the actor and singer, the SLP can often offer vocal hygiene and voice therapy techniques that the professional can use in normal day voice usage when not acting or singing.

The SLP will often work closely with the counselor, psychologist, or psychiatrist for patients with psychogenic voice problems. Working on voice symptoms alone may often need to be supplemented with psychological therapy to deal with underlying emotional problems that may be driving the voice problem. While loss of voice (aphonia) can often be treated successfully by symptomatic voice therapy, the vocal gains may only be temporary or reoccur in particular environmental situations. Similarly, long-term dysphonias without identifiable physical causes often resist successful resolution because the voice symptoms serve the patient in some way. Mutational falsetto, or continuing to use a higher sounding voice after puberty (puberphonia), is often thought to be a psychogenic voice disorder among our psychology colleagues. However, the experience of most SLPs is the higher voice in the postpubertal male usually can be changed in one or two voice therapy visits. Most young men seem to be trapped by habit in using the higher voice and are dramatically relieved with the discovery of the adult male voice. On occasion, the SLP may still refer these adolescents for some counseling or psychological therapy.

The majority of functional voice disorders are the result of the voice patient using excessive effort and are classified as muscle tension dysphonia (MTD). Both children and adults with MTD often abuse, overuse, or misuse their voices. The primary focus of the SLP with these patients is to identify their vocal excesses; once identified, vocal misuse can be reduced and often eliminated by voice therapy alone (Cohen and Garrett, 2007). We will be citing in Chapters 7 and 8 numerous other successful voice therapy outcome studies, similar to the seminal study of Benninger and Jacobson (1995). They followed 115 MTD patients who eventually developed vocal nodules or polyps from continued vocal excesses. After receiving appropriate voice therapy to reduce these excesses, 94% experienced resolution of their problem. The authors concluded that with appropriate voice modification and therapy provided by the SLP that "nodules will generally resolve with return of normal vocal function" (p. 326). Voice therapy for patients with MTD is usually a collection of voice techniques that facilitate the easy balance of respiratory, voice, and resonance behaviors.

Progress in voice therapy can be determined from pre- and posttreatment measures of respiratory function, acoustic comparisons, and voice quality and resonance changes. Self-perception by the voice patient (Bogaardt et al., 2007) regarding any change in voice and its impact on quality of life adds needed outcome data. Useful outcome data also come from follow-up contacts and measures by the SLP over a specified period of time.

SUMMARY

We have looked at voice and the larynx as part of the biological viability of the individual, as a tool in emotional expression, and as complicated and extensive factors in spoken human communication. We have seen that there appear to be four causal factors in the development and maintenance of voice disorders: organic, neurogenic, psychogenic, and excessive muscle action. The child or adult with a voice problem is evaluated by the SLP, who uses instrumental and noninstrumental approaches for various respiratory and acoustic measures in attempting to identify causal factors and define aspects of voice production. "Diagnostic probes," the application of trial therapy approaches, are then used to determine the efficacy of a particular therapy technique for improving the patient's voice productions. The patient's self-perception of the handicapping impact of the voice disorder on his or her life is then recorded. If evaluation measures indicate that the patient can profit from therapy, the SLP then provides needed voice therapy. At the conclusion of voice therapy, therapy success is determined by comparing pre- and posttherapy measures, providing needed outcome data.

Thought Questions

1. What are some typical voice problems that could develop from one of the four causes presented in the chapter? Could some of the voice disorders overlap?
2. In answer to the need for evidence-based practice in remediation of voice disorders, can you think of different ways to "prove" that particular voice therapy techniques are effective? Can a combination of therapy techniques be studied for their effectiveness in reducing or eliminating a voice problem?
3. Describe how different authors have described and categorized different etiologies of voice disorders. Generate your own rubric and write a rationale for each category.

chapter 2

The Normal Voice

Learning Objectives

- List the five aspects of voice
- Describe the three processes of normal voice production
- Identify the major anatomical structures responsible for normal voice
- Explain how these structures work together in the production of normal voice
- Recognize changes in the larynx and voice across the lifespan

This chapter describes the normal voice and its characteristics. It is important to understand the range of the normal voice in order to be able to diagnose and plan treatment for a disordered voice. Few things are so difficult to define or understand as "What is normal and what constitutes normal limits?" Voice therapy is often "antagonistic" therapy. We are trying to undo what patients have done to their voices through "overworking" the normal mechanism. In order to help someone return to the range of normal and abandon the abnormal functions, one must know the characteristics of the normal voice. To be effective in voice evaluation and therapy, clinicians must have a good working knowledge of the structures involved in phonation. Also, they must have knowledge of the normal functioning of these structures.

NORMAL ASPECTS OF VOICE

Normal voice may be characterized by five aspects. First, the normal voice must be loud enough to be heard. We may refer to this as adequate carrying power, which is a key component of speech intelligibility. This means that the normal voice can be heard and speech can be understood over the noise of most everyday environmental sounds such as the TV, air conditioning, computer typing, and so on. Second, the normal voice must be produced in a manner that is hygienic—that is, without vocal trauma and resulting laryngeal lesions. Third, the normal voice should have a pleasant quality. Fourth, the normal voice should be flexible enough to express emotion. We often say a great deal with the emotional tone of our voice. The sentence "I am so happy for you" can be either sincere or sarcastic just by the tone of voice, while the words remain the same. The expression, "Oh, wonderful," can be said with excitement or with scorn. Lastly, the normal voice should represent the speaker well in terms of age and gender. We should not be surprised to meet someone for the first time after speaking to him or her on the phone. Our voice should not portray us as either older, younger, or as less mature than we are. Nor will we likely be pleased if we are mistaken for the opposite gender. The normal voice could be said to represent the speaker faithfully.

Using these five aspects of loudness, hygiene, pleasantness, flexibility, and representation, we can begin to address the area of normal voice. A normal voice for a seven-year-old boy will be quite different from that of a 70-year-old female, but both can be normal and adequately loud, hygienic, pleasant enough to not be distracting, sufficiently flexible to express the speaker's emotion, and appropriate for the speaker's age and gender.

This chapter presents the structures and functions that underlie normal voice—the anatomical structures and physiological functions necessary for normal respiration, phonation, and resonance. A current view of the clinical physiology of these events accompanies this discussion.

NORMAL PROCESSES OF VOICE PRODUCTION

Separating the normal speaking voice into three individual processes (respiration, phonation, and resonance) for purposes of study is helpful, but we must remember that the three components of voice production are highly interdependent. For example, without the expiratory phase of respiration there would be no phonation or resonance. Without adequate movement of the velopharyngeal mechanism, there would be an imbalance of oral–nasal resonance. Moreover, these three processes are constantly and simultaneously changing. Let us first consider the structures and function of respiration, particularly as related to production of voice.

Respiration

Humans have learned to use respiration for the purpose of phonation, making speech possible. Both speaking and singing require an exhalation (outgoing airstream) capable of activating vocal fold vibration. When training their voices, speakers or singers frequently focus on developing conscious control of the breathing mechanism. This conscious control, however, must not conflict with the physiological oxygen requirements of the individual. When a problem occurs with respiration, it is often the conflict between physiological needs and the speaking–singing demands for air that causes faulty usage of the vocal mechanism. Our dependence on a constantly renewed oxygen supply imposes certain limitations on how many words we can say, how many phrases we can sing, or how much loud emphasis we can use on one expiration.

Respiratory Anatomy. For quiet breathing, inspired air enters through the nostrils to the nasal cavities and into the nasopharynx through the open velopharyngeal port before entering the oropharynx. For mouth breathers and for speaking purposes, the air enters through the open mouth and passes through the oral cavity into the oropharynx. The air then flows through the hypopharynx and into the larynx, passing between the ventricular or false vocal folds and between the true vocal folds down into the trachea or windpipe. During quiet breathing, the adult male glottis (area between the vocal folds) is about 13 mm (0.5 inches) wide at its broadest point, and the glottis remains essentially unchanged from inhalation to exhalation (Zemlin, 1998, p. 146). At the bottom end of the trachea is the tracheal bifurcation, otherwise known as the carina, where the airway divides into the two bronchial tubes of the lungs (see Figure 2.1). The bronchial tubes further branch into divisions known as the bronchioles, and they eventually terminate in the lungs in little air sacs known as alveolar sacs. Some of the bronchioli are visible in the upper picture of Figure 2.1, but most of the bronchioli and all the alveoli are covered by the pleural membrane that covers the lungs.

The lungs lie within the thoracic cavity. The thorax can move in several ways. For example, the rib cage wall expands for inspiration of air and collapses for expiration. The ribs connected to the 12 thoracic vertebrae and their adjoining muscles play an important role in respiration. Sometimes the accessory muscles in the neck assist in deep inspiration when they contract because they elevate the shoulders and increase the vertical dimension of the thorax. At the base of the thorax is the diaphragm, an important composite of muscle, tendon, and membrane that separates the thoracic cavity from the abdominal cavity. As the diaphragm contracts, it descends and increases the vertical dimension of the thorax; as the diaphragm relaxes, it ascends back to its higher position. The diaphragm has direct contact with the lungs, and only the pleural space comes between the lungs and the diaphragm. The shape of the diaphragm, its superior contour, can be seen on the lower surface of the cadaver lung in Figure 2.1. The relaxed diaphragm is high in the chest within the rib cage, and the stomach and liver lie directly below it. As the diaphragm contracts and descends, it pushes from above on the contents of the

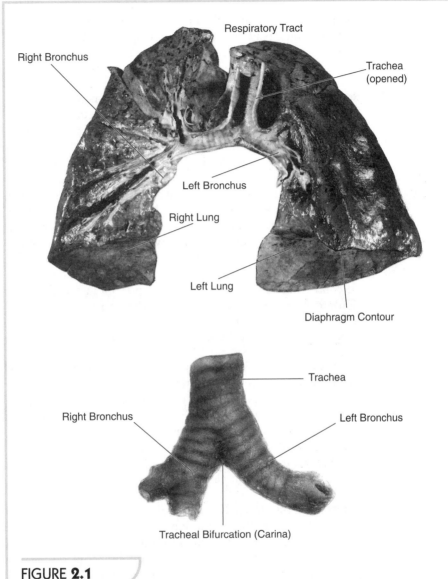

Respiratory Tract

Right Bronchus

Trachea
(opened)

Left Bronchus

Right Lung

Left Lung

Diaphragm Contour

Trachea

Right Bronchus

Left Bronchus

Tracheal Bifurcation (Carina)

FIGURE **2.1**

Lungs and Tracheal Bifurcation

An illustration of the tracheal bifurcation that introduces air into the lungs by way of the left and right bronchi. At the bottom end of the trachea, known as the carina, the airway divides into the two bronchial tubes. The bronchial tubes further branch into divisions, the bronchioles, and they eventually terminate in the lungs in little air sacs, the alveolar sacs. Some of the bronchioli are visible in the upper picture, but most of the bronchioli and all the alveoli are covered by the pleural membrane that covers the lungs.

abdomen below, often displacing the abdominal wall by pushing it outward on inspiration. The abdominal wall is composed primarily of the abdominal muscles that sometimes play an active role in expiration. This is especially true in singing, in loud speech, when laughing (thus the term "belly laugh"), or when producing a very long phrase.

Respiratory Function.   The respiratory tract functions much like a bellows. When we move the handles on the bellows apart, the bellows becomes larger and the air within it becomes less dense than the air outside it. The outside air rushes in due to the lower pressure of the less dense air in the bellows and the greater pressure in the more dense outside air. The inspiration of air into the bellows is achieved by active enlargement of the bellows's body. Similarly, in human respiration, the inspiration of air is achieved by active movement of muscles that enlarge the thoracic cavity. When the thorax enlarges, the lungs within the thorax enlarge. The air within the lungs becomes less dense than atmospheric air, and inspiration begins. The air is expired from the lungs by decreasing the size of the chest, thus compressing the air and forcing it to rush out. In human respiration, however, much of expiration is achieved by passive collapse of the thorax and not by active muscle contraction. This is an extremely important fact and can be valuable information for voice clinicians. Much of expiration is passive. Hixon and Hoit (2005) have described human respiration as having two types of forces that are always present: passive, nonvolitional forces and active, volitional forces.

Passive Forces.   Much of the power required for normal speech can be supplied by the passive forces of respiration (passive exhalation). These forces include the natural recoil of muscles, cartilages, ligaments, and lung tissue, the surface tension of a special film that lines the alveoli, and the pull of gravity. These forces reduce the size of the thorax during expiration (in a manner analogous to the recoil of a stretched spring) and thus contribute to outward airflow from the lungs, which may be used in speech. The mechanism of passive force can be understood by examining the concept of relaxation pressure.

Relaxation Pressure.   The most efficient and most pleasing voice is produced at mid-air-pressure levels and mid-lung-volume levels of air. To demonstrate this, simply take about a half-breath and produce an /i/ vowel for five seconds at a medium loudness level. Then listen to the vocal quality. Now take a very deep breath and produce the same /i/ vowel for five seconds at medium loudness. The vocal quality will generally be poorer because of the increased effort required to control the greater air volume and higher air pressure. Finally, produce the same /i/ vowel for five seconds at medium loudness immediately after releasing three-fourths of your air supply. Again, the vocal quality will suffer as you try to compensate for the low air pressure and low lung volume, oftentimes by hyperadduction of the vocal folds.

This exercise demonstrates how vocal quality is affected by extremely high or low air pressure at high or low lung volume (see Figure 2.2). It translates into an excellent clinical stimulation technique. We can often change the vocal quality of

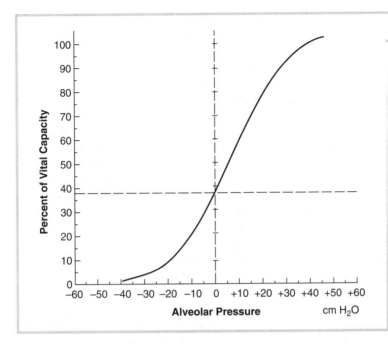

FIGURE **2.2**

The Relaxation Pressure Curve

The passive forces of exhalation tend to generate force during inhalation that works to restore the lung and rib cage system to the normal resting state or equilibrium. After active inhalation, these passive forces of exhalation rebound to provide some of the expiratory force needed for speech. There is a nearly linear relationship between relaxation pressure and lung volume in the range between 20% and 70% of the vital capacity. This curve represents the pressure generated by the passive factors of the respiratory system.

FA.22

our dysphonic patients by instructing them to use the midrange of air pressure and lung volume. Teaching a shortened phrasing pattern may be important to teaching breath-stream management. Except in singers or actors, this generally is all the respiration training that needs to be given by the speech–language pathologist. All the emphasis placed on breathing exercises and respiration training in the past seems unproductive and unnecessary for nearly all of our patients with dysphonia. The clinical facilitating technique of glottal fry (discussed in Chapter 7) makes use of this information because glottal fry is produced with little air pressure and little airflow.

Active Forces. Additional power required for normal speech can be supplied by the active forces of respiration (active exhalation), made up of the more than 20 muscles within the chest wall, their patterns of movement, and the amount of air contained with the lungs. As described by Hixon and Hoit (2005, p. 18), the more air the lungs contain, the greater the force that can be produced to decrease the size of the thorax (i.e., the greater the expiratory force that can be generated). By contrast, the less air the lungs contain, the greater the force that can be produced to increase the size of the thorax (i.e., the greater the inspiratory force that can be generated).

A key problem for many voice disordered patients is the tendency to squeeze the glottis closed in order to produce the needed power, rather than to increase air pressure and airflow by contracting the abdominal muscles. We can better understand this mistake by a simple analogy. If we are watering flowers in a garden and we want to reach the far row of plants, we can either place a thumb over the end of the hose and squirt the water further (increase the power), or we can increase the water power by turning the faucet on further. When we squeeze the glottis closed, we are "putting a thumb over the end of the hose." When we contract the abdominal muscles, we are "turning the faucet further on" and increasing the airflow. Even though squeezing the glottis tends to increase the vocal power, vocal quality is diminished because the voice sounds strained. If this method is habitual, the excessive effort becomes the basis of a hyperfunctional voice disorder. Such effort may lead to laryngeal changes that can result in abnormal voice. When we need increased power to speak louder, to stress words, or to extend a phrase when singing or speaking, we should use the larger muscles of the abdomen and "turn on the faucet" controlling the source of air. Thus, the pressure at the valve (the larynx) is not excessive, and vocal quality is improved with delicate laryngeal tissue not subjected to stress and strain, which produces laryngeal edema and laryngitis. Vocal quality is not diminished, and adverse tissue change is avoided. Voice clinicians can use this water analogy to teach patients how to monitor breath control by properly using expiratory reserve volume (see the definition of terms later in this section) via the abdominal muscles, rather than using excessive glottal valving in the larynx.

Muscles of Respiration.   We now need to consider the muscles of respiration (see Figures 2.3 and 2.4). When discussing these muscles, it is helpful to think of three major categories: (1) the muscles of the rib cage, (2) the diaphragm, and (3) the muscles of the abdominal wall. Thinking of the muscles of respiration in this way makes it easier to discuss the movements that occur due to the passive and active forces discussed previously, as well as the adjustment capabilities of the respiratory system for speech purposes.

The respiratory system is capable of a wide variety of adjustments. The behavior of the system components during speech depends on body position (upright versus lying down) and the nature of the speaking task (sustained vowels versus conversational speech or reading aloud) (Hixon and Hoit, 2000). For running speech in the upright body position, the rib cage wall is active during both inspiration and expiration (Hixon, Mead, and Goldman, 1976). During inspiration, muscles of the rib cage wall raise the rib cage and stiffen this structure in a manner that optimizes the function of the diaphragm. During expiration, muscles of the rib cage wall act in conjunction with those of the abdominal wall to generate the expiratory forces needed to drive speech production. Most often, expiratory muscles of the rib cage wall are used. The diaphragm is the principal muscle of inspiration. During expiration the diaphragm is usually inactive. The abdominal wall is also active during both inspiration and expiration. During inspiration the abdominal wall serves as a platform from which the diaphragm functions (Hixon and Abbs, 1980). During expiration, muscles of the abdominal wall act in conjunction with those of the rib cage wall to generate the expiratory forces needed to drive speech production.

Figure 2.5, the simple tracings of a pneumotachometer, shows the relative time for inspiration–expiration for a passive tidal breath, for saying the numbers "1, 2,

---

FIGURE **2.3**

A List of Muscles of Respiration

Muscles of the Rib Cage Wall
Sternocleidomastoid
Scalenus group (anterior, medial, posterior)
Pectoralis major
Pectoralis minor
Subclavius
Serratus anterior
External intercostals
Internal intercostals
Transversus thoracis
Lattisimus dorsi
Serratus posterior superior
Serratus posterior inferior
Lateral iliocostals
Levatores costarum
Quadratus lumborum
Subcostals

Muscles of the Diaphragm
Diaphragm

Muscles of the Abdominal Wall
Rectus abdominus
External oblique
Internal oblique
Transversus abdominis

3, 4, 5," and for singing the musical passage, "I don't want to walk without you, baby," from the old song by that title. Note that the inspiratory time during normal tidal breathing is much longer than the quick inspiration for speech and singing, indicated by the rapid rise of the tracing from a resting baseline in an almost vertical move. In the tidal breath the rise from the baseline is gradual and sloped rather than vertical.

We will now define the terms we will use in following discussions to describe aspects of respiration. Methods for evaluating respiratory volumes and capacities will be discussed in Chapter 6.

- *Lung volumes and capacities* refer to the amount of air in the lungs at a given time and how much of that air is used for various purposes, including speech (Solomon and Charron, 1998). Lung volumes include *tidal volume, inspiratory*

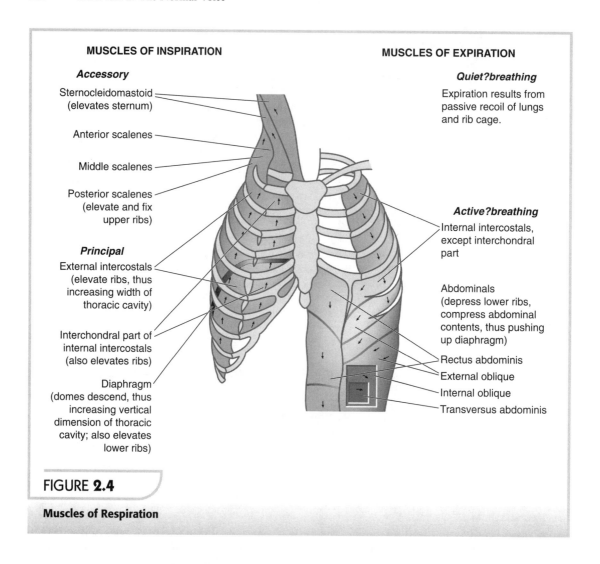

FIGURE 2.4

Muscles of Respiration

reserve volume, expiratory reserve volume, and residual volume. Lung capacities combine various lung volumes and include *inspiratory capacity, vital capacity, functional residual capacity,* and *total lung capacity.* Lung volumes and capacities vary depending on the patient's age, gender, level of physical exertion, and vocal training. Data reported by Hoit and Hixon (1987) and Hoit and colleagues (1989, 1990) indicate that, in general, lung volumes and capacities increase from infancy through puberty and then remain stable until advancing age, when they decrease slightly (see Table 2.1).

- *Tidal volume* (TV) is the amount of air inspired and expired during a typical respiratory cycle. It is determined by the oxygen needs of the individual. The term *tidal volume* is descriptive in that the movement of air in and out of the lungs is analogous to the flow and ebb of an ocean tide (Hixon and Hoit, 2005, p. 36).

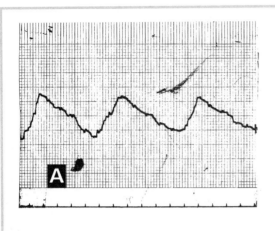

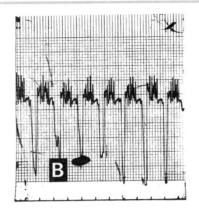

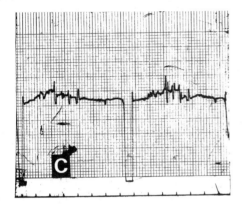

FIGURE **2.5**

Pneumotachometer Tracings Measure Airflow over Time

Note the relative time for inspiration as opposed to expiration for three conditions: tracing A (three tidal breaths) produces an inspiration–expiration time ratio of about 1:2; tracing B (counting from one to five on eight trials) produces a ratio of about 1:3; tracing C (singing twice, "I don't want to walk without you, baby") yielded an inspiration–expiration ratio of approximately 1:10.

- *Inspiratory reserve volume* (IRV) is the maximum volume of air that can be inspired beyond the end of a tidal inspiration.
- *Expiratory reserve volume* (ERV) is the maximum volume of air that can be expired beyond the end of a tidal expiration.
- *Residual volume* (RV) is the volume of air that remains in the lungs after a maximum expiration. No matter how forceful the expiration, the residual volume cannot be forced from the lungs and averages between 1000 and 1500 cc

TABLE **2.1**	Group Means of Seven Age Groups of Subjects for Some Lung Volumes and Capacities (in cubic centimeters)						
	Subjects' Age Group						
	7	10	13	16	25	50	75
Males							
TLC	2120	3140	4330	6200	6740	7050	6630
VC	1670	2510	3550	5080	5350	5090	4470
FRC	980	1400	1970	2940	3120	3460	3440
ERV	530	770	1180	1810	1730	1500	1280
Females							
TLC	2070	2980	3740	4980	5030	5310	4860
VC	1580	2340	2999	3780	3930	3600	2940
FRC	970	1430	1690	2560	2420	2930	2590
ERV	480	780	940	1350	1320	1220	670

Source: Adapted from Hoit and Hixon (1987); Hoit, Hixon, Altman, and Morgan (1989); and Hoit, Hixon, Watson, and Morgan (1990).

in the young adult male. To estimate the residual volume, indirect measurement methods must be used.

- *Inspiratory capacity* (IC) is the maximum volume of air that can be inspired. It is the sum of the TV and IRV.
- *Vital capacity* (VC) is the total amount of air that can be expired from the lungs and air passages following a maximum inspiration. It includes all of the lung volumes except the RV.
- *Functional residual capacity* (FRC) is the volume of air contained in the lungs and airways at the end of a resting tidal exhalation. It is the sum of the ERV and RV.
- *Total lung capacity* (TLC) represents the total volume of air contained in the lungs and airways after a maximum inspiration. It is the sum of all four lung volumes (TV + IRV + ERV + RV).

In normal speech breathing, the relative timing of inspiration–expiration is only slightly longer for expiration. Humans appear to have a slight bias toward longer expirations, which is apparently quite compatible with the need to extend expiration for purposes of speech. Influences on speech breathing include the speaker's body position, body type, and age, as well as the type of utterance being produced, interactions between the speaker and the listener, the background noise in the setting, and so forth. As summarized by Hixon and Hoit (2005, pp. 105–106): (a) speech breathing while upright is different from speech breathing while lying down due to the effect of gravity on relaxation pressure and chest wall movements; (b) body type influences speech breathing because of the effect of body fat on the movements of the abdominal wall and rib cage wall; (c) advanced age (seventh or eighth decade of life) brings changes in laryngeal valving, which result in larger lung volumes and rib cage wall excursions and greater average expenditures of air per syllable; (d) speech breathing patterns are highly variable until age three with refinements throughout childhood and adolescence; and (e) cognitive–linguistic factors affect when an inspiration occurs, how long the following expiration will be, how often silent pauses will occur, and how much speech is produced per breath group. The speech–language pathologist must take these factors into consideration when conducting a speech breathing evaluation (more on this topic in Chapter 6). For example, when breath support or perhaps breath control is a problem in a voice disordered patient, it is often related to failure to take breaths at appropriate places. At other times, the tendency to push too hard in extending the expiratory reserve volume results in a strained vocal quality. Understanding lung volumes and capacities, and the difference between breathing for life versus breathing for speech is the foundation for identifying those voice disordered patients whose dysphonia is due in part to abnormal respiratory function.

Anatomy of Phonation

The larynx, positioned atop the trachea, is the gateway to the respiratory tract. The larynx serves important biological functions, which include allowing air into and out of the lungs for life-sustaining breathing, protecting the airway from infiltration of food or liquid during swallowing, protecting the airway from infiltration of foreign bodies, and fixing the thorax during activities demanding highly elevated abdominal pressures (such as forced bowel and bladder evacuation, childbirth, and heavy lifting). Central to these functions is the ability of the vocal folds to *abduct* (move away from each other starting together at midline) or *adduct* (move toward each other ending together at midline), essentially serving as a valve between the speech tract and the respiratory tract. Using this valve to generate voice (*phonate*) has required the development of intricate neural controls that permit us to set the vocal folds into precise vibration for speaking and singing. Vocal fold vibration is possible because (1) the vocal folds are located within a fixed laryngeal framework; (2) muscles within the larynx (intrinsic laryngeal muscles) facilitate vocal fold abduction and adduction; (3) some of these intrinsic laryngeal muscles cause changes in the elastic properties of the vocal folds, affecting their rate of vibration; and (4) an outgoing airstream also affects vocal fold vibration. The myoelastic-aerodynamic theory of phonation, described later in this chapter, takes these factors into account. First, however, we turn to providing an overview of laryngeal anatomy, including changes affecting voice across the lifespan.

The Laryngeal Framework.   The larynx is a constricted tube with a smooth surface. It is located deep within the strap muscles of the neck. It is situated vertically at the level of vertebrae C4–6 in adults, but is higher in children, at the level of vertebrae C1–3. The larynx is approximately 44 mm long (1.7 inches) in adult males and approximately 36 mm long (1.5 inches) in adult females. The circumference of the larynx in adults is approximately 120 mm (5 inches). There is a framework of cartilages, ligaments, membranes, and folds that gives the larynx form. Connected to this framework are extrinsic and intrinsic laryngeal muscles that facilitate movement of either the laryngeal frame (in the case of the extrinsic muscles) or the vocal folds within (in the case of the intrinsic muscles).

Ligaments and membranes connect the larynx superiorly to the hyoid bone, inferiorly to the cricoid cartilage, and anteriorly to the epiglottis. These attachments of the larynx loosely position it at midline in the neck. Because the larynx is not rigidly fixed in the neck it is capable of limited up and down and side-to-side movements. To illustrate, put the first three fingers of your hand on your larynx and swallow—you should feel the larynx elevate and move forward slightly and then glide back to its resting position. Going further, if you apply a little firmer grip you can move the larynx from side to side. Also, if you raise your tongue within the oral cavity, or protrude your tongue, you will feel the larynx elevate slightly; this is partially because the base of the tongue inserts into the hyoid bone and as it contracts it lifts the hyoid bone slightly. The vertical and horizontal movements of the larynx are considered normal, and lack of such movements during a head and neck examination can be indicative of neurological damage, degenerative changes, blunt force trauma, or the presence of a tumor or other mass.

The Extrinsic Laryngeal Muscles.   The extrinsic laryngeal muscles have one attachment to the larynx and another attachment to some structure external to the larynx. Along with the hyoid bone, they are located in an area of the neck called the anterior triangle, which is bounded by the mandible, the sternocleidomastoid muscles, and the midline platysma muscle. The individual extrinsic laryngeal muscles are described anatomically as being part of one of two groups: the suprahyoids (inserting into the hyoid bone from the skull above) or the infrahyoids (inserting into the hyoid bone from the larynx or sternum below). It is clinically useful, however, to understand how each muscle contributes to elevation (raising) or depression (lowering) of the hyoid bone and larynx, as listed below:

Elevators	Depressors
Digastrics	Omohyoid
Geniohyoid	Sternohyoid
Mylohyoid	Sternothyroid
Stylohyoid	Thyrohyoid
Genioglossu	
Geniohyoid	
Hypoglossus	
Thyropharyngeus	

The raising and lowering of the larynx is observable and noted mainly during the pharyngeal stage of swallowing, serving primarily to help protect the airway from aspiration of food or liquid. To illustrate, take your index finger and place it on your Adam's apple. Swallow and you will feel the larynx raise and then return to its resting position. The extrinsic laryngeal muscles also come into play slightly during production of higher and lower pitches (especially in untrained singers). To illustrate, again place your index finger on your Adam's apple and count from 1 to 10 at your normal pitch and loudness—you should not feel any appreciable raising or lowering of the larynx. Repeat this exercise, but when you get to the numbers 6 through 10 raise your pitch dramatically—you should feel the larynx rise. Conversely, if you lower your pitch dramatically, your larynx will lower. A good speaking voice does not apparently require much active muscle involvement of the extrinsic laryngeal muscles. Trained singers keep the height of the larynx nearly constant while singing a range of high and low notes (Sataloff, 1981).

Laryngeal Cartilages.   There are five major laryngeal cartilages important for voice production and airway protection: the cricoid, the thyroid, the paired arytenoids, and the epiglottis. These are shown in Figures 2.6 through 2.8. Two other

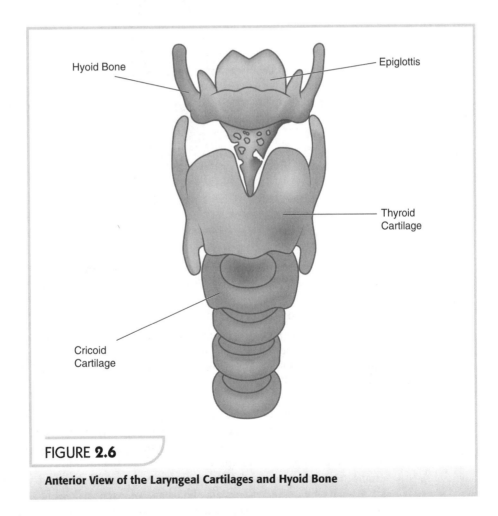

Hyoid Bone

Epiglottis

Thyroid
Cartilage

Cricoid
Cartilage

FIGURE **2.6**

Anterior View of the Laryngeal Cartilages and Hyoid Bone

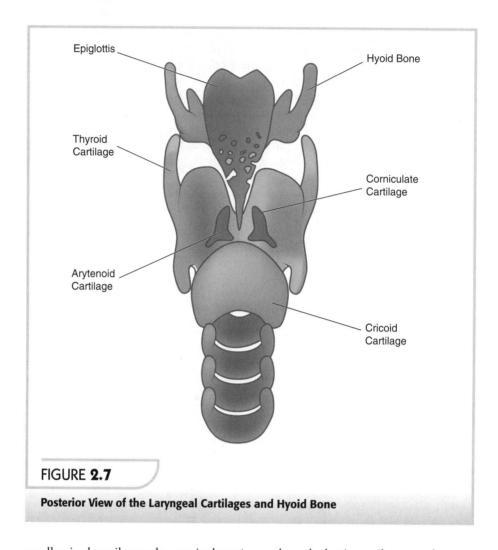

Epiglottis

Hyoid Bone

Thyroid
Cartilage

Corniculate
Cartilage

Arytenoid
Cartilage

Cricoid
Cartilage

FIGURE **2.7**

Posterior View of the Laryngeal Cartilages and Hyoid Bone

small paired cartilages, the corniculates (cone-shaped, elastic cartilages on the apex
of the arytenoids extending into the aryepiglottic folds) and the cuneiforms (cone-
shaped, elastic nodules located in the aryepiglottic folds) apparently play only a
minimal role in the phonatory functions of the larynx. The larynx develops in utero
from paired branchial arches, so slight asymmetries in structure are often observed,
particularly as one ages (Lindestadt, Hertegard, and Bjorck, 2004). Such asymmetries typically do not affect voice, though.

The cricoid, thyroid, and arytenoid cartilages are intricately connected to one
another by joints, ligaments, membranes, and muscles (described in later sections).
The cricoid is the second largest of the three cartilages and is a signet-shaped ring
connected to the first tracheal ring. The two pyramid-shaped arytenoid cartilages
sit atop its high posterior wall. The base of each arytenoid cartilage has two
concave and smooth surfaces, called processes, to which muscles attach. One of these

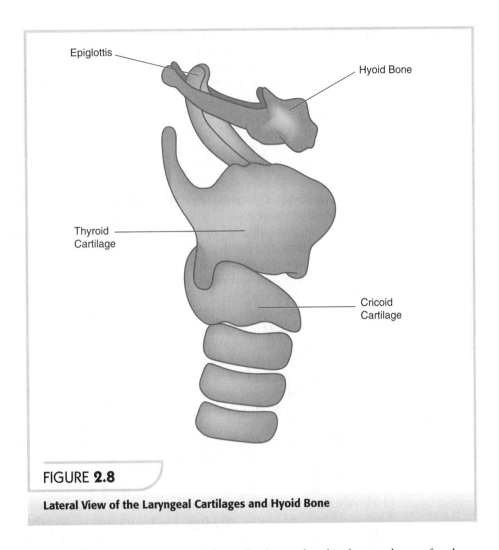

FIGURE **2.8**

Lateral View of the Laryngeal Cartilages and Hyoid Bone

surfaces, the muscular process, is laterally-directed and is the attachment for those intrinsic laryngeal muscles that cause the arytenoid cartilage to rock, rotate, and slide on the cricoid cartilage. The other process, the vocal process, is anteriorly-directed and is the posterior attachment for the vocal ligament and vocalis muscle. The remaining major cartilage, the thyroid cartilage, is the largest of the three listed. It has several parts: two laminae, a superior thyroid notch, two superior horns, two inferior horns, and two oblique lines. The two laminae fuse anteriorly in the midline and form the laryngeal prominence (commonly called the Adam's apple). In postpubertal males the angle of the laryngeal prominence is approximately 90° and in females the angle is approximately 120°. If you feel your Adam's apple with your middle finger oriented horizontally and then place your index finger right next to it you should feel a v-shaped notch between the laminae—this is the superior thyroid notch, present because the laminae are incompletely fused. The superior horns are posterior points of attachment for ligaments connecting the thyroid cartilage to the hyoid bone above. The inferior horns are also posterior points of attachment and connect the thyroid cartilage to the cricoid cartilage below via a joint. Each lamina also contains an oblique line, a ridge that descends diagonally from superior to inferior; this ridge is a line of attachment for some of the extrinsic laryngeal muscles and the inferior pharyngeal constrictor muscle. Similar to cartilage throughout the skeletal system, all the laryngeal cartilages are coated with a tough leathery covering (the perichondrium) that gives the larynx a waxy look. This perichondrium is thicker externally than internally.

Extrinsic Laryngeal Ligaments and Membranes.   There are also ligaments and membranes that connect parts of the larynx to adjacent support structures. Some of these ligaments and membranes connect laryngeal cartilages to the epiglottis, some connect laryngeal cartilages to the hyoid bone, some connect the epiglottis to the hyoid bone or tongue, and some connect laryngeal cartilages to the trachea. It is helpful in gaining an understanding of some of these ligaments and membranes to refer again to Figures 2.6–2.8 and note that there are spaces between some of the major laryngeal cartilages and their adjacent external structures. For example, the medial and lateral thyrohyoid ligaments, along with the thyrohyoid membrane, connect the thyroid cartilage to the hyoid bone (see Figure 2.9). The cricotracheal ligament and cricotracheal membrane connect the cricoid cartilage to the uppermost tracheal ring. The cricothyroid membrane connects the cricoid and thyroid cartilages (see Figure 2.9). One can appreciate the thyrohyoid space (for example) with palpation (touch). To illustrate, place your thumb on your neck, just above the thyroid notch and just below your chin, and gently press inward. What you are feeling is underlying muscles, medial ligaments, and membranes—that is, you should appreciate that the thyroid cartilage is not fused with the hyoid bone above it. If you keep your thumb in place and swallow, you will feel a tightening of the muscles and ligaments and a narrowing of the space as the larynx elevates. You will also feel this tightening if you go from producing a voice at your normal pitch to one at a much higher pitch. Keep in mind too that we have previously described the larynx as a closed tube. Therefore, there must be membranes spanning the space between cartilages. The interested reader is referred to Zemlin (1998) for a complete listing and description of all the extrinsic laryngeal ligaments and membranes.

The Laryngeal Cavity.   The laryngeal inlet (aditus laryngis) is the entrance into the larynx (see Figure 2.10). It is a triangular opening, wider in front than in back, that slopes obliquely down and back. Its boundaries are the epiglottis in the front, the aryepiglottic folds on each side and the arytenoid cartilages behind. Its shape is variable, depending on the position of the arytenoid cartilages and the epiglottis. The laryngeal vestibule is immediately beneath the inlet and contains two protruding sets of mucosal folds—the ventricular folds (more commonly referred to as the false vocal folds) and the true vocal folds (more commonly referred to simply as the vocal folds). (We will describe these folds in a later section). The area

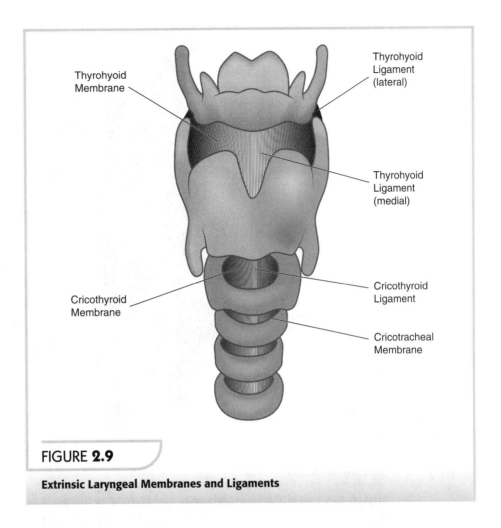

Thyrohyoid Membrane

Thyrohyoid Ligament (lateral)

Thyrohyoid Ligament (medial)

Cricothyroid Membrane

Cricothyroid Ligament

Cricotracheal Membrane

FIGURE **2.9**

Extrinsic Laryngeal Membranes and Ligaments

between the false vocal folds and the true vocal folds is the ventricular space; within this pocketlike space are sacs that secrete mucous to coat the surface of the vocal folds below. The area between the vocal folds is the rima glottidis; the glottis refers to the vocal folds and the space in between them. The laryngeal cavity can thus be divided into the supraglottic space ("above glottis") and subglottic space ("below glottis"). The subglottis is narrower than the supraglottis but eventually widens as it joins the tubular trachea. The laryngeal cavity is lined with a wet mucosa continuous with the mucosa of the tongue, pharynx, and trachea. This mucosa covers the laryngeal cartilages, membranes, ligaments, and muscles and is rich with sensory receptors and mucous-secreting glands. Irritation or drying of this lining can often contribute to a hoarse voice quality. In a more serious condition, the epithelial cells constituting this lining can become malignant, necessitating possible removal of all or part of the larynx.

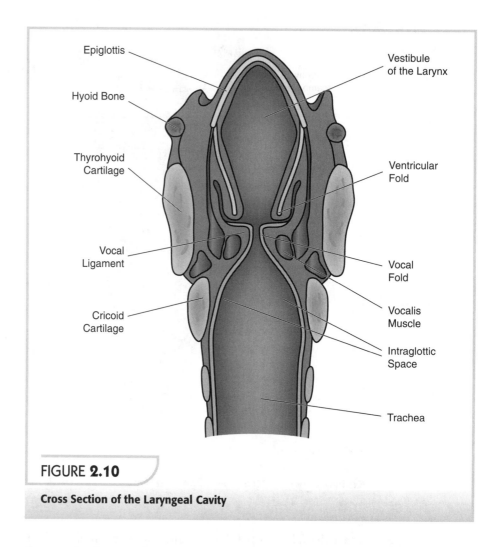

Epiglottis

Hyoid Bone

Thyrohyoid Cartilage

Vocal Ligament

Cricoid Cartilage

Vestibule of the Larynx

Ventricular Fold

Vocal Fold

Vocalis Muscle

Intraglottic Space

Trachea

FIGURE **2.10**

Cross Section of the Laryngeal Cavity

Laryngeal Joints. The two laryngeal joints, the cricothyroid joint and the cricorarytenoid joint (see Figure 2.11), are both synovial joints (filled with a lubricating fluid) that achieve movement at the point of contact of the articulating cartilages. Without these two joints, the vocal folds would not be able to approximate (make contact) nor change their length. The cricothyroid joint is formed between the inferior horns of the thyroid cartilage and the posterior cricoid arch. Rotation at this joint results in the thyroid cartilage tilting downward and also gliding forward and back relative to the cricoid, providing the major adjustment for change in pitch. The cricoarytenoid joints are formed between the superior borders of the cricoid cartilage and the arytenoid cartilages. The movement at the joint is described primarily as a rocking-gliding motion. The rocking motion at this joint primarily results in the vocal processes of the arytenoid cartilages swinging downward and

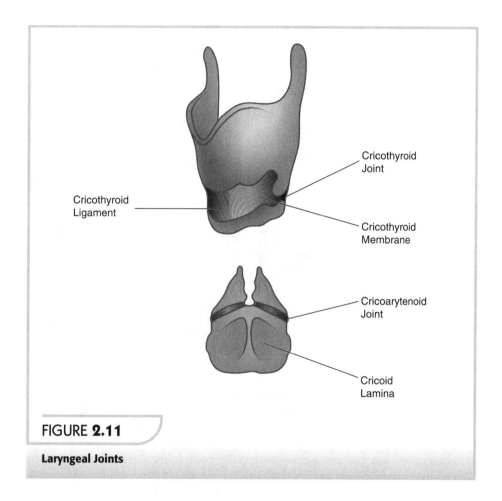

Cricothyroid Joint

Cricothyroid Membrane

Cricothyroid Ligament

Cricoarytenoid Joint

Cricoid Lamina

FIGURE **2.11**

Laryngeal Joints

inward (for adduction), or upward and outward (for abduction). The gliding motion primarily results in changes in vocal fold length. Arthritis or trauma can result in limited or absent motion of the arytenoid cartilages, resulting in vocal fold immobility (Speyer, Speyer, and Heijnen, 2008).

Intrinsic Laryngeal Ligaments and Membranes. There are ligaments and membranes which connect the laryngeal cartilages to each other. Beneath the mucous membrane on each side of the larynx is a broad sheet of fibrous tissue containing many elastic fibers—it is sometimes referred to as the fibroelastic membrane of the larynx. This membrane (see Figure 2.12) has an upper portion called the quadrangular membrane and a lower portion called the conus elasticus (the triangular membrane). The dividing line between these upper and lower membranes is the ventricular space. The paired quadrangular membrane originates in the lateral margins of the epiglottis and adjacent thyroid cartilage (at a midpoint between its

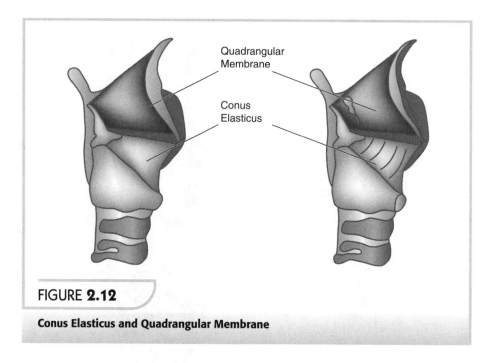

Quadrangular
Membrane

Conus
Elasticus

FIGURE **2.12**

Conus Elasticus and Quadrangular Membrane

upper and lower borders) and attaches to the corniculate cartilage and the lateral surface of the arytenoid. The free superior margins of the quadrangular membranes form the aryepiglottic folds, which drape an underlying aryepiglottic muscle. The free inferior borders of the quadrangular membranes form the ventricular ligaments, also known as the false vocal folds. The conus elasticus connects the cricoid cartilage with the thyroid and arytenoid cartilages via the medial and lateral cricothyroid ligaments. The free superior borders of the conus elasticus form the vocal ligaments.

The Intrinsic Laryngeal Muscles.   The intrinsic laryngeal muscles connect the laryngeal cartilages to each other. Collectively, the contraction or relaxation of these muscles results in either the adduction, abduction, tensing, or relaxing of the vocal folds. These muscles are innervated by various branches of the Vagus nerve (cranial nerve [CN] X). The following brief descriptions identify key muscles in Figure 2.13.

Posterior Cricoarytenoids.   This paired muscle is the lone abductor muscle. Its fibers originate from a middle depression on the posterior surface of the cricoid and insert into the posteromedial surface of the muscular process of the arytenoid on either side (right-sided fibers go to the right muscular process and so on). Contraction of this muscle draws the muscular process posteriorly, which pivots the arytenoid cartilage laterally and abducts the vocal fold. This muscle is particularly active during more active abduction, such as when needed for a quick or deep inhalation.

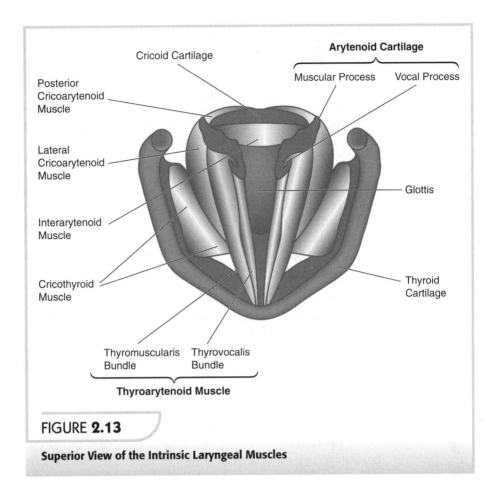

Cricoid Cartilage

Arytenoid Cartilage

Muscular Process   Vocal Process

Posterior Cricoarytenoid Muscle

Lateral Cricoarytenoid Muscle

Interarytenoid Muscle

Cricothyroid Muscle

Glottis

Thyroid Cartilage

Thyromuscularis Bundle   Thyrovocalis Bundle

Thyroarytenoid Muscle

FIGURE **2.13**

Superior View of the Intrinsic Laryngeal Muscles

Lateral Cricoarytenoids. This paired muscle functions as a direct antagonist to the posterior cricoarytenoid muscle as it plays its adductor role. Its fibers originate from the arch of the cricoid and insert into the anterolateral surface of the muscular process of the arytenoid on either side. Contraction of this muscle draws the muscular process anteriorly, which pivots the arytenoid cartilage medially and adducts and lowers the position of the vocal folds.

Transverse Arytenoid. This unpaired muscle is also an adductory muscle. Its fibers originate from the posterior surface of the arytenoid cartilage on one side and insert into the corresponding surface of the opposite arytenoid cartilage. Contraction of this muscle draws the body of each arytenoid cartilage together, adducting and compressing the vocal folds.

Oblique Arytenoids. This paired muscle is also an adductory muscle. Its fibers originate from the muscular process of the arytenoid cartilage on one side and insert into the posterior surface of the arytenoid cartilage on the opposite side. Contraction of this muscle draws the apex of each arytenoid cartilage together, adducting the vocal folds.

Thyroarytenoids. This paired muscle forms the bulk of the muscular portion of the vocal folds. Both anatomically and functionally, this muscle has two components: a medial muscle called the thyrovocalis (or simply, vocalis) and a bulkier lateral portion called the thyromuscularis (or simply, muscularis). Fibers of the vocalis originate on the inner surface of the thyroid cartilage near the thyroid notch and insert on the lateral surface of the vocal process of the arytenoid. Fibers of the muscularis originate on the thyroid cartilage just lateral to those of the vocalis and insert on the muscular process of the arytenoid. Contraction of the vocalis draws the cricoid and thryoid cartilages further apart, tensing the vocal folds when balanced by the antagonistic contraction of the cricothyroid muscle. Contraction of the muscularis draws the arytenoid cartilages forward, relaxing and adducting the vocal folds.

Cricothyroid. This muscle is made up of two components: the pars recta and the pars oblique (*pars* = part). Both are vocal fold tensors. The fibers for each component originate from the arch of the cricoid cartilage and end in two distinctly different insertions. The lower fibers (pars oblique) insert near the thyroid lamina and the inferior horn of the thyroid cartilage. The upper fibers (pars recta) insert into the lower surface of the thyroid lamina. When the pars recta contracts, the thyroid cartilage is tilted downward; when the pars oblique contracts, the thyroid cartilage is drawn forward. As a result, the distance between the anterior thyroid cartilage and the arytenoid cartilages is increased—because the vocal folds are passively strung between the thyroid and arytenoid cartilages, their length increases, their tension increases, and their mass per unit of length decreases. This results in faster vibration, which is perceived by the listener as an increase in pitch.

The Vocal Folds. The ventricular folds (false vocal folds) are two thick, membranous folds, each enclosing a narrow band of fibrous tissue, the ventricular ligament (see Figure 2.10). This ligament is attached to the thyroid cartilage (immediately below the attachment of the epiglottis) and to the arytenoid cartilage (a short distance above the vocal process). The lower border of the ventricular folds is the upper boundary of the laryngeal ventricle. The space between the ventricular folds is called the rima vestibuli. The ventricular folds should not adduct during normal phonation; in the rare and clinically significant cases when they adduct during phonation, the result is called ventricular phonation.

The vocal folds (true vocal folds) are also two membranous folds, each enclosing a narrow band of elastic tissue, the vocal ligament. This ligament (see Figures 2.10, 2.13, and 2.14) is attached to the thyroid cartilage (midway between its upper and lower borders) and to the vocal process of the arytenoid. The upper border of the true vocal folds is the lower boundary of the laryngeal ventricle. The space between the vocal folds is called the rima glottidis. Laterally, the vocalis

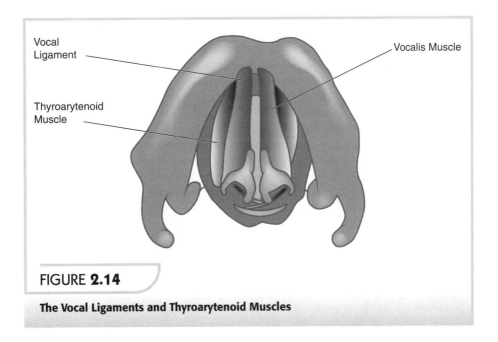

Vocal Ligament

Vocalis Muscle

Thyroarytenoid Muscle

FIGURE **2.14**

The Vocal Ligaments and Thyroarytenoid Muscles

muscle lies parallel with it. The vocalis is covered by mucous membrane, which is extremely thin and closely adherent to its surface. In adults the vocal folds are approximately 20 mm long (0.8 inches). The anterior three-fifths of the vocal fold is described as being more membranous while the posterior two-fifths is described as being more cartilaginous. The membranous part produces voice when vibrating; the cartilaginous part is where the vocal fold attaches to the vocal process of the arytenoid cartilage. During quiet breathing the posterior glottis is approximately 8 mm wide (0.3 inches), but that width may double during deep inhalation.

Each true vocal fold is composed of mucosa and muscle; interwoven throughout are blood vessels. From top to bottom, the vocal fold has five layers (see Figure 2.15): (1) superficial epithelium, (2) superficial lamina propria, (3) intermediate lamina propria, (4) deep lamina propria, and (5) vocalis muscle. The superficial epithelium and superior and intermediate lamina propria are composed of elastin fibers, which allow for stretching. The deep layer of the lamina propria is composed of collagen fibers, which prohibits stretching. The vocalis fibers make up the bulk of the vocal fold. Alternative descriptions, such as the cover-body concept (Hirano, 1981) place these five layers under three headings: (1) the cover (epithelium and superficial lamina propria), (2) a transitional zone (intermediate and deep layers of the lamina propria), and the body (vocalis muscle). Regardless of which description one uses, it is clear that the vocal fold does not comprise the same tissue from top to bottom—that is, there is a loosely adherent cover, an underlying vocal ligament providing some stiffness and support, and a further underlying bulky muscle. The cover gives the vocal fold a glistening white appearance and vibrates most markedly

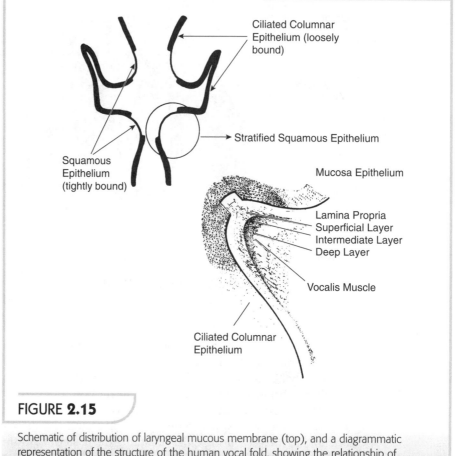

FIGURE **2.15**

Schematic of distribution of laryngeal mucous membrane (top), and a diagrammatic representation of the structure of the human vocal fold, showing the relationship of epithelium to adjacent tissues, the lamina propria (three layers), and vocalis muscle.

Source: From Zemlin, W. R. (1998). *Speech and Hearing Science: Anatomy and Physiology* (4th ed). Boston: Allyn and Bacon.

during phonation. During a laryngostroboscopic examination the cover can be seen moving during vocal fold vibration, a phenomenon known as the mucosal wave (Hirano and Bless, 1993). Even when the vocalis muscle is weak or paralyzed, the cover may still vibrate passively (and to a more limited degree) because of exhaled air flowing over it. However, if the vocal fold is stiff and edematous (swollen) the mucosal wave may be absent or markedly decreased.

Laryngeal Blood Supply and Lymphatic Drainage.   A dual blood supply flows to and from each side of the larynx (see Figure 2.16). The two major arteries

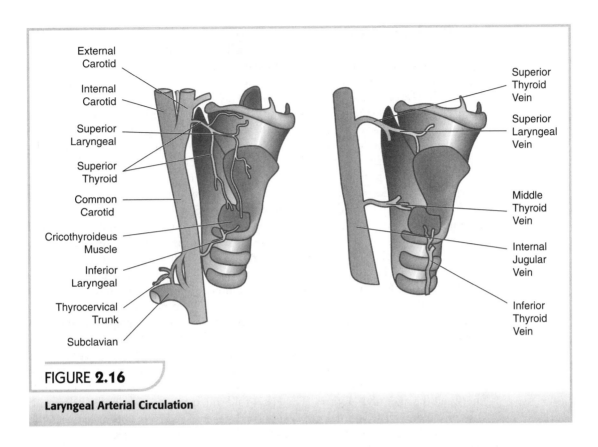

External Carotid

Internal Carotid

Superior Laryngeal

Superior Thyroid

Common Carotid

Cricothyroideus Muscle

Inferior Laryngeal

Thyrocervical Trunk

Subclavian

Superior Thyroid Vein

Superior Laryngeal Vein

Middle Thyroid Vein

Internal Jugular Vein

Inferior Thyroid Vein

FIGURE **2.16**

Laryngeal Arterial Circulation

supplying the larynx are the inferior and superior laryngeal arteries, branches of the thyroid artery. The two veins draining the larynx are the inferior and superior laryngeal veins. The inferior arteries and veins serve the upper larynx (i.e., the arytenoid cartilages, the false vocal folds and the laryngeal ventricle); the superior arteries and veins serve the lower larynx (i.e., the piriform sinus and the quadrangular membrane). The laryngeal lymphatic vessels drain into the cervical lymph nodes. Abnormalities in laryngeal blood flow can be observed clinically most dramatically in the case of a vocal fold hemorrhage, resulting in immediate and severe dysphonia.

Changes in the Larynx across the Lifespan. The larynx changes from birth through adolescence and adulthood and into the geriatric years. These changes can be observed during examination of both the external and internal larynx. Many of the differences heard in the voice over the lifespan can be attributed to fundamental changes in laryngeal anatomy and physiology. Understanding this process helps the speech–language pathologist work most effectively with voice disordered patients of all ages.

The pediatric larynx is not just a smaller version of the adult larynx. The marked differences between the two primarily involve the position of the larynx, the size and configuration of the laryngeal cartilages, and the size and fine structure of the vocal folds (the interested reader is referred to Sapienza, Ruddy, and Baker, 2004, for a complete description of the developing pediatric larynx). The pediatric larynx is situated higher in the neck than that of an adult, descending to the adult position after puberty. With this descent comes a lengthening and widening of the pharynx, contributing to changes in the resonance of the voice. The whole laryngeal framework in children is much softer than in adults, which makes it less susceptible to blunt trauma; by the same token, however, the larynx is more susceptible to collapse and compromise of the airway. The pediatric hyoid bone assumes a much lower vertical position and may overlap the thyroid cartilage. Additionally, there is no Adam's apple; this thyroid prominence does not appear until puberty. The angle of the thyroid laminae in newborns is approximately 120°, close to that of an adult female but wider than that of an adult male. The cricothyroid space in the developing larynx is a narrow slit and difficult to appreciate with palpation (touch). Finally, the length and fine composition of the pediatric vocal folds are also quite different. The length of the vocal fold in newborns is 2.5–3.0 mm (0.01–0.12 inches), growing rapidly with puberty and reaching an adult length of approximately 17–21 mm (0.7–0.8 inches) in adult males and 11–15 mm (0.4–0.6 inches) in adult females (Hirano, Kurita, and Nakashima, 1983). The membranous part of the newborn vocal fold is approximately the same length as the cartilaginous part. There is no vocal ligament in newborns; an immature one develops between the ages of 1–4 years. The vocal fold mucosa is thinner in newborns and young children. The lamina propria is a single layer; two layers appear between the ages of 6–12 years; and a fully differentiated covering is only apparent at the conclusion of puberty.

As a person ages into the 60s and beyond, structural changes across physiological systems impact the accuracy, speed, range, endurance, coordination, stability, and strength of muscular movements (the interested reader is referred to Chodzko-Zajko, 1997, for a review of normal aging and human physiology). Changes in laryngeal anatomy and physiology, coupled with changes in the nervous, respiratory, and supralaryngeal systems, can account for many of the changes heard in the senescent ("older") voice (the interested reader is referred to Zraick, Gregg, and Whitehouse, 2006, for an extensive review of speech and voice changes in geriatric speakers). Some of the age-related changes in the larynx include hardening of the laryngeal cartilages, atrophy and degeneration of the intrinsic laryngeal muscles, deterioration of the cricoarytenoid joint, degeneration of glands in the laryngeal mucosa, degenerative changes in the lamina propria, and degenerative changes in the conus elasticus (Kendall, 2007; Linville, 2001; Thomas, Harrison, and Stemple, 2007). These changes can lead to what is commonly referred to as "presbyphonia"—an age-related voice disorder characterized by recognizable perceptual changes in the pitch, pitch range, loudness, and quality of the older speaker's voice (Roy, Stemple, Merrill, and Thomas, 2007). Presbyphonia will be described further in Chapter 8.

Principles of Phonation

To provide further detail about laryngeal functioning for voice production, we first summarize the myoelastic-aerodynamic theory of phonation (van den Berg, 1958), followed by brief descriptions of the major laryngeal adjustments needed to accomplish phonation. An overview of voice registers is then presented. We conclude with discussions of the mechanisms for changing vocal pitch, loudness, and quality. It is our hope that the reader will use the material presented in this chapter as a basis for understanding not only normal voice production, but abnormal voice production as well.

The Myoelastic-Aerodynamic Theory of Phonation.   According to van den Berg (1958), the myoelastic-aerodynamic theory of phonation "deals with the control of the larynx by the higher centers of phonation" (p. 227). Generally regarded as the most accurate model to explain the mechanics of vocal fold vibration, the major elements of this theory are embedded in its title. *Myo* refers to involvement of muscles, *elastic* to the ability of those muscles to return to their original state, *aero* to airflow and pressure, and *dynamic* refers to movement and change. The major principles of this theory can be summarized as follows: (1) the vocal folds adduct (come to midline) by contraction of certain intrinsic laryngeal muscles; (2) when fully approximated there is an increase in subglottal air pressure relative to supraglottal air pressure; (3) the increased subglottal air pressure causes the vocal folds to separate first on their inferior border and then their superior border, eventually abducting completely (but not necessarily widely); (4) when abducted, the velocity of airflow between the vocal folds increases and the pressure between the vocal folds decreases (the Bernoulli principle); (5) the decreased air pressure, coupled with the elastic recoil of the vocal folds, causes them to move back toward midline; and (6) the vocal folds approximate first on their inferior border and then their superior border, eventually adducting (but not necessarily tightly or forcefully). Thus, the vocal folds have completed one cycle of vibration (closed-open-closed) due to *both* myoelastic and aerodynamic forces, not simply repetitive muscle contraction. This cycle of vibration will repeat so long as sufficient subglottal air pressure (on the order of 3–5 cm H_2O at minimum) can build up to blow the vocal folds apart again. This cycle is repeated approximately 125 times per second, or 125 Hertz (Hz), in the habitual phonation of an adult male, approximately 225 Hz in an adult female, and approximately 265 Hz for a prepubertal child.

Laryngeal Adjustments for Speech.   The larynx is capable of making remarkably fast and accurate phonatory adjustments during speech. To illustrate, examine the following two written phrases: "He went to seven zoos" and "I wore seven shoes." When saying these phrases aloud one can appreciate that each phrase consists of a combination of voiced and voiceless phonemes (sounds), in different sequences. In order for these phrases to "sound right" when spoken aloud, the larynx must adjust to the phonetic demands placed on it. That is, the laryngeal musculature must adjust in such a manner that the voice turns on when it should, stays on when it should, and turns off when it should. On top of that, the voice that is produced must be acceptable in terms of pitch, loudness, and quality.

Moore and von Leden (1958) have described three types of vocal onset (or attack): breathy (aspirate), simultaneous (easy, gentle), and glottal. To illustrate, consider the two phrases in the previous paragraph and place your right index finger on your Adam's apple and your left index finger just in front of (but not touching) your lips. Now, say the first word of each phrase ("He" versus "I"), paying close attention to the sensations on each finger during each utterance. When saying "He" you should feel exhaled air on your left finger prior to feeling vibration of the vocal folds on your right finger, an example of breathy vocal attack—that is, air begins to flow before the vocal folds are adducted. When saying "I" you should feel the opposite sensation; that is, exhaled air on your left finger is felt after vibration of the vocal folds is felt on your right finger. This is an example of glottal attack—air begins to flow after the vocal folds are firmly adducted (much like in a cough). A third type of attack, called simultaneous vocal attack, can be appreciated by examining the word "zoos" in the first sentence. During production of the /z/ phoneme in the initial word position, you should feel exhaled airflow and vocal fold vibration at the same time. These three types of attack (breathy, glottal, and simultaneous) are all normal. Problems arise, however, when a particular type of attack (typically, glottal or breathy) is misused. For example, hard glottal attack is a misuse of normal glottal attack. This abnormal laryngeal adjustment is often associated with the "drill sergeant's" voice—a voice where the onset of each word is greatly punctuated in terms of attack and loudness. In another example, breathy phonation is often associated with the "Marilyn Monroe" voice—a voice that is light and airy throughout an utterance, regardless of linguistic content. Simultaneous attack is considered the most optimal means of initiating phonation because it places less stress and strain on the vocal folds. In Chapter 7 we present facilitating approaches to reduce hard glottal attack.

Looking again at the word "zoos" in the first sentence, one can also appreciate two additional laryngeal adjustments—sustained phonation and termination of phonation. Once simultaneous attack begins the vocal folds must be actively held in a position within the airstream that allows their continued vibration. Placing your two index fingers in position again, you should feel ongoing airflow and vocal fold vibration throughout the utterance. Compare this to production of the word "vice," in which vocal fold vibration ceases just prior to production of the final /s/ phoneme.

Voice Registers.　Consider for a moment whether your voice quality changes as you speak or sing at various pitch levels within your overall pitch range. Chances are it does. Voice quality near the bottom of your pitch range is likely very different from that near your habitual speaking pitch, and both are likely very different from voice quality near the top of your pitch range. You probably also perceive a consistent voice quality within each of these three broad areas of your range, but not across them. That is, there may be abrupt changes in voice quality as you move through your range (particularly if you are an untrained singer). The concept of vocal register addresses these vocal phenomena. A vocal register is defined as a series of consecutive pitch values of approximately equivalent vocal quality (Hollien, 1974). There is a rich history of considerable debate about how to label, define, and differentiate among registers (see Laver, 1980; Titze, 1994; and Cleveland, 1994 for discussions reflecting current ideas and Luchsinger and Arnold, 1965, for historical reference). There is a general consensus that at least three recognizable registers exist: modal, glottal fry (or pulse), and falsetto. Each of these registers is characterized physiologically by different modes (or patterns) of vocal fold vibration (Laver, 1980). Thus, any change to the pattern of vocal fold vibration may result in a perceived change in voice quality.

The patterns of vocal fold vibration largely result from the degree of longitudinal tension on the vocal folds, the degree of medial compression of the vocal folds, and the degree of adductive force. Active longitudinal tension is achieved through the contraction of the vocalis muscle, whereas passive longitudinal tension is achieved through contraction of the cricothyroid muscle. Medial compression is obtained by contracting the lateral thyroarytenoid muscles. The adductive force is caused by contraction of the interarytenoid muscles and the lateral cricoarytenoid muscles. Each register differs in terms of these physiological parameters (Laver, 1994).

Modal phonation is the register that we use for most conversational speech. The span of frequencies in this register for adult women is approximately 150–500 Hz and for adult men, approximately 80–450 Hz, with habitual speaking pitch falling in the low-to-mid part of the range. There is moderate longitudinal tension, moderate medial compression, and moderate adductive force. Vocal fold vibration is periodic, with very little audible frication (breathiness). The minimum subglottal pressure needed to maintain this pattern of vibration is approximately 3–5 cm H_2O. Average airflow rate is between 100–350 cc/sec. According to Cleveland (1994) singers may divide the modal register into a lower and heavier chest voice and a higher and lighter head voice.

The glottal fry (or pulse) voice usually occupies the frequencies below the modal register, though there may be some overlap between the two registers in adult males. The span of frequencies in this register for both women and for men is approximately 35–90 Hz. There is minimal longitudinal tension on the vocal folds, which are short and thicker, with a lax cover, moderate medial compression of the vocal folds, and mild adductive force. Vocal fold vibration is characterized by a double (or sometimes triple) closure pattern for each cycle (Chen, Robb, and Gilbert, 2002). The vocal folds close, bounce open, and then rapidly close again before finally opening to complete the cycle (Behrman, 2007). This generates a syncopated secondary beat perceived as a crackling sound, much like bacon frying in a pan of oil or the sound of a stick being dragged along a picket fence. The minimum subglottal pressure needed to maintain this pattern of vibration is approximately 2 cm H_2O, a value often seen at the end of long phrases. Average airflow rate is between 12–20 cc/sec. Excessive use of pulse phonation can be harmful to the vocal fold mucosa. The facilitating approaches of respiration training and pitch change, discussed in Chapter 7, are often effective in helping patients eliminate chronic use of glottal fry phonation. We also describe the use of glottal fry as a facilitating approach to eliminate muscle tension dysphonia.

The falsetto voice usually occupies the frequencies above the modal register, though there may be some overlap. Falsetto is most easily recognized in the adult male voice at a speaking pitch of 300–600 Hz. There is moderately high longitudinal tension on the vocal folds; they are long and stiff, thin along the edges, and often bow-shaped. There is moderately high medial compression of the vocal folds and high adductive force. The posterior cartilaginous portion of the glottis is so tightly adducted that little or no posterior vibration occurs while the anterior portion vibrates rapidly. The vocal folds make contact only briefly as compared to modal phonation, which gives falsetto its characteristic "breathy" quality. At times there may also be a posterior chink during the production of falsetto that contributes to the breathy quality. The amplitude of vocal fold excursion (lateral movement) is reduced. As a result of the limited lateral movement, the mucosal wave is confined to the medial edge of the vocal folds. The minimum subglottal pressure needed to maintain this pattern of vibration is less than that for modal phonation. This voice is perceived as not only being high-pitched, but thin and airy, with very little attack.

Teachers of voice strive to blend the various registers, so that the difference in quality of voice becomes almost imperceptible as the singer transitions from one register to the next. Some singers seem to have only one register; no matter how they change their pitch, their voice always seems to have the same quality, with no discernible break toward the upper part of the pitch range. This is no small accomplishment and requires considerable voice training. It is a highly regarded attribute in the professional singing voice.

How We Change Pitch.   Vocal pitch is a perceptual attribute correlated with the frequency (rate) of vocal fold vibration. As fundamental frequency changes the listener perceives a change in pitch. The primary biomechanical determinants of the rate of vocal fold vibration are (1) the length of the vocal folds, (2) the tension of the vocal folds, and (3) the mass of the vocal folds per unit of length. There are also changes in subglottal pressure that occur as one changes frequency. All these factors interact with one another to achieve a target frequency of vibration.

As the vocal folds lengthen, their tension increases and their mass per unit of length is decreased (think of a rubber band that becomes thinner as it is stretched). As a result the vocal folds vibrate faster. Which muscles contribute to this change, and how? The primary intrinsic laryngeal muscle involved in pitch change is the cricothyroid muscle. When this muscle contracts there is an increase in the distance between the anterior thyroid cartilage and the arytenoid cartilage. The thyrovocalis also contributes to pitch change. When it contracts the cricoid and thyroid cartilages are drawn further apart, tensing the vocal folds (when balanced by the antagonistic contraction of the cricothyroid muscle). As the vocal folds become shorter, less tense, and thicker, they vibrate slower. This change in frequency of vibration is perceived as a lowering of pitch. The thyromuscularis is the primary muscle responsible for this change. When it contracts the arytenoid cartilages are drawn forward, relaxing and adducting the vocal folds.

Near the upper end of the natural pitch range, increased elasticity of the vocal folds results in increased glottal resistance, requiring increased subglottal air pressure to produce higher frequency phonations. Increased tension of the vocal folds requires greater air pressure to set the folds into vibration. As van den Berg (1958) has written, the average person must slightly increase subglottal air pressure in order to increase voice pitch; however, because increasing subglottal pressure has an abducting effect on the vocal folds, the folds must continue to increase in tension (longitudinal tension) to maintain their approximated position. Although the primary determinants of vocal frequency are the length, mass, and tension adjustments of the vocal folds, increases in frequency are usually characterized by increasing subglottal pressures, increased medial compression of the vocal folds, and increased glottal airflow rates.

How We Change Loudness.   Vocal loudness is a perceptual attribute correlated with the intensity of the sound wave generated during phonation. As intensity changes the listener perceives a change in loudness. The primary biomechanical determinants of intensity are (1) subglottal pressure, (2) medial compression of the vocal folds, and (3) the duration, speed, and degree of vocal fold closure. There also are supraglottal adjustments that contribute to changes in vocal loudness.

Hixon and Abbs (1980) have written: "Sound pressure level, the primary factor contributing to our perception of the loudness of the voice, is governed mainly by the pressure supplied to the larynx by the respiratory pump" (p. 68). To illustrate, place your fingertips on your rib cage and feel what happens as you count aloud from 1 to 10 at a normal and constant loudness level. Repeat this exercise, steadily increasing loudness as you say the numbers 6 through 10. What you likely felt was an expansion of your rib cage. More air in the lungs will result in a greater buildup of subglottal air pressure when the vocal folds adduct, particularly the longer they remain adducted. As vocal intensity increases, the vocal folds tend to remain closed for longer periods of time during each vibratory cycle. When the vocal folds are eventually blown open they abduct more widely. This allows more and more air molecules to escape—air that is explosively turbulent and which generates more acoustic power (think of the sound of a hairdryer and how much louder the air is coming out of the nozzle when the dryer is set to a higher fan speed compared to a lower fan speed).

How We Change Voice Quality.   Voice quality is a perceptual attribute related to the sound of the voice beyond its pitch and loudness (Behrman, 2007). The "quality" of one's voice is what distinguishes it from other voices of similar pitch and loudness. Changes in voice quality appear to result from changes at two levels of the speech production system: (1) the glottal source and (2) the resonant characteristics of the vocal tract. The principles of voice quality change are not as well understood as those of pitch and loudness change. Further complicating matters is the subjective nature of voice quality judgments—what sounds acceptable to one listener may not be acceptable to another. On a related note, even when two listeners agree about the quality of a particular voice they each may use a different term to describe that voice. Moreover, there is considerable debate about which objective measures of voice quality correlate with subjective measures.

Abnormal voice quality may be a hallmark feature of dysphonia, regardless of etiology. In our clinical practice we see patients who present with a voice that is breathy, rough, strained, harsh (strained + rough), or hoarse (strained + rough + breathy). Each of these vocal qualities can result from either functional, organic, or neurological causes, or some combination of causes. Most of the facilitating approaches described in Chapter 7 can be used to improve voice quality, particularly the abnormal voice qualities that result from vocal hyperfunction.

Breathy voice quality is often associated with incomplete glottal closure. When the vocal folds are loosely or incompletely approximated, turbulent airflow contributes noise to the vocal signal. Intensity is diminished. Rough voice quality is often associated with aperiodic vocal fold vibration. The irregular mucosal wave movement adds spectral noise. Intensity may be increased. Strained voice quality is often associated with considerable medial compression of the true (and perhaps false) vocal folds. Strained voice quality is also often associated with aperiodic vocal fold vibration, which adds spectral noise. Intensity may be increased. The four spectrograms in Figure 2.17 contrast the breathy voice, the harsh voice, the hoarse voice, and the normal voice. Each of the spectrograms was produced by the same normal speaker prolonging an /i/.

Perkins (1983) has added constriction and vertical as well as horizontal focus to the concept of voice quality production. He describes the feeling of constriction on a continuum of open (the yawn) to closed (the swallow). The clinical facilitation technique of yawn–sigh discussed in Chapter 7 demonstrates the clinical value of these physiological configurations of the supraglottal vocal tract. Imagery or feeling is used to determine the vertical focus of the voice, "the perception associated with the placement of the focal point of the tone in the head" (Perkins, 1983, p. 113). At the low end of the vertical focus, speakers or singers feel their voice is being squeezed out of the throat, whereas at the high end the focus seems to be high in the head. The sensation is described as if the tone were "floating in the head." Vocal efficiency seems to occur best at the higher end of the vertical placement. The clinical facilitation technique of focus discussed in Chapter 7 makes use of these observations. It has been our experience that subjects given these instructions relative to the imagery of constriction and verticality produce voices with greater aperiodicity (hoarseness) at the low end of the vertical scale and greater vocal clarity at the high end. In time Perkins's construct of constriction and horizontal as well as vertical focus may well have greater measurement potential and utilization.

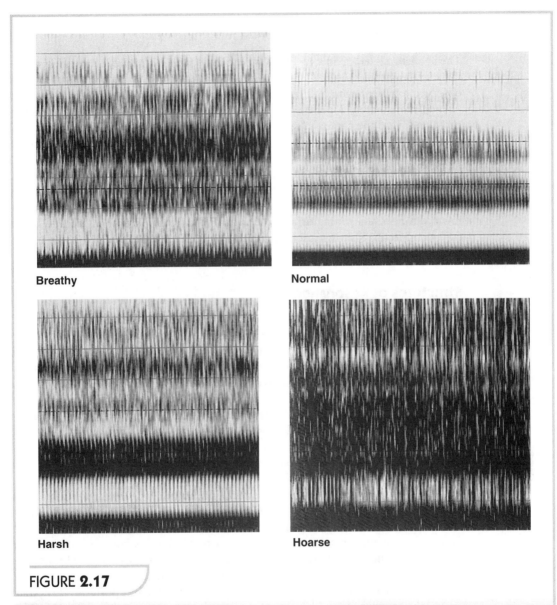

Breathy

Normal

Harsh

Hoarse

FIGURE **2.17**

Spectograms

Four spectograms of the same speaker producing the /i/ vowel under four conditions: breathy, normal, harsh, and hoarse. The relative spacing of the formants stays the same as the signal source changes.

RESONANCE

The acoustic signal produced by the vocal folds would be a weak-sounding reedy voice without the additional component of resonance. Years ago one of the authors observed a patient who had been cut from ear to ear with a massive wound that opened immediately superior to his thyroid cartilage. Before the wound was sutured, we heard the patient's feeble attempts at phonation. Much of his airflow and sound waves escaped through the wound. The result was a voice that was truly unique. Someone even likened it to the thin bleat of a baby lamb. Apparently, what is perceived as the quality, timbre, richness, fullness, and loudness of the voice is largely produced by the supraglottal resonators. Even though the structures of the chest and trachea may play some role in resonance, this role is not as clearly defined as that of the supraglottal resonators of the pharynx, oral cavity, and nasal cavity. Figure 2.18 shows a line drawing and cadaver head that demonstrate the F-shaped vocal tract.

Structures of Resonance

The vocal tract begins, for all practical purposes, at the level of the glottis. The airflow and sound waves probably have some beginning passage in the ventricular space (B in Figure 2.18) between the true folds (A) and the ventricular folds (C). In Figure 2.18 the cavities of the vocal tract have been shaded darker. The epiglottis (D), by its concavity, probably serves as a deflector or sounding-board resonator as sound waves travel between the aryepiglottic folds (E) into the hypopharynx (F). The hypopharynx is the cavity directly above the esophagus (G). Its anterior border comprises the structures and opening of the larynx; its sides and back wall are composed of the inferior pharyngeal constrictors. Superior to the inferior pharyngeal constrictors are the middle pharyngeal constrictors (H). The oropharynx (J) begins at the tip of the epiglottis and extends to the level of the velum and hard palate. The small angular spaces between the front of the epiglottis and the back of the tongue (L) are called the valleculae (I). Cutting away the mandible (K) in a lateral view is the great body of the tongue, which occupies most of the oral cavity and forms the constantly changing floor of that cavity. The hard palate is designated (O), with the soft palate or velum (N) forming the roof of the oral cavity. The lips, teeth, and cheeks play obvious front and lateral roles in shaping the oral cavity. The middle and superior pharyngeal constrictors form the lateral and posterior muscular wall of the oropharynx (J). The site of the velopharyngeal closure, necessary for the separation of the oral and nasal cavities required for oral resonance, is the Passavant's pad (M) area of the superior pharyngeal constrictor; most people do not have much Passavant area enlargement. As shown in Figure 2.18, superior to the velopharyngeal contact point, the posterior pharyngeal wall makes a sharp angulation forward, forming the superior wall of the nasopharynx (P) and continuing on as the superior wall of the nasal cavity. We make no further structural breakdown of the nasal cavities (Q) as a prelude to our discussion of resonance. Note that

Figure 2.18 also shows the lateral walls, pillars of fauces, and muscles of the palate, pharynx, and tongue. If we look again at the overall lateral view of the vocal tract, we see that the total darkened areas look something like a large letter F. The vocal tract in the photograph resembles an F because the velopharyngeal port is open, connecting the oral and nasal cavities together. If the port were closed at the velopharyngeal contact point (M), the vocal tract opening available for voice resonance would resemble the letter r, formed only by the pharynx and the oral cavity opening above the surface of the tongue.

Mechanism of Resonance

In humans the larynx is situated at approximately the 5th cervical vertebra, thus creating a resonating chamber to filter and amplify the acoustic signal. Some areas of the vocal tract, depending on their configuration, are compatible with the periodic vibration coming from the vocal folds and amplify the fundamental frequency and its harmonics. For example, a fundamental frequency of 125 Hz will resonate harmonic frequencies at 250, 375, 500, and so on (each subsequent harmonic frequency is a whole number multiple of the fundamental). For a more detailed description of vocal tract acoustics, the reader is referred to sources such as Daniloff (1985), Borden, Harris, and Raphael (1994), Minifie (1994), and Kent and Read (2002). The continuous vocal tract tube is constantly interrupted at various sites from the intrusion and movement of various structures. Some of the interruptions or constrictions may be severe, such as carrying the tongue high and forward in the oral cavity. Any movement of mandible, tongue, or velum, for example, will greatly alter the opening of the oral cavity. Some of the movements have no effect on the fundamental or sound source; some of them filter or inhibit the fundamental. What finally comes out of the mouth or the nasal cavity perceived as voice has become a complex periodic signal with the same fundamental frequency as the vocal fold source, but highly modified in its overall sound characteristics. We can hear several familiar voices all saying the same few words at the same fundamental frequency and still be able to differentiate each voice and assign it to each familiar person. Even if we do not know the speaker, we can fairly accurately tell the approximate age and the gender of the speaker. Perhaps even more importantly, by filtering the glottal tone we can tell if the person has a cold, is upset or angry, tired, frightened, or the meaning could even be changed by the change in quality or emphasis while saying the same words. The vocal characteristics related to the individualization of each person's vocal tract will have given each voice its own unique characteristics (vocal quality) as the result of the amplification and filtering unique to each vocal tract.

The F configuration of the supraglottal vocal tract is constantly changing. What happens in any one portion of the tract influences both the total flow of air and sound wave through the total tract and the sound that eventually issues out from the mouth (or nose). By action of the pharyngeal constrictors and other supraglottal muscles, the overall dimensions of the pharynx are always changing. The membranes of the pharynx and the degree of relaxation or tautness of the pharyngeal

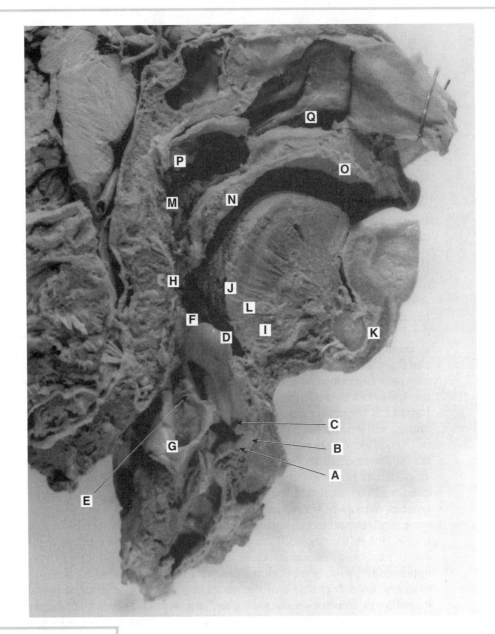

FIGURE 2.18

The F-Shaped Vocal Tract

The F-shaped vocal tract is shown in both the photograph of a cadaver head on the left and the line drawing on the right. Letters A through Q identify various structures of the vocal tract: (A) True folds; (B) ventricular space; (C) ventricular folds; (D) epiglottis; (E) aryepiglottic folds; (F) hypopharynx; (G) inferior pharyngeal constrictors and upper esophageal sphincter; (H) middle pharyngeal constrictors; (I) valleculae; (J) oropharynx; (K) mandible; (L) tongue; (M) Passavant's pad; (N) soft palate (velum); (O) hard palate; (P) nasopharynx; (Q) nasal cavity.

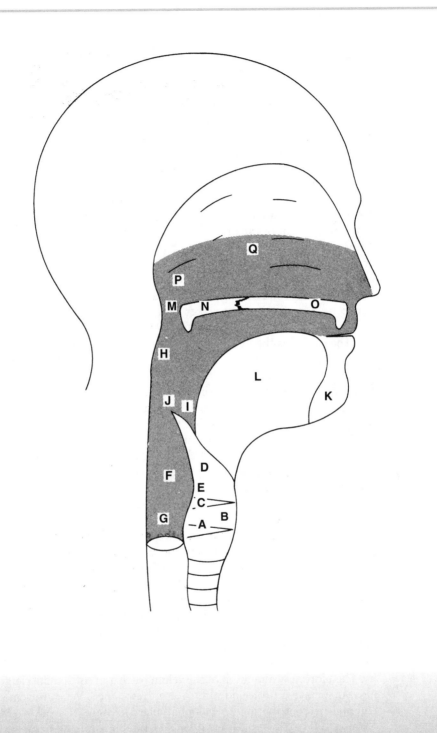

constrictors have noticeable acoustic filtering effects. Higher frequency vocalizations seem to receive their best resonating effects under a fairly high degree of pharyngeal wall tension. Lower frequencies appear to be better amplified by a pharynx that is somewhat larger and more relaxed. This appears to be related to the short wavelength of high frequency sounds and the long wavelength of the low frequency components.

The oral cavity, or mouth, is as essential for resonance as the pharynx. Of all our resonators, the mouth is capable of the most variation in size and shape. It is the constant size–shape adjustment of the mouth that permits us to speak or, more accurately, allows us to be understood. Our vowels and diphthongs, for example, are originated by a laryngeal vibration, but shaped and restricted by the size and shape adjustment of the oral cavity. The mouth has fixed structures (teeth, alveolar processes, dental arch, and hard palate) and moving structures (tongue, velum, cheeks, mandible, and lips). We are most concerned with the moving structures, primarily the tongue, velum, and mandible, in our study of voice resonance. It is the mouth and other supraglottal resonators that give the perception of a regional dialect to help identify the speaker and, more importantly, that allows for the formation of distinguishable vowels.

The tongue is the most mobile articulator, and it possesses both extrinsic and intrinsic muscles to move it. Each of the extrinsic muscles can, on contraction, elevate or lower the tongue at its anterior, middle, or posterior points and extend it forward or backward. The intrinsic muscles control the shape of the tongue by narrowing, flattening, lengthening, or shortening the overall tongue body and elevating or lowering the tongue tip. The various combinations of intrinsic and extrinsic muscle contractions can produce an unlimited number of tongue positions with resulting size–shape variations of the oral cavity. In addition to the tongue movements, the lowering and closing of the mandible contributes to the formation of specific vowels. The relationships of these cavities to vowel formants have been well described in several references, such as the Peterson and Barney study (1952) and Kent and Read (2002).

The structural adequacy and normal functioning of the velum are also important for the development of normal voice resonance. The elevation and tensing of the velum, as well as some pharyngeal wall movement, are vital for achieving velopharyngeal closure. A lack of adequate palatal movement, despite adequacy of velar length, can cause serious problems of excessive nasality. Although the velum probably serves as a sounding-board structure in resonance, it plays an obviously important role in separating the oral cavity from the nasal cavity (Abdel-Aziz, 2008). The movement and positioning of the velum changes the size and shape of three important resonating cavities: the pharynx, the oral cavity, and the nasal cavity. Therefore, any alteration of the velum (such as a soft-palate cleft or velar weakness) may have a profound influence on resonance. Velar movement is only one component contributing to velopharyngeal closure (Dworkin, Marunick, and Krouse, 2004). Closure patterns that separate the oral and nasal cavities from one another may include velar action coupled by posterior pharyngeal wall movement or velar action with active lateral and posterior pharyngeal wall movement. Watterson and McFarlane (1990) describe five classes of velopharyngeal closure and their various effects on speech and voice. Regardless of the type of closure pattern (velar-posterior-lateral pharyngeal wall), the site of closure is generally in the Passavant's area (designated as M in Figure 2.18). More will be said of nasal resonance and treatment of hypernasality and hyponasality in Chapter 9.

SUMMARY

This chapter reviewed the respiratory, phonatory, and resonance aspects of voice and also discussed the five aspects of voice—loudness, hygiene, pleasantness, flexibility, and representation. We found that the outgoing airstream is the primary driving force of voice. The efficient user of voice develops good expiratory control. The value and magnitude of respiratory volumes were discussed. A description of the physiology of phonation reviewed the structures and mechanisms of normal phonation, including frequency, intensity, and quality shaping mechanisms. Supraglottal structures and functions specific to quality and resonance were also reviewed. The entire vocal tract contributes to the amplification and filtering of the fundamental frequency into the final unique voice of any speaker. Understanding these processes underpins the provision of effective voice therapy for patients with a variety of dysphonias.

Thought Questions

1. Discuss the interdependent nature of the five aspects of voice.
2. Discuss the function of the laryngeal muscles responsible for pitch changes. Which muscles are they?
3. What determines pitch?
4. Describe the anatomy and physiology of phonation, including the principles of the Bernoulli effect.
5. What is the mucosal wave and what is one condition that might compromise its movement?
6. Cite average fundamental frequencies for men, women, and children. Why are they different?
7. Can large men produce a falsetto? Explain your answer.

chapter 3

Organic Voice Disorders

LEARNING OBJECTIVES

- Describe and define the roles of different kinds of specialists who are interested in voice

- Identify the major organic causes of voice disorders

- Explain the medical and behavioral approaches to these organic disorders

Voice is the sound produced by the vibrating vocal folds. This sound is shaped by the vocal tract into a unique acoustic form that allows the listener to recognize the speaker. Voice disorders result from faulty structure or function somewhere in the vocal tract, in the processes of respiration, phonation, articulation or resonance. When one or more aspects of voice such as loudness, pitch, quality, or resonance are outside of the normal range for the age, gender, or geographic background of the speaker, we say a voice disorder exists. In Chapter 2 we discussed the aspects of voice that characterize or identify normal voice. When one or more of these aspects is outside the normal range, the voice is disordered. For example, if the voice is too loud or too soft or is produced with trauma to the mechanism, sounds strange, is unpleasant, is unable to express emotion or meaning by pitch variations, or leads the listener to misjudge age or gender, the voice is said to have a defect. Long ago Van Riper and Irwin (1958) said that speech is defective if it interferes with communication, draws undue attention to itself, or causes the speaker to be somehow maladjusted. The same may be said for voice.

When the voice changes in any negative way, it is said to be disordered or dysphonic. Such changes have many different common names: hoarseness, harshness, huskiness, stridency, thinness, to name only a few. Unfortunately, there is little common agreement about what these terms mean among different listeners. In this text, we use a more generic term, *dysphonia*, which means any alteration in normal phonation. The lack of a common vocabulary for the various parameters of voice production and voice pathology is perhaps related to the number of different kinds of specialists who are concerned with voice—the laryngologist, the singing teacher, the speech–voice scientist, the speech–language pathologist, and the voice-and-diction teacher. The laryngologist is primarily interested in identifying the etiological and pathological aspects for purposes of treatment; the singing teacher uses imagery in an attempt to get the desired acoustical effect from the voice student; the speech–voice scientist has the laboratory interest of the physiologist or physicist; the speech–language pathologist often attempts to use the knowledge and vocabulary of all three of these disciplines to bring about voice improvement through treatment of the voice; and the voice-and-diction teacher assesses the dynamics of voice production and uses whatever is necessary to get the best voice. It is no wonder that interdisciplinary communication among voice specialists breaks down, considering the number of individuals involved.

Tolerance by the public or an indifference to voice problems makes the early identification of voice pathologies difficult. Hoarseness that persists longer than several days is often identified by the laryngologist as a possible symptom of serious laryngeal disease, and it may be. Hoarseness is certainly the acoustic correlate of improper vocal fold functioning, with or without true laryngeal disease. The distinction between organic disease of the larynx and functional misuse has been a prominent dichotomy in the consideration of phonatory disorders. It is important for the laryngologists, in their need to rule out or identify true organic disease, to view the laryngeal mechanism by laryngoscopy in order to make a judgment about organic–structural or neurological involvement. In the absence of observable structural deviation or neurological involvement, the laryngologist generally describes the voice disorder as functional. It has become important for the speech–voice pathologist to view the larynx as part of the voice evaluation and in designing the voice therapy (McFarlane and Lavorato, 1984; McFarlane, Watterson, and Brophy, 1990; Watterson and McFarlane, 1991). Indeed, ASHA (American Speech-Language-Hearing Association) affirms the practice of visualization of the larynx by both otolaryngologists and speech–language pathologists (1998a). It is an important milestone for speech–language pathologists to be able to count laryngeal visualization and imaging as within their scope of practice.

In Chapter 1 we introduced four distinct categories of voice disorders—organic, neurogenic, psychogenic and muscle tension related. This chapter introduces voice disorders related to organic causes.

CANCER

Cancer or *carcinoma* in the vocal tract is a life-threatening disease that requires serious medical–surgical management. Lip and intraoral cancers rarely contribute to changes in voice, but they may have obvious negative effects on articulation. Extensive oral lesions involving the tongue, perhaps even requiring partial or total surgical removal of the tongue (glossectomy), or palatal and velar cancer can seriously affect articulation, vocal resonance, and, of course, swallow. The American Cancer Society estimated 28,000 new cases of oral or pharyngeal cancer in the United States for the year 2002.

Some of the identified causes of oral cancer include smoking (particularly pipe smoking), use of smokeless tobacco, chronic infections, herpes, repeated trauma to the irritated site, and *leukoplakia* (whitish plaque). Often patients first experience chronic lesions in the mouth or on the tongue that do not seem to heal. Usually continuous pain near the lesion site brings the patient to the physician. The majority of these oral lesions are treated successfully with microsurgery (removal of small lesions) and radiation therapy. The primary goal of surgery–radiation therapy is to eradicate the primary lesion so that it does not spread (metastasize) to another adjacent or remote body site. Sometimes carcinoma is detected in the nasal sinuses and at sites within the pharynx, although such lesions are relatively rare. The most serious vocal tract malignancies, however, are those that involve the larynx, which by their position in the airway, present a serious potential threat to airway adequacy. Laryngeal cancer comprises approximately 6% of all malignancies diagnosed annually in the United States, according to the American Cancer Society.

In general, there are three classifications of laryngeal cancers, depending on the site of the lesion: *supraglottal*, involving such structures as the ventricular and aryepiglottic folds, the epiglottis, the arytenoid cartilages, and the walls of the hypopharynx; *glottal*, from the anterior commissure to the vocal process ends of the arytenoids; and *subglottal*, involving the cricoid cartilage and trachea. The treatment combines radiation therapy and surgery for small to moderate lesions; extensive cancer requires perhaps a hemilaryngectomy, a supraglottal laryngectomy, or total laryngectomy. We discuss these later in this chapter, and we consider laryngeal cancer, rehabilitation after laryngectomy, and the role of the speech–language pathologist in some detail in Chapter 8.

CONGENITAL ABNORMALITIES

Laryngomalacia

Laryngomalacia refers to the failure of cartilage to stiffen with development, resulting in an epiglottis that is too pliable and collapses into the airway. Laryngomalacia accounts for 75% of all congenital anomalies of the larynx and is the most prevalent cause of stridor in the neonate (Andrews and Summers, 2002;

Elluru, 2006). In most children with the condition, symptoms are evident at birth or within the first few hours or days of life. Laryngomalacia is diagnosed and managed by an otolaryngologist, who normally confirms the condition using transnasal fiberoptic laryngoscopy (O'Sullivan, Finger, and Zwerdling, 2004). Children with laryngomalacia rarely present with acute airway compromise, and Andrews reports that it is common for children to outgrow laryngomalacia by 18 months. However, for those 5% who require surgical intervention, this may be arranged in a semi-elective fashion within one to two weeks of presentation (Elluru, 2006). Supraglottoplasty is currently the preferred intervention, replacing tracheostomy (Denoyelle et al., 2003).

Subglottal Stenosis

Subglottic stenosis is the narrowing of the subglottic space. It can be congenital or acquired. Congenital stenosis results from an interruption of the cricoid cartilage or arrested development of the conus elasticus during embryological development (Weinrich, 2002). It is defined as a lumen 4.0 mm in diameter or less at the level of the cricoid (Cotton, Gray, and Miller, 1989). Acquired stenosis may occur following endotracheal intubation either related to lifesaving procedures or surgery. In some children, prolonged intubation can result in scarring, hypertrophy, and stenosis. Just as some individuals are susceptible to hypertrophic scarring of the skin, some infants appear to be prone to scarring and stenosis in response to intubation trauma (Faust, 2003). In both cases, if the stenosis is severe, air is not exchanged and tracheostomy may be necessary.

Walner and Cotton (1999) introduced levels of stenosis grading that help determine levels of intervention by the speech–language pathologist. For children with Grades I or II subglottal stenosis—that is, stenosis corresponding to 0–50% and 51%–70% respectively, careful observation rather than intervention may be appropriate. Stenosis of grades III or IV, on the other hand, which correspond to 71% to 99% and 100% respectively, will often present with either tracheal dependency or stridor and exercise intolerance. Children in these latter categories may require endoscopic or surgical intervention, usually with voice intervention to follow (Weinrich, 2002).

Tracheoesophageal Fistulas and Esophageal Atresia

Tracheoesophageal fistulas (TEF) are openings that occur between the esophagus and trachea. Esophageal atresia is an abnormal occlusion of the esophagus. TEF is associated with vascular compromise to the developing esophagus. TEF with a distal esophageal pouch occurs in 80 to 85% of affected patients and results in gastric distention, direct tracheal aspiration, and reduced diaphragmatic excursion (Sataloff, 1997b). TEFs can also be proximal; in some cases, double TEFs have been reported. The standard intervention is surgery, followed by voice and feeding therapy by the speech–language pathologist.

CONTACT ULCERS (GRANULOMAS)

Laryngeal
Images
Photo
Gallery

As we mentioned in Chapter 2, the total length of the glottis can be divided into thirds: the anterior two-thirds is muscular (vocalis portion of the thyroarytenoids) and covered by a membrane, and the posterior third is cartilaginous (arytenoids) and covered by a membrane. Contact ulcers are small ulcerations that develop on the medial aspect of the vocal processes of the arytenoid cartilages due to irritation. When granulated tissue forms over these ulcers as a protective mechanism, they are called contact ulcer granulomas. Figure 3.1 illustrates a moderately large contact ulcer granuloma.

The typical symptoms of contact ulcers are deterioration of voice after prolonged vocalization (vocal fatigue), accompanied by pain in the laryngeal area or sometimes pain that lateralizes out to one ear. Watterson, Hansen-Magorian, and McFarlane (1990) also found hoarseness or roughness reported 75% of the time and throat clearing in 65% of the 57 cases of contact ulcers they studied. Laryngoscopy usually reveals bilateral ulcerations with heavy buildup of granulation tissue along the approximating margins of the posterior glottis. Greene (1980) labeled the toughened membranous tissue changes on the posterior glottis as *pachydermia*, citing the work of Kleinsasser (1979), and wrote that "contact ulcers are not actually ulcers or granulomas but consist of 'craters' with highly thickened squamous epithelium over connective tissue with some inflammation (edema)" (p. 147).

Contact ulcers are multifactorial in nature and are considered a chronic inflammatory disease of the larynx. They seem to result from one of three causes or a combination of these: hard glottal attack along with throat clearing and coughing, laryngopharyngeal reflux, and endotracheal intubation.

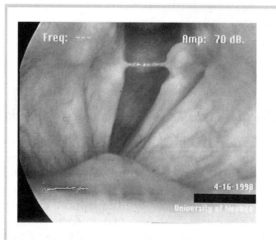

FIGURE **3.1**

Left Contact Ulcer with Granuloma, Young Adult Male

Contact ulcers (granulomas) are associated with hard glottal attack, laryngopharyngeal reflux, tracheal intubation, or a combination thereof.

The first cause is excessive slamming together of the arytenoid cartilages during production of low-pitched phonation coupled with excessively hard glottal attack and perhaps increased loudness with frequent throat clearing and coughing. The speaker is usually a hard-driving person who speaks in a loud, controlling low pitch, often with words punctuated by sudden onset. However, Watterson, Hansen-Magorian, and McFarlane (1990) found that hard glottal attack was reported only 26% of the time by diagnosing clinicians, while pain was reported in 56% of the total of 57 cases studied. Indeed we now feel that those patients who develop contact ulcers and granuloma due to faulty vocal functioning alone are in the minority. These individuals may experience co-occurring organic factors such as laryngopharyngeal reflux (LPR).

In LPR, the second etiology, stomach acid is forced up the esophagus and exits the upper esophageal sphincter, thus irritating the area between the arytenoids or the vocal fold covering. Patients with contact ulcers who also demonstrate marked irritation of LPR tissue are candidates for a thorough examination of the gastrointestinal tract (Koufman, 1991). Maier, Lohle, and Welte (1994) advocate ambulatory 24-hour pH monitoring for patients suspected of having this disorder. If LPR is detected, the patient may best be treated with antireflux medications, antacids, diet management, and voice therapy. Other behavioral changes, such as elevating the head of the bed and reducing the size of meals and eating several hours before going to bed, are helpful in reflux management. Also of note is that posterior commissure irritation may also stem from coughing as a result of postnasal drip. In this case, the patient should be referred to an otolaryngologist. See Reflux later in this chapter for further investigation into the relationship between postnasal drip and LPR.

Maier, Lohle, and Welte (1994) and Emami, Morrison, Rammage and Bosch (1999) found that the majority of their patients with contact ulcers who received an antireflux regimen and voice therapy experienced a complete remission of the contact ulcers. In another group of patients, when the ulcers and granulomas were removed surgically, more than 90% of these patients experienced recurrence unless voice therapy was performed. This was also found by Hirano and colleagues (2002), who reported that for 23 surgeries performed to remove contact granulomas, 10 of the 23 recurred. After surgical removal of the offending lesion, Hirano suggests that voice therapy is usually needed to help the patient regain a normal voice.

Leonard and Kendall (2005) reported the effects of a unique behavioral voice therapy program in patients who had failed other treatments for vocal process granulomas related to LPR. The researchers introduced a "phonoscopic" approach, whereby the patient observed his or her larynx endoscopically while voicing, and altered vocal fold vibration so that a small gap remained between the vocal processes. Of the 10 patient who received intervention, eight experienced full or a marked reduction in the granuloma.

Endotracheal intubation is a third cause of contact ulcers in a small number of cases, especially where large, protective granulomas are the presenting picture following the removal of the endotracheal tube. Any patient who is intubated during surgery or for airway preservation risks having a traumatized laryngeal membrane with the subsequent development of granuloma. The risk is particularly greater in children and women, who have smaller airways and are thus more often traumatized by large tubes (Whited, 1979). The physician places a tube down the pharynx into the airway, between the open (it is hoped) vocal folds, and on into the trachea. If the tube is larger than the glottal opening, the patient runs the risk of trauma. Ellis and Bennett (1977) have recommended that, in order to prevent intubation granuloma or hemangioma, patients should be intubated with tubes one size smaller than what would be needed for a snug fit.

Tracheal intubation often leads to postintubation granuloma (Balestrieri and Watson, 1982). Certainly, children and adults who have been intubated for whatever reason should receive a postintubation laryngeal examination. Any change in postsurgical voice should be investigated for intubation trauma with resulting irritation and granuloma. These complications from intubation may not appear immediately but rather develop over time (McFerran et al., 1994). No voice therapy should be initiated until a laryngeal examination is completed. If postsurgical granulomas are identified along the posterior glottis, medical–surgical treatment will promote healing and preserve the airway.

The focus of voice therapy for patients with contact ulcers and/or granuloma is to take the effort out of phonation. The patients must learn to use a voice pitch that can be produced with relatively little strain (which usually means pitch needs to be elevated), to speak with greater mouth and jaw relaxation, to speak at lower levels of volume, and to eliminate all traces of excessively hard glottal attack. Contact ulcers are rare today, according to Watterson, Hansen-Magorian, and McFarlane (1990); these cases comprise about 1% of total voice cases. Those patients who do have contact ulcers, however, seem to respond fairly well to voice therapy that is systematically employed.

In the past we generated a vocal hygiene program for a 38-year-old music salesman who reported pain in the laryngeal area following an upper respiratory infection accompanied by excessive coughing and throat clearing. Endoscopy revealed a collection of granular tissue at the vocal process of the left arytenoid cartilage with slight erythema at the vocal process of the right arytenoid cartilage. The patient stringently followed a program that eliminated vocally abusive behaviors, increased hydration, and reduced reflux. He also used confidential voice, reduced hard glottal attack, and engaged in vowel blending exercises. Posttherapy endoscopy revealed 80% reduction in the granular material and no additional reports of pain.

In addition to the three etiologies described above, surgery on the vocal folds will sometimes produce a reactive tissue irritation leading to the formation of granulomas. The most common reactive lesion is Teflon granuloma of the larynx (Varvares, Montgomery, and Hillman, 1995), usually caused by possible "overinjection, injecting too close to the vocal fold margin, or injecting too deeply." Teflon injection is usually reserved to give greater bulk to the paralyzed vocal fold in unilateral adductor paralysis, permitting better approximation of the normal fold with the paralyzed fold. This results in a better-sounding voice. However, if the voice begins to deteriorate several months after injection, the possibility of Teflon granuloma should be investigated. Other surgical traumas, such as removal of cysts or altering the glottal margin, have as a possible side effect the development of reactive tissue granuloma. From the perspective of the speech–language pathologist, if surgical revision of the larynx has resulted in a better voice, and then months or years afterwards the voice deteriorates, the larynx should be reexamined using endoscopy or stroboscopy in an attempt to identify possible reactive granuloma. Surgically induced irritation with resulting granuloma require medical–surgical resolution of the problem.

The speech–language pathologist should be alert to the fact that any inflammatory disease of the larynx, such as tuberculosis, syphilis, or sarcoidosis, can lead to granulomatous tissue changes (Pillsbury and Sasaki, 1982). Such tissue changes may produce voice symptoms. The overall management of voice problems related to inflammatory disease is pharmacologic.

CYSTS

DVD

Laryngeal
Images
Photo
Gallery

Cysts in the larynx are usually unilateral, occurring on the vocal folds (inner margin, superior or inferior surface) or anywhere on the ventricular folds. They are often caused by an abnormal blockage of the ductal system of laryngeal mucous glands (Case, 2002), but there are other causes. Cysts may be congenital or acquired. The cyst often appears soft and pliable, in contrast to the hard, fibrotic structure of a vocal nodule. The speech–language pathologist who identifies any kind of laryngeal lesion should refer the patient to an otolaryngologist. This is especially true for cysts because their management requires surgical excision rather than voice therapy per se. Courey et al. (1996) studied 41 benign laryngeal lesions (nodules, polyps, cysts, and corditis) and identified seven squamous cysts and seven mucous cysts. All 14 cyst lesions were found on histological examination to be benign. Depending on the site of the lesion, the patient may or may not experience dysphonia. Sataloff (1997a) writes that, because cysts rarely resolve spontaneously, they should be removed surgically using a small superficial incision along the superior edge of the vocal fold, without disrupting the glottal margin. Voice therapy postsurgically is usually confined to helping the patient eliminate any voice compensations (such as increased glottal attack) that may have been used to minimize negative voice effects caused by the cyst.

ENDOCRINE CHANGES

Occasionally patients' voice problems are related to some kind of endocrine dysfunction. Endocrine disorders often have a major impact on developing larynges and cause excesses in fundamental frequency, so that an individual's voice is either too low or too high in pitch. For example, in hypofunction of the pituitary gland, laryngeal growth is retarded. A pubescent child with such a problem will experience a continued high voice pitch. Such a pituitary problem can prevent normal development of progesterone by the ovaries (in girls) and testosterone by the testes (in adolescent males). The resulting lack of secondary sexual characteristics (including a change in voice) is treated by endocrine therapy designed to stimulate normal pituitary function. The opposite problem, caused by some tumors of the pituitary gland, results in a "precocious puberty as well as acromegaly" (Strome, 1982, p. 18). Hypofunctioning of the adrenal glands (Addison's disease) can also contribute to lack of secondary sex characteristics, including a prepubescent voice in males. Sometimes tumors in the adrenal system cause adrenal hormone excesses, causing virilization and a deepening of the voice.

Hypothyroidism, insufficient secretion of thyroxin by the thyroid gland, can produce many physical changes over time, including increased mass of the vocal folds, which, in turn, lowers pitch. Aronson (1990) describes the dysphonia of hypothyroidism as "characteristically hoarse, sometimes described as coarse or gravelly, and of excessively low pitch" (p. 60). Such symptoms can usually be well controlled by thyroid hormone therapy. In hyperthyroidism (excessive thyroid function), vocal symptoms are less severe, and the patients experience jumpiness and irritability, which result in a breathy voice that may lack sufficient loudness.

Premenstrual vocal syndrome, as described by Greene (1980) and Abitbol and colleagues (1999), is characterized by vocal fatigue, reduced pitch range, hypophonia, and loss of certain harmonics. The syndrome usually begins four to five days before menstruation in 33% of women. Videostroboscopic examination reveals congestion, microvaries, vocal fold thickening, and reduced vibratory amplitude. Some female opera singers avoid heavy singing obligations several days before and after menstruation. Two recent studies (Amir et al., 2006; La et al., 2007) suggest that oral contraceptive pills may reduce the irregularity of vocal fold vibration in professional and nonprofessional singers during menstruation.

The climacteric (menopause) is a time when some women may experience vocal changes, particularly a lowering of fundamental frequency. Because of the secretion of excessive androgenic hormones after the menopause, the glottal membrane becomes thicker, increasing the size-mass of the folds, and producing a lowering of voice pitch (Gould, 1975) and sometimes vocal roughness. It would appear that, in any case in which the larynx is under- or overdeveloped for the age and sex of the patient, some endocrine imbalance might be suspected. If some kind of hormonal imbalance is discovered, the primary treatment, if possible, would be hormonal therapy. Voice therapy can be of help to the patient in developing the best vocal performance possible with the changing (because of hormone therapy) mechanism. Most of the techniques presented in Chapter 7 are appropriate when applied to these patients for direct alteration of voice parameters such as pitch, loudness, and quality.

HEMANGIOMA

Hemangiomas are similar to contact ulcers and granulomas, differing only in type of lesion. Whereas a granuloma is usually a firm granulated sac, a hemangioma is a soft, pliable, blood-filled sac. Like granulomas, hemangiomas often occur on the posterior glottis, frequently associated with vocal hyperfunction, hyperacidity, or intubation. This blood-filled lesion, when identified, should be removed surgically (with cold steel or laser). As soon as glottal healing permits, a vocal hygiene program and voice therapy should be initiated.

HYPERKERATOSIS

Patients often come to their dentist or otolaryngologist because they are concerned about some oral or pharyngeal lesions they have observed. Once professionally identified, these lesions are often biopsied and found to be either malignant (cancerous) or nonmalignant (benign). Laryngeal examination may also locate and subsequently identify, by biopsy, additive lesions in the pharynx or larynx. Hyperkeratosis, a pinkish, rough lesion, is often the identified lesion, a nonmalignant growth that may be the precursor of malignant tissue change (Isenberg, Crozier, and Dailey, 2008). Hyperkeratotic growths are reactive lesions to continued tissue irritation. Therefore, hyperkeratotic lesions must be watched closely over time for any change in appearance. Favorite sites of hyperkeratosis include under the tongue, on the vocal folds at the anterior commissure, and posteriorly on the arytenoid prominences. Their effect on voice may be negligible or severe, depending on the site and the extent of the lesion. We once had an eight-year-old girl voice patient with hyperkeratosis of the vocal folds who had experienced the secondhand smoke of both parents for those eight years.

It is generally believed that chronic irritants to the oral and laryngeal membranes over time are the primary etiologies of hyperkeratosis. Consequently, the most effective treatments are eliminating the sources of tissue irritation, that is, ceasing smoking and, in cases of laryngopharyngeal reflux, prescribing a proton-pump inhibitor and encouraging lifestyle modifications. Sataloff and colleagues (1996) report on a case of severe hyperkeratosis mimicking cancer. The 50-year-old patient had smoked for 30 years and presented with complaints of persistent cough, throat clearings, and other symptoms of laryngopharyngeal reflux (LPR). Surprising to the authors, pathology revealed hyperkeratosis, inflammation, and viral changes suggestive of papilloma, but there was no carcinoma. The patient's voice improved after surgery, vocal hygiene, antireflux therapy, and smoking cessation. Garcia, Krishna, and Rosen (2006) described a case of tenacious hyperkeratosis that persisted in spite of aggressive antireflux therapy. After two months on a regimen, the patient still presented with surface irregularities and keratosis of both vocal folds. Biopsy was negative for malignancy, but the pathologist reported several areas of mild to moderate dysplasia (tissue changes). The dose of panto-prazole was increased to 40 mg twice a day, and ranitidine and GERD behavior modifications continued. Four months later, strobovideolaryngoscopy revealed an absence of keratosis and vocal fold inflammation.

INFECTIOUS LARYNGITIS

Some of the same people who experience traumatic laryngitis after only minor abuse/misuse of the voice also experience infectious laryngitis when they have an upper respiratory infection (URI). The case histories of such people often contain multiple entries of loss of voice, dysphonia, or laryngitis. In other individuals, in-fectious laryngitis is a very rare event that occurs as one of the symptoms of a severe head and chest cold. Infectious laryngitis often develops in a patient who has had a fever, headache, runny nose (rhinorrhea), sore throat, and coughing. Although most problems of infectious laryngitis are viral in origin, the more severe problems (often accompanied by high fever and a very sore throat) may be caused by bacterial in-fections. Bacteria-caused laryngitis can often be dramatically treated, with relatively quick resolution, through antibiotic therapy. Unfortunately, most laryngitis experi-enced during a URI that is viral in origin does not respond to antibiotics. Amanta-dine appears to be useful against influenza (Wingfield, Pollock, and Gunert, 1969); however, it may not be effective against all types of viruses, and side effects include xerostomia and xerophonia, among others (Sataloff, 1997b). Increased resistance among Americans to amantadine and other influenza-specific antiviral drugs un-derscores the need for novel prevention and treatment strategies (Rothberg, Haessler, and Brown, 2008). Strome (1982) recommends voice rest, humidification, increased fluid intake (hydration), reduced physical activity, and analgesics.

From a voice conservation point of view, absolute voice rest—no attempts at spoken communication, including voice or whisper—should be initiated by the pa-tient with such a laryngeal infection. Whispering should be discouraged, because most people produce a glottal whisper by placing the vocal folds in close approx-imation to one another, which, in effect, produces a light voice. The irritated, swollen tissues continue to touch and to vibrate. What infectious laryngitis patients need is total voice rest for a period of two or three days, with the vocal folds in the open, inverted-V position, and increased fluids (hydration).

LARYNGECTOMY

One of the primary functions of the human larynx is to prevent aspiration into the airway. The larynx contains three valve sites: the true folds, the ventricular folds (false folds), and the aryepiglottic folds, each of whose valving action allows them to shut off the airway to prevent the inhalation of liquids, foods, saliva, mucus, and any other stray foreign bodies that may be headed through the larynx into the airway. When the larynx is so compromised by disease (such as advanced cancer) or trauma that it cannot safely perform its valving role, the patient becomes a candidate for a laryngectomy, the total removal of the larynx. Total laryngectomy alters respiration, swallowing, and speech. To maintain an airway, an opening is created in the trachea (tracheostomy) through which the laryngectomee (a patient who has had the operation) breathes all pulmonary (lung) air in and out.

Esophageal speech has historically been the method of choice for alaryngeal communication. In this method, air is either injected or inhaled by mouth into the pharyngoesophageal (PE) segment and immediately expelled, setting the PE segment into vibration. Blom and Singer introduced a new tracheoesophageal puncture technique and use of a valved appliance called a tracheoesophageal prosthesis (TEP) in 1979. The prosthesis permits pulmonary air to flow from the trachea through a prosthetic shunt into the esophagus, facilitating the production of esophageal "voice" without extensive special training. Some laryngectomees prefer an artificial larynx to esophageal speech. The artificial larynx, also known as the electrolarynx, introduces sound for speech by placing the instrument against the external throat or oral structures or inserting a tube or fitted prosthetic electrolarynx into the mouth while speaking. We describe the use of and training for other vibratory voicing sources and forms of alaryngeal voice in Chapter 8.

Except in cases of traumatic injury to the larynx requiring an emergency laryngectomy, most laryngectomy operations are scheduled only after some counseling has been completed by the surgeon, the speech–language pathologist, and sometimes a laryngectomee. We describe pre- and postoperative counseling, evaluation, and training of the patient with a total laryngectomy in some detail in Chapter 8.

A brief note should be made here of the first successful transplantation of the larynx, trachea, pharynx, and thyroid and parathyroid glands, performed at Cleveland Clinic, in 1998. The patient's larynx was severed 20 years earlier in a motorcycle accident and until the transplant he had used an external device (Cooper Rand Electrolarynx) to speak. Douglas Hicks, Ph.D., a speech–language pathologist, has followed the patient since the operation in 1998. At 40 months postoperation, a news brief reported that the patient had a human sounding voice with inflection, pitch range, and qualities unique to the recipient. He also swallowed normally. However, he still required a tracheostomy. In spite of this success, the 1998 transplant has been the only true laryngeal transplant reported in peer-reviewed literature to date. That full clinical trials have not been conducted is due to several barriers, notably patient selection, difficulties with recurrent laryngeal nerve and superior laryngeal nerve reinnervation, vascular anastomosis, immunosuppression, and cost benefits (Birchall and Macchiarini, 2008).

LEUKOPLAKIA

Leukoplakia are whitish patches that are additive lesions to the surface membrane of mucosal tissue and that often extend beneath the surface into the subepithelial space. Although the lesions are classified as benign tumors, similar to hyperkeratosis, they are considered to be *precancerous lesions and must be followed closely.* Within the vocal tract, common sites for leukoplakia are under the tongue and on the vocal folds. It is important to note that it is difficult or impossible to distinguish between leukoplakia and cancer of the larynx by visual inspection alone. The primary etiology of these white patches is continuous irritation of membranes. The most common cause is heavy smoking; a heroic effort must be initiated to prevent continued irritation, such as absolute insistence that the patient quit smoking and emotional support for the patient. More recently, laryngopharyngeal reflux (LPR) has been a suggested cause (Beaver et al., 2003), as has human papillovirus (Makowska, Bogacka-Zatorska, and Rogozinski, 2001). Continued irritation and subsequent growth of leukoplakia often leads to squamous cell carcinoma.

Although leukoplakia on or under the tongue have only minimal effects on voice, leukoplakia on the vocal folds may dramatically alter voice. The added lesion mass to the vocal folds lowers voice pitch and frequently causes hoarseness and sometimes hypophonia. Because leukoplakia are also random in size and location, they often cause the vocal folds to be asymmetrical, which may result in diplophonia as each fold vibrates at a different frequency because of its different size or mass. Leukoplakia that occupy space on the glottal margin may prevent optimal approximation of the folds, contributing to breathiness, reduced loudness, and overall dysphonia. The treatment of leukoplakia is medical–surgical (Sieron et al., 2001), and voice therapy only contributes to developing the best voice possible. In spite of lesion effects, a functional aspect of the dysphonia can often be lessened with therapy. These functional aspects may be the only vocal symptoms and thus voice therapy is important to restore normal voice.

PAPILLOMA

Laryngeal
Images
Photo
Gallery

Recurrent respiratory papillomatosis is the most common benign laryngeal neoplasm in children and the most common cause of pediatric hoarseness (Derkay, 2001). It is estimated to have an incidence of 4.3 per 100,000 pediatric patients (Andrus and Shapshay, 2006). Papillomas are wartlike growths, viral in origin, that occur in the dark, moist caverns of the airway, frequently in the larynges of young children. Other extralaryngeal sites are the oral cavity, trachea, and the bronchi. Papillomas can represent a serious threat to the airway, limiting the needed flow of air through the glottal opening. The majority of papillomas occur in children under the age of six; for this reason, hoarseness and shortness of breath in preschool children should be evaluated promptly. Although the majority of papillomas stop recurring about the time of puberty, approximately 20% persist beyond puberty (Andrus and Shapshay, 2006). We have seen adults who developed papillomatosis in adulthood without ever having it in childhood. When papillomas occur in the larynx, their additive mass often contributes to dysphonia. For this reason, the voice clinician should be particularly alert to any child who demonstrates dysphonia. Any child with continued hoarseness for more than 10 days, independent of a cold or allergy, should have the benefit of a laryngeal examination to identify the cause of the hoarseness.

If papillomas are identified, the treatment is usually medical–surgical. Treatment is considered palliative, not curative, because of the resiliency of the human papillomavirus (HPV) genome in the tissue. Treatment includes excision by a microdebrider (Roy and Vivero, 2008), laser surgery, conventional excision surgery, radiation therapy, and interferon therapy (Lundquist et al., 1984). Surgical intervention is required whenever the papilloma growths begin to interfere with the airway. If the lesion mass does not interfere with respiration or voicing, it is usually tolerated. According to Wetmore, Key, and Suen (1985), there may be complications from continued surgical procedures for papilloma. These authors followed 40 patients (26 children; 14 adults) who collectively had received a total of 122 laser surgeries for papilloma over six and a half years. Eleven of twelve patients who had undergone more than six operations over this time period experienced anterior glottal webs with persistent vocal fold edema as complications, and their vocalization was seriously affected. Dedo and Jackler (1982) report that laser surgery was clearly the superior procedure for removal of recurring papilloma in 109 patients; with the laser approach, they report that almost half of their patients eventually reached remission and had no recurrence of the lesions. Despite the possible complications from continuous surgery from recurring papilloma, the lesions must be removed when they begin to impinge on the airway. Eventually, when the individual has developed the immunological state needed to resist the virus-inspired papilloma, the papilloma will no longer recur, according to Kleinsasser (1979).

Lundquist and colleagues (1984) report a medical approach to the treatment of the viral-caused papilloma: injecting the patients intramuscularly with interferon. In following 17 juvenile patients receiving interferon therapy over a several-year period, Lundquist and colleagues found that "nine were totally cured, four had no more tumor growth but were still being treated, three experienced diminished tumor growth, and one refused further treatment" (p. 386). While interferon has some serious side effects (persistent flulike symptoms), these treatments have produced good voice results and have reduced or eliminated the papilloma. Those patients that we have seen postinterferon therapy have generally experienced significant reduction in the papilloma and have been able to engage in voice therapy.

Rosen and colleagues (1998) reported preliminary results of a trial using indole-3-carbinol for the treatment of recurrent respiratory papillomatosis. This substance is found in high concentrations in cabbage, brussels sprouts, broccoli, and cauliflower and is an approved FDA nutritional supplement. Eighteen months after treatment with the natural substance (indole-3-carbinole), one-third of the subjects had total cessation of the papilloma growth, another one-third had reduced growth, and one-third had no clinical response to the treatment.

Researchers in Toronto reported outcomes for papilloma treated with intralesional cidofovin following CO_2 laser removal. Initially, patients showed a marked improvement in the disease; however, the disease relapsed to a significant extent (El Hakim, Waddell, and Crysdale, 2002). Further studies are required for this and other approaches to papillomatosis.

The speech–language pathologist is sometimes asked to see a toddler or young child with obstructive papilloma who has had to have an open tracheostomy to permit adequate respiration. Developing functional communication with such a child and fostering normal language growth are the primary concerns of the clinician. Teaching the child to occlude the open stoma with a finger or fitting the child with a one-way valve that covers the stoma (to permit vocalization without finger occlusion) usually permits some voicing. In older children or adults who are being treated surgically for recurring papilloma, helping them to develop the best voice possible with the compromised laryngeal mechanisms is a realistic goal in voice therapy. Some work on respiration control (such as voicing with larger lung volumes of air) or working on loudness and pitch may improve vocal function.

PUBERTAL CHANGES

At about age nine, before the onset of puberty, the larynges of boys and girls are anatomically about the same size, and they produce about the same voice pitch (265 Hz). Pubertal growth changes in girls begin around nine, with the onset of puberty, and gradual pubescent changes occur over a four- to five-year period. In boys, puberty begins around 11 to 12, and dramatic growth changes occur over the four- to five-year pubertal period. However, noticeable laryngeal growth and the dramatic change in vocal fundamental frequency occur in the last year of puberty: The "average time from onset to completion of adolescent voice change is three to six months, one year at most" (Aronson, 1990, p. 45). By age 17, adolescents of both sexes have usually reached their full adult development (Offer, 1980). As we discuss elsewhere (see Chapters 2 and 5), the voice pitch levels of males and females drop dramatically after puberty (the male voice drops at least a full octave; the female voice drops almost half an octave). Laryngeal and airway growth does not happen overnight. Although the changes are gradual, over a four-year period, marked laryngeal growth (particularly in boys) occurs in the last six months of change. During this time of rapid laryngeal growth, boys may experience temporary dysphonia and occasional pitch breaks that are not cause for parental or clinical concern. Because these mass changes in puberty tend to thwart any serious attempts at singing or other vocal arts, middle school is often a poor environment for choral music. A boy who is a soprano in September may well be the choir baritone by June. Until children experience some stability in laryngeal and airway growth, the demands of singing might well be inappropriate for their rapidly changing mechanisms. Even though it has become common to involve young singers in more sophisticated musical tasks, the facts still remain that adolescents are particularly susceptible to vocal fatigue while singing and many are not trained in the proper technique of singing and are not cognizant of the physical limits of their voice (Jamison, 1996). Because of the rapid changes, attempting to develop optimum pitch or modal-pitch levels in adolescents should be avoided.

REFLUX

Over the past 20 years, there has been a growing acknowledgment that occult gastroesophageal reflux disease (GERD) and laryngopharyngeal reflux (LPR) are etiologic factors in a high percentage of patients with laryngeal complaints (Sataloff, 1997b). In adults, an estimated 4 to 10% of chronic nonspecific laryngeal disease seen in otolaryngologic and voice clinics is associated with GERD or LPR (Gilger, 2003). GERD is the passage of gastric juices from the stomach into the esophagus. If these contents move superiorly and exit the upper esophageal sphincter, the disorder is identified as LPR, as the contents spill into the pharynx. LPR is synonymous with extraesophageal reflux (EER), another commonly accepted term for reflux upstream from the stomach (Sasaki and Toolhill, 2000). In addition to being associated with chronic oral–pharyngeal dysphagia (Logemann, 1998), LPR has been implicated in the occurrence of erythema, edema, contact ulcers and granulomas, laryngitis, chronic rhinitis, sinusitis, globus pharyngeus, respiratory compromise, otitis media, laryngomalacia, and subglottic stenosis, to name a few (Arvedson, 2002; Koufman, 1991; Sataloff, 1997b).

The symptoms of acid reflux vary considerably among voice patients, ranging from no symptoms to mild heartburn to extreme burning or choking in the larynx, awakening the patient from a deep sleep. Typical symptoms of LPR/EER may include morning hoarseness, sour taste in mouth with bad breath, frequent throat clearing and coughing, and severe symptoms occurring when the head is lower than the abdominal area (such as in shoe tying, diving, or tumbling). Among the physical findings on laryngeal examination are posterior glottal redness, contact ulcers, pharyngeal irritation, and arytenoid hyperplasia with possible granuloma. The patient on questioning may be unaware of any symptoms related to LPR/EER; we have found that this is especially true among children.

At present, 24-hour esophageal pH monitoring is considered the most definitive study of LPR/EER, even for children (Faust, 2003). Esophageal pH monitoring involves passing a thin catheter transnasally into the esophagus. A special sensor records each reflux incidence over a 24-hour period. After the catheter is removed, the recorder is attached to a computer so that data it has gathered can be interpreted. A more recent advance in pH monitoring involves the placement of an acid-sensing capsule that is introduced to the esophagus via a catheter, and then the catheter is removed. The capsule transmits reflux events for two days to a recorder, and then detaches from the esophagus and is passed in the stool. Koufman (1991) reported on 225 patients with suspected reflux. Eighty-eight percent of the patients underwent 24-hour pH probe testing, with 62% of those demonstrating abnormal studies. Of these, 30% demonstrated LPR.

Based on the knowledge that a negative pH probe test does not rule out reflux, some authorities are now advocating esophageal biopsy to rule in the disease. This approach can be performed in infants as young as two weeks of age (Coletti, Christei, and Orenstein, 1995; Stroh, Faust, and Rimell, 1998). Upper gastrointestinal endoscopy is another diagnostic procedure. In addition to these instrumental assessments, a simple questionnaire for determining the presence of reflux and the type of reflux present has been developed and refined by Belafsky, Postma, and Koufman (2002b), known as the Reflux Symptom Index (RSI).

Reflux treatment can be divided into three categories: behavioral, pharmacological, and surgical, or a combination of these treatments. We have found good results with behavioral therapy alone in reducing or eliminating LPR as measured by post-pH-probe testing, endoscopic evaluation, and acoustic and perceptual measures. Behavioral therapy involves following a vocal hygiene program that includes elevating the head of the bed, remaining upright for at least 60 minutes after meals, avoiding spicy foods, not exercising after eating, and cutting down on caffeine, carbonated drinks, and alcohol, especially in the afternoons and evenings. We even recommend that patients avoid drinking excessive quantities of water right before bed because this can raise the level of acid in the stomach. Other treatment recommendations for controlling reflux are avoiding activities that compress the abdomen, weight loss, wearing looser clothing around the waist, and eliminating smoking. Following these management suggestions for reflux can often produce a dramatic lessening of symptoms, both in voice and pharyngeal–laryngeal mucosal irritation.

For those patients who do not readily respond to behavioral therapy, a combination of antireflux therapy with a proton-pump inhibitor (PPI) and a prokinetic agent has been shown to result in rapid symptomatic and endoscopic improvements in the majority of patients (Arvedson, 2002; Hamdan et al., 2001). A study by Park and colleagues (2005) found that PPIs taken twice a day (BID) appear to be more effective than once a day (QD) in achieving clinical symptom response. Greater acid suppression was achieved at four months compared with two months. In addition to LPR, PPIs have been used in the treatment of postnasal drip (PND). Pawar and colleagues (2007) studied the effects of PPI on patients having postnasal drainage with no objective evidence to support a sinonasal or infectious etiology. Findings supported the potential benefits of PPI therapy to reduced PND frequency, hoarseness, and chronic cough.

Surgical laparoscopic fundoplication has been shown to be effective in treatment of LPR for patients who show poor response to PPI (up to 120 mg/day). Five years after laparoscopic surgery, a corpus of 445 patients with previous poorly controlled GERD revealed reduced acid reflux, lower esophageal sphincter pressure, and symptom control. The authors report that the patients also revealed a significant improvement in both the physical and mental health component of a quality of life assessment (Anvari and Allen, 2003).

The speech–language pathologist usually encounters the dysphonic patient with LPR/EER initially at the time of the voice evaluation. If the signs of posterior laryngeal irritation are present, the patient is referred to the otolaryngologist. They will work as a team to plan a successful reflux management regimen and a voice therapy program that can produce optimal vocal function. Helping the patient reduce throat clearing and nonproductive coughing (more often habit than mucus-producing), developing easy glottal attack, changing throat focus to facial mask focus, and sometimes elevating voice pitch one or two half notes are among the facilitating approaches that help the reflux patient maintain a good, functional voice.

SULCUS VOCALIS

Sulcus vocalis may be either congenital or acquired and of unknown etiology, although vocal abuse and laryngopharyngeal reflux may play a role in the acquired form (Belafsky, Postma, and Koufman, 2002a). A study by Xu and colleagues (2007) suggested 5% sulcus vocalis among children referred for voice disorders. Figure 3.2 demonstrates a severe complete sulcus vocalis.

Although Ford and colleagues (1996) cite the earliest mention of sulcus vocalis in the literature (Giacomini in 1892), there has been a lot of clinical confusion over the years as to both the etiology and description of the disorder. *Sulcus* is a generic term that means furrow or indentation. In sulcus vocalis, on endoscopy or stroboscopy, we see a furrowed medial edge of the vocal fold, usually bilaterally symmetrical. The spindle configuration may involve all or any segment of the edge of the fold. The furrow may be confined to the superficial layer of the mucosa or penetrate into the vocal ligament and muscle (Giovanni, Chanteret, and Lagier, 2007). The patient presents clinically with some degree of dysphonia, often referred with a confusing array of previous diagnoses such as bowing, presbylaryngis, paralysis, or thyroarytenoid atrophy (Hirano et al., 1990).

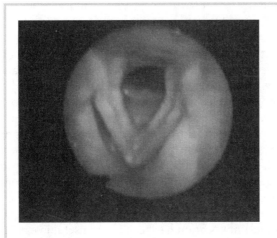

FIGURE **3.2**

Sulcus Vocalis

This 68-year-old male represents a complete bilateral sulcus vocalis, appearing as a reduplication of the vocal folds, giving him *two sets of vocal cords and two ventricles.* The arytenoid cartilages appear to be split as well.

One of the more definitive studies of sulcus vocalis was done by a Wisconsin group (Ford et al., 1996), finding in two studies (normative and clinical) that sulcus vocalis can be seen in three forms. They first identified among 116 control subjects 9 subjects who displayed *physiological sulcus*, an indentation of the vibrating fold without "histopathologic change in the lamina propria." Although these subjects showed some fold indentation, their voices were judged as normal. Among 20 clinical cases with a diagnosis of sulcus vocalis, they found two other distinct types (congenital or acquired from irritation) having clear involvement of the lamina propria with spindle or posterior gaps between the two involved folds. All of these clinical cases showed some compromise in mucosal wave, resulting in audible dysphonia of varying degrees.

The speech–language pathologist today sees more patients with sulcus vocalis than in former years. With mirror examination, many of these abnormalities were missed. However, videostroboscopy permits close examination of vocal fold cover abnormalities. With sulcus vocalis, when the folds are abducted, we can often identify the fold furrow; on adduction with phonation, we can see the compromised mucosal wave produced by the stiff, compromised lamina propria and glottal incompetence, with air leakage through the midline of the anterior two-thirds of the folds. Vocal quality reveals a strained quality with little pitch change and low intensity with difficulty speaking loudly without fatigue. Individuals may experience periods of aphonia and increased tension in the laryngeal muscles (Giovanni et al., 2007)

The primary treatment for sulcus vocalis is surgical, followed by voice therapy. One surgical approach is described by Hirano and Bless (1993) as a sulcusectomy in which an incision is made on each fold above the sulcus, usually for the length of each fold; the upper and lower borders of the sulcus are then sutured together, securing a mechanical coupling of the two parts as healing progresses. A second surgical approach is injecting collagen, fat, or fascia into the sulcus, usually in the middle of the offended vocal fold (Dursun et al., 2008; Pinto et al., 2007). Collagen is one of the components of Reinke's space and it can be injected in the deep layers of the lamina propria (Ford et al., 1995). A third surgical approach for correcting sulcus vocalis is a mucosal slicing technique, making many microvertical slices across the sulcus, as described by Pontes and Behlau (1993). Medialization thyroplasties (Isshiki et al., 1996) and strap muscle transposition (Su et al., 2004) have also been suggested to reduce glottal incompetence.

After surgery, glottal function needs reassessment by the speech–language pathologist. Improved function may still require that old habits of the patient need to be identified and corrected, particularly in reducing vocal hyperfunction. Although voice therapy after surgery for sulcus vocalis is highly individualized, we introduce techniques that seek to adjust the balance between proper glottal closure, pitch, and loudness. Pitch shifts, loudness changes, lateral digital pressure, and experimentation with firmer glottal closure are productive techniques. Auditory feedback with real-time amplification has been found useful in establishing easy-onset phonation after surgery with this patient group.

WEBBING

A laryngeal web growing across the glottis between the two vocal folds inhibits normal fold vibration, often producing a high-pitched rough sound during vibration and seriously compromising the open glottis. Webs may be congenital or acquired. A congenital web, which is detected at the time of birth, is the result of the glottal membrane failing to separate in embryonic development. Depending on the size of the web, the baby will produce stridor (inhalation noises), shortness of breath, and often a different high-pitched (squeal) cry. Approximately three-fourths of all laryngeal webs cross the glottis (Strome, 1982). Testing for chromosome 22q deletion is suggested, as this may be associated with velocardiofacial syndrome (Miyamoto et al., 2004). The presence of a congenital web requires immediate surgery, often followed by a temporary tracheostomy; usually, an infant larynx will recover over a period of four to six weeks.

Acquired webs result from some kind of bilateral trauma of the medial edges of the vocal folds. Anything that might serve as an irritant to the mucosal surface of the folds may be the initial cause of the webbing. Because the two vocal folds are so close together at the anterior commissure, any surface irritation due to prolonged infection or trauma may cause the inner margins of the two fold surfaces to grow together. To explain further, one principle of plastic surgery is that, when approximated together, offended tissue surfaces will tend to grow and fuse together. This same principle explains why webbing occurs. The offended surface of the two approximated folds tends to grow together, in this case forming a thin membrane across the glottis. Webbing grows across the glottis in an anterior to posterior fashion, usually ceasing about one-third of the distance from the anterior commissure, where the distance between the two folds becomes too great. Severe laryngeal infections sometimes cause enough glottal irritation to precipitate web formation. Bilateral surgery of the folds, perhaps for papilloma or nodules, can also be followed by a web (Wetmore, Key, and Suen, 1985). External trauma to the folds, such as a direct hit on the thyroid cartilage that causes it to fracture, may damage the folds behind it, thus creating enough glottal irritation for a web to develop. Laryngeal or tracheal surgery is the most frequent event producing the postsurgical acquired web. Whatever causes the original bilateral irritation, as a part of healing, both folds grow together anteriorly, forming a glottal web sometimes called a *synechia*.

Laryngeal web may cause severe dysphonia as well as shortness of breath, depending on how extensively the webbing crosses the glottis. The treatment for the formation of a web is surgery. The webbing is cut, freeing the two folds. To prevent the surgically removed web from growing again, a vertical keel is placed between the two folds and kept there until complete healing has been achieved. The laryngologist fixates the keel, which is shaped very much like a boat rudder and is about the size of a fingernail, between the folds, preventing them from approximating. The patient is then on voice rest as long as the keel is in place, because its presence inhibits normal fold vibration. When the keel is removed, often in six to eight weeks, the patient generally requires some voice therapy to restore normal phonation. If there was extensive damage to the larynx from the trauma, it may well be impossible after healing and voice therapy to ever develop the same kind of normal voice the patient had before the accident. The prognosis for voice recovery after webbing and its surgical treatment is highly individualized, depending on the extent of the trauma and the size of the resulting web. We have had patients who were able to speak and sing with a normal voice following surgical reduction of the web and a course of voice therapy.

We reported on the importance of differential diagnosis in the case of a 13-year-old girl who was referred to our clinic with chronic shortness of breath and stridor (Von Berg and McFarlane, 2002b). The patient presented with a history of pneumonia and pneumatocile (ulceration of the lung), followed by tracheostomy and mechanical ventilation, as an infant. Ten years later she continued to complain of shortness of breath, especially during times of stress and exercise. Although paradoxical vocal fold movement, asthma, and unilateral vocal fold paralysis were certainly considerations, a definitive diagnosis was confirmed with endoscopy that revealed a subglottic web occluding two-thirds of the airway. The web was consistent with the patient's medical history, complaints, and clinical assessment. It became apparent that after reconstructive laryngeal surgery and decannulation as a baby, the raw edges of the vocal folds had fused together and formed a web that remained for the next 10 years. The patient was referred for surgical intervention for the web.

Summary

Organic voice problems may result from various laryngeal disorders, such as papilloma, granuloma, webbing, and other disorders. For each of the various organic voice disorders, we discussed medical management and the role of the speech–language pathologist in evaluation and therapy.

Thought Questions

1. Describe why a child might present with an acquired sublottal stenosis. Describe a stenosis grading scale and the corresponding interventions. What type of vocal quality would you expect a child to present with after intervention? What types of facilitating techniques might be appropriate to address these changes in vocal quality?

2. What are the three potential etiologies of contact ulcers and granulomas, and how is each addressed?

3. Describe the approaches recommended for vocal fold cysts. Are these approaches similar to lesions stemming from vocal hyperfunction (Chapter 5)?

4. What are the similarities among, and differences between, hyperkeratosis and leukoplakia?
5. Describe the various medical approaches to papilloma. Access and summarize one peer-reviewed manuscript that describes an approach.
6. Describe two assessment techniques used to diagnose reflux. Explain how reflux can contribute to respiratory compromise, sinusitis, contact ulcers, and other pathologies of the upper aerodigestive tract and airway.
7. Define the difference between a laryngeal web and sublottal stenosis. Describe the typical dysphonias that might accompany these conditions.

4

Neurogenic Voice Disorders

LEARNING OBJECTIVES

- Describe the central and peripheral nervous systems' roles in the innervation of the vocal mechanism

- Identify the major role of each cranial nerve involved with voice production

- Recognize the changes in voice and speech associated with each neurogenic disorder

- Explain the various approaches to the disorders and be able to describe the peer-reviewed literature describing efficacy of the approach

In Chapter 2 we reviewed the normal anatomy and physiology required for voice. We considered the causes and treatment of a number of voice disorders in Chapter 3 and will consider other causes in Chapter 5. In this chapter, we review the neurological structures and processes that must function in coordinated balance to produce what we perceptually consider as normal voice. By gaining an appreciation of the neurophysiological bases of voice, we can then begin to recognize and pinpoint the causes of neurogenic dysphonias. As Duffy (2005) suggests, changes in speech can be the first or only manifestation of neurogenic disease. Recognition of these changes can have a significant impact on medical diagnosis and care. Indeed, on numerous occasions the voice clinician has been the first to identify the salient features of myasthenia gravis, Parkinson's disease, and even progressive supranuclear palsy. Only through early detection and differential diagnosis are the voice professional and the patient's health care team able to generate an intervention program that directly addresses the patient's deficits.

To understand the complexities of neurogenic dysphonias, it is necessary to have an understanding of the innervation of the larynx and resonators from the central and peripheral nervous system structures. A comprehensive discussion of the neuroanatomy and neurophysiology of phonation is beyond the scope of this book; readers are directed to excellent texts by Brookshire (2007), Duffy (2005), Yorkston and colleagues (1999), and Darley, Aronson, and Brown (1975) for a discussion of speech science, anatomy and physiology, and motor speech disorders. However, we do offer a working view of the central and peripheral nervous systems and innervations of the muscles necessary for voice.

A WORKING VIEW OF THE NERVOUS SYSTEM

The central nervous system (CNS) and the peripheral nervous system (PNS) coordinate all laryngeal operations, from the elevation of the larynx for swallowing, to the triple valving closure (true vocal folds, ventricular folds, and aryepiglottic folds) required for a cough, to the delicate nuance sung by the operatic lyric soprano. We know far less about the neural controls required for human singing and talking than we do about the neural governing in all mammals (including the human) of such laryngeal vegetative functions as breathing, coughing, or swallowing. The human not only has all the sensory–motor structures and functions of most mammal species, but has added abilities to subdue or augment response (for example, suppress crying when the situation is not appropriate), or to use phonatory functions for expression of emotions, in verbal and nonverbal communication, or artistic expression. The expanded cerebral cortex unique to the human species has much to do with the enabling of the human to use voice in a controlled sequential pattern as heard or said in spoken language, or in the exact pitch and loudness requirements of singing, or in the voicing cues (inflection, loudness changes, etc.) we use in spoken communication.

The Central Nervous System (CNS), the Cortex, and Its Projections

The central nervous system is composed of the brain and spinal cord and is housed in the bony, protective structures of the cranium and vertebral column. Sophisticated sensory–motor function, such as formulation of speech and voice, appears to be directed by the cerebral cortex, a six-layer composite of millions of neurons, interconnected by their dendrites and axons. Researchers suggest that both the frontal and temporal lobes are primarily involved with the production of voice, although these areas do not represent the only structures involved in sensory–motor programming for voice. The motor cortex for laryngeal control is in the inferior and lateral aspects of the motor cortex and primary motor strip. The third frontal convolution, or Broca's area, in the left hemisphere, has much to do with preplanning a motor speech act, including voice response. For example, in regional cerebral blood flow studies, Broca's area shows greater density of blood just before something is said. The actual production of the utterance at the cortical level activates bilaterally at specific locations along the precentral gyrus. The projections from the cortex are polysynaptic, passing to the midbrain and then to the brain stem.

It appears that the insula (older cortex phylogenetically) medial to the temporal lobe plays an active role in motor planning for voice and speech (Dronkers, 1996; Dronkers, Redfern, and Shapiro, 1993). Later review by Bennett and Netsell (1999) suggests that the insula may be involved in far more than motor planning and that it may be associated with all aspects of speech and language processing. The temporal lobes, in turn, provide cortical input for audition. Heschl's gyrus, the primary auditory cortex, bilaterally receives tonotopic frequency input from the medial geniculate bodies of the thalamus. New research investigating the relationship of linguistic (phonetic) and extralinguistic (voice) information in preattentive auditory processing suggests a parallel and contingent process (Strouse et al., 1998).

Speech comprehension is associated with Wernicke's area, which communicates directly with Broca's convolution via the bundle of association fibers known as the arcuate fasciculus. The actual execution of voice may be dependent on temporal cortical connections to lower brain centers, such as from the temporal planum of the cortex to the pulvinar body of the thalamus (Minckler, 1972).

Pyramidal and Extrapyramidal Tracts

The pyramidal and extrapyramidal tracts are part of the CNS. The pyramidal tract is composed of long axons that extend from the cortical neurons located in the primary motor strip and travel uninterrupted until they reach their corresponding cranial nerve nuclei in the brain stem. As illustrated in Figure 4.1, the pyramidal tract is composed of white matter nerve fibers (corticobulbar and corticospinal) that pass in a bundle between the basal ganglia and the thalamus, which is called the internal capsule.

One way to think of the pyramidal tract is that it functions like a neural turnpike, permitting the transmission of impulses from the cortex to the cranial nerve nuclei without interruption of local neural traffic. Conversely, the extrapyramidal tract (Figure 4.2) is similar to a country road, with fibers stopping in many locations, bringing neural transmissions to synapse with the basal ganglia, across to the thalamus and the subthalamus, and to the cerebellum, among other structures. The extrapyramidal tract enables extensive checking and balancing of sensory and motor information with its many interconnections between the cortex, thalamus and the basal ganglia. It is suggested that the many checks and balances afforded by the extrapyramidal system are crucial for maintaining posture, tone, and associated activities that provide a foundation for skilled movements executed by the pyramidal tract.

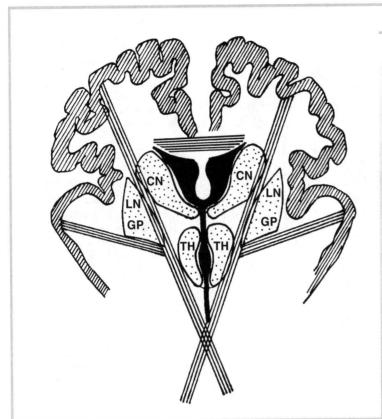

FIGURE **4.1**

A Schematic View of the Pyramidal Tract

The pyramidal tract is like a neural turnpike with fibers descending uninterrupted via the internal capsule from their cortical origins to their terminations at cranial nerve nuclei in the brain stem. This line drawing shows basal ganglia (including CN, caudate nucleus; LN, lenticular nucleus; GP, globus pallidus); and TH, thalamus. Pyramidal fibers are depicted as ▭▭▭.

Thalamus, Internal Capsule, and the Basal Ganglia.   The subcortical areas occupied by the thalamus, which is medial in the hemisphere, the internal capsule that runs laterally adjacent to it, and the more lateral basal ganglia are known collectively as the corpus striatum, which gets its name from the contrast of the gray matter nuclei and the white matter projections between them. The corpus striatum is the site of most of the sensory–motor integrations of the cerebrum. The thalamus is to sensation what the basal ganglia are to motor behavior.

Even the thalamus has its posterior (pure sensory) and anterior (sensory influenced motor) divisions. The posterior thalamus is known as the pulvinar body, which receives neural impulses from the auditory tract via the medial geniculates, the most inferior–posterior of the pulvinar. From the medial geniculates, after some central mixing within the thalamus, the auditory fibers radiate in a bundle superiorly to the primary auditory cortex, Heschl's gyrus. Similarly, the visual fibers come into the lateral geniculate bodies of the pulvinar section of the thalamus,

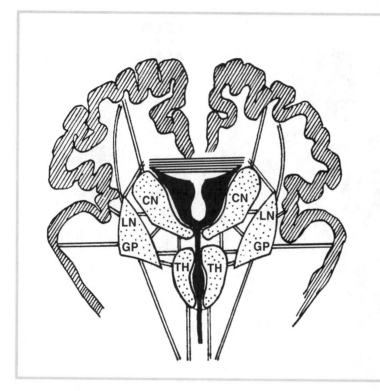

FIGURE **4.2**

A Schematic View of the Extrapyramidal Tract

The line drawing of the extrapyramidal tract depicts its neural fibers like a neural country road, starting and stopping at various cortical, basal ganglia, and thalamic sites and ending (or starting) at lower brain stem sites. These extrapyramidal fibers are depicted as ═════. This line drawing shows the basal ganglia (including CN, caudate nucleus; LN, lenticular nucleus; GP, globus pallidus); and TH, thalamus.

undergo central mixing, and exit in a bundle and go directly to the primary visual cortex in the occipital lobes.

There is also some speculation (Boone, 1997, 1998; Minckler, 1972) that afferent–efferent fibers between the lateral wall of the pulvinar body and the temporale planum play an important role in auditory comprehension of the spoken word and some control in producing vocal response. Within the main thalamic body there appears to be much integration of sensory information occurring, getting organized for some kind of motor response via the anterior nuclei and ventral anterior nuclei of the thalamus. From the anterior thalamus, sensory projections go either directly to the sensory cerebral cortex or to nuclei within the basal ganglia.

While there are some basal ganglia–thalamic connections crossing within the internal capsule, the main body of the internal capsule is largely composed of the descending–ascending neural projections of the pyramidal tract. The internal capsule area of the brain is highly susceptible to cerebral vascular accidents (CVAs), primarily because much of its blood supply is furnished by an artery known as the *lenticular striata* (often called the *artery of apoplexy*), which for some reason seems to be blocked by thrombosis more than other cerebral arteries. Such blockage of blood would cause white matter projections to die, resulting in contra-unilateral symptoms of paralysis (note that such a high-level lesion would not cause contralateral vocal fold paralysis). Any lesion (disease, CVA, or trauma) to the internal capsule could cause contralateral sensory–motor symptoms of skeletal muscles, classified as upper motor neuron lesions. Sensory loss could include hypothesias and motor loss would be seen in hemiparesis or hemiplegia (paralysis with spasticity).

The basal ganglia utilize the sensory information provided by the thalamus. The main nuclei of the basal ganglia are the caudate nuclei and the lenticular nuclei, which includes the putamen and globus pallidus. Bilateral innervations of both smooth and striated muscle occur within both the caudate and lenticular nuclei, and, at this level, we first see bilateral innervation of velar, pharyngeal, and laryngeal muscles. The basal ganglia utilize the continuous, multiple sensory information from the thalamus in organizing appropriate motor responses (including vocalization).

Neurotransmitters. It should be acknowledged at this point that the transmission of neural impulse between various nuclei via white matter nerves is facilitated by several enzymes, known as *neurotransmitters*. At the termination of nerves within the cerebrum, where neural synapses occur, serotonin functions as a nervous system neurotransmitter. The sympathetic nervous system employs epinephrine and norepinephrine to aid in the transmission of neural impulses for innervation of smooth muscle, glands, and viscera. The basal ganglia are dependent on dopamine as the primary neurotransmitter. The facial, neck, and skeletal muscles are dependent on acetylcholine as the chemical mediator between the muscle's nerve nucleus and the muscle body itself. While neural transmission can be altered or stopped by isolated lesions to the gray body or its nerve connections, many of the diseases of the CNS cause inhibition or overproduction of neurotransmitter solutions.

For example, it is well known that degenerative changes in the substantia nigra cause a deficiency in a chemical neural transmitter known as dopamine in the caudate nucleus and putamen. The disturbed basal ganglia and extrapyramidal control circuit results in a hypokinetic dysarthria observed in Parkinson's disease, discussed later in this chapter. The symptoms of Parkinson's are vastly ameliorated with levodopa, a synthetic dopamine.

The Brain Stem and the Cerebellum. The projection fibers from both the pyramidal and extrapyramidal tracts extend anteriorly into the pons and posteriorly via the cerebral peduncle terminating into the medulla oblongata. This cortical to lower center tract includes both afferent and efferent fibers. There are neural connections from the midbrain to the pons and on to the cerebellum and connections from the peduncle area into the cerebellum. The medial hypothalamus is the lowest structure of the midbrain, under which are the lesser (in number) gray bodies and myelinated nerve tracts (innumerable) that comprise the brain stem. The hypothalamus forms the lateral walls of the central third ventricle and connected to it are some gray bodies hugging the third ventricle aqueduct, containing important vegetative respiratory areas known as the periaqueductal gray (Davis et al., 1996). Hypothalamic fibers, pyramidal, and extrapyramidal projections communicate anteriorly in the brain stem to the pons, while posterior fibers form the cerebral peduncle, which extends down, forming the medulla. The medulla extends from the lowermost portion of the pons with its upper portion forming the floor of the fourth ventricle.

The cerebellum wraps around the pons and cerebral peduncle and has many interconnections with the pons, cerebral peduncle, medulla, and spinal cord. The cerebellum functions as the great regulator of the extrapyramidal tract, coordinating sensory information (proprioceptive, kinesthetic, tactile, auditory, visual) with coordinated motor response. Lesions to the cerebellum from trauma or disease cause speech symptoms of incoordination, known as ataxic dysarthria. The voice–speech symptoms of cerebellar lesions are prosodic slowdown (scanning speech), changes in resonance, and inarticulate speech, all sounding like the speech of someone highly intoxicated.

Eighty percent of the descending projection fibers coming from the cerebral peduncle cross over (decussate) to the other side in the medulla just below the brain stem; 20% remain ipsilateral. Of great importance to voice is the nucleus ambiguus in the superior medulla, located just below the pyramidal decussation. As the medulla extends downward, it begins to narrow into the spinal column. The same posterior–sensory/anterior–motor organization continues in the medulla and down into the spinal cord. Posterior nerve tracts and gray nuclei (left and right) are sensory in nature while the anterior white matter tracts and anterior horn nuclei (left and right) execute motor function.

Let us consider briefly at this point what constitutes an upper motor neuron lesion or a lower motor neuron lesion. Functionally, an upper motor lesion produces symptoms of spasticity, such as in a CVA in which the patient may experience hemiplegia (one-sided spastic paralysis of extremities). A lower motor lesion, such as the cutting of the recurrent laryngeal nerve, causes unilateral vocal fold flaccid paralysis. Upper motor neuron function begins at the cerebral cortex and ends at the nucleus ambiguus; lower motor neuron function begins at the nucleus ambiguus and travels down the spinal cord, ending at the lowest spinal nucleus. Also included as lower motor neuron structures are the nerves exiting from the pons and medulla (such as the cranial nerves) and the nerves that carry sensory and motor impulses to and from the various spinal nuclei for their particular muscles. The autonomic motor system and these cerebrospinal nerves, including their associated sensory receptors, constitute what is known as the peripheral nervous system (PNS).

The Peripheral Nervous System (PNS)

We will limit our discussion of the peripheral nervous system primarily to those cranial nerves that have direct impact on voice, and, in particular, two branches of cranial nerve X, the vagus, that innervate the larynx: the superior and recurrent laryngeal nerves.

While cranial nerves V, VII, and VIII have direct impact on speech, they do not appear primary in the production of voice. Cranial nerve V, trigeminal, emerges from the pons with its primary motor fibers innervating the muscles of mastication; the sensory components that might influence voice are the tactile sensations of the nose and oral mucosa. Cranial nerve VII, facial, leaves the lower portion of the pons and terminates in its motor innervation of facial muscles; its sensory components include taste in the anterior two-thirds of the tongue and sensation to the soft palate. Cranial nerve VIII, acoustic, has its cochlear division ending in the dorsal and ventral cochlear nuclei in the superior medulla; leaving the cochlear nuclei, the auditory pathways begin and continue to various neural stations, ending in Heschl's gyrus in the temporal lobe. As mentioned earlier in this chapter and throughout the text, the auditory system appears to play a primary role in voice production and control.

Cranial Nerves (IX, X, XI, XII).   We will give special attention to cranial nerves IX, X, XI, and XII as each has some role in phonation and voice resonance. For each nerve, we will look at origin and insertion with a brief statement relative to nerve function, especially as it relates to voice.

Cranial Nerve IX, Glossopharyngeal.   Originating laterally in the medulla, the nerve passes through the jugular foramen coursing between the internal carotid artery and the external jugular vein and subdivides into its numerous branches that go to various innervation sites. Its functions include taste in the posterior third of the tongue and sensation to the fauces, tonsils, pharynx, and soft palate. Its primary motor innervation is to the superior pharyngeal constrictor in the pharynx and to the stylopharyngeus muscle.

Cranial Nerve X, Vagus.   The vagus nerve, in addition to its many functions of control of the autonomic nervous system involving thoracic and abdominal viscera, has two important branches that innervate the larynx, the superior laryngeal nerve (SLN) and the recurrent laryngeal nerve (RLN). In the next section of this chapter, we will present in greater detail the origins and functions of the SLN and the RLN. The vagus nerve originates in the nucleus ambiguus in the medulla from which it emerges laterally and courses its way, continually branching along the way, with particular branches terminating at the various innervation sites from the pharynx to the abdominal viscera. Affecting voice are the sensory components of the vagus with sensory innervation of the pharynx and larynx; motor aspects affecting voice include innervation of the velum, base of tongue, superior, middle, and inferior pharyngeal constrictors, larynx, and autonomic ganglia of the thorax (affecting the respiratory aspects of phonation).

Cranial Nerve XI, Spinal Accessory.   Cranial nerve XI is a motor nerve that has innervation of the neck accessory muscles as its primary function. It is composed of two sections, the cranial portion and spinal portion. The cranial branch originates in the nucleus ambiguus and emerges from the side of the medulla with five successive small rootlets. Some fibers are distributed to the superior branches of the vagus nerve, innervating the levator veli palatini and uvula. Fibers from the spinal portion of the nerve originate from the anterior horn of the spinal cord and merge with lower spinal portion fibers to innervate the major muscles of the neck, such as the sternocleidomastoid and the trapezius muscles. Lesions to cranial XI can cause obvious problems of resonance and in the contribution of neck accessory muscles to respiration.

Cranial Nerve XII, Hypoglossal.   The hypoglossal nerve is a motor nerve innervating (as the name suggests) the extrinsic and intrinsic muscles of the tongue as well as some of the neck strap muscles. The nerve originates in its own nucleus, the hypoglossus nucleus, in the lower medulla, exiting laterally and entering the hypoglossal canal in the occipital bone, descending and then moving laterally into its many innervation sites. The muscles it innervates are the omohyoid, sternothyroid, styloglossus, hyoglossus, genioglossus, geniohyoid, sternohyoid, and all of the intrinisc muscles of the tongue. Cranial nerve XII has much to do with positioning of the larynx, that is, depression or elevation of the total laryngeal body, and is essential for all intrinsic movements of the tongue. Its primary impact on voice is on resonance and quality.

Superior and Recurrent Laryngeal Nerves.   As the vagus nerve leaves the nucleus ambiguus and exits laterally from the superior medulla and descends down the neck, it soon begins a series of branches. The first and most superior nerve branch off the vagus is the pharyngeal branch that contains both sensory and motor branches that supply the mucous membrane and selected muscles of the pharynx and soft palate. The next branch off the vagus bilaterally is the superior laryngeal nerve.

The superior laryngeal nerve branches off the vagus at about the level of the carotid sinuses in the neck (above which begins the carotid artery bifurcation) and angles medially toward the superior larynx. The superior laryngeal nerve divides into two branches (internal and external). The internal branch provides sensory innervation to the mucous membrane at the base of the tongue and to the mucous membrane of the supraglottal larynx. The external branch provides motor innervation to part of the lower pharyngeal constrictor and to the cricothyroid muscles. Although presented briefly in Chapter 2, let us consider the function (and symptoms of disorder) of the cricothyroid muscle:

Cricothyroid (CT).   Like all intrinsic laryngeal muscles (except the transverse arytenoids), the cricothyroid muscles are paired (L and R). The muscle is divided into two parts, the recta and the obliqua. Contraction of the cricothyroid muscles increases the distance between the cricoid and thyroid cartilages, increasing the length of the vocal folds, which decreases their cross-sectional mass. This action results in an increase of vibratory frequency and is heard as a rise in pitch. This stretching action also contributes to an adducting action of the vocal folds. Lesions to the CT are relatively rare and are seldom due to trauma but more often are related to some form of viral neuropathy (Tucker and Lavertu, 1992). Inability to elevate vocal pitch is the primary symptom of CT disease or trauma; in the case of unilateral CT paralysis, there may also be extreme hoarseness and occasional diplophonia (because of the disparate tension between the two vocal folds).

The next nerve branching off the descending vagus nerve is the recurrent laryngeal nerve (RLN). The RLN branches off the vagus considerably below the level of the larynx, almost at the level of the middle of the trachea. The right RLN loops "behind the right common carotid and subclavian arteries at their junction and courses vertically to the larynx" (Zemlin, 1998, p. 375). The left RLN leaves the vagus at a lower level than the right RLN, looping under and behind the aortic arch before making its vertical ascent to the larynx. Of some relevance to its frequent accidental cutting during surgery is its precarious location in the neck, ascending to the larynx in a groove between the trachea and the esophagus; the RLN then divides into three branches that enter the larynx through the cricothyroid membrane. The RLN is vital to the abductory–adductory function of the larynx as it innervates the five intrinsic muscles of the larynx, as first introduced in Chapter 2. At this point, however, we will reintroduce the five intrinsic muscles of the larynx that are innervated by the RLN, with a brief description of their function and voice symptoms if they do not receive their innervations:

Thyroarytenoid (TA).   The thyroarytenoid muscle is the main mass of the vocal fold. The muscle originates on the posterior side of the thyroid cartilage, which is known as the *anterior commissure*. The medial portion of the muscle is often described as the *vocalis muscle,* inserting posteriorly in the vocal process of the arytenoid. The larger muscle portion of the TA, known as the *thyromuscularis,* leaves the inner thyroid cartilage wall and extends posteriorly to the anterior surface of the arytenoid muscular process. The TA muscle mass, its ligament, and its cover (known collectively as the *vocal fold*) when adducted serves as the primary protective valve of the airway. Airway protection appears to be the primary role of the larynx and the TA is certainly a primary valve in this protection. Second, the vibrating mass of the vocal fold produces phonation. Changes in pitch are related to changes in tension of the thyroarytenoid muscle, either from its internal muscle contraction or stretching from external causes. TA contraction also contributes to medial vocal fold adduction. Flaccid paralysis of this muscle resulting from cutting or trauma to the RLN will in time lead to vocal fold atrophy resulting in weakness in vocal fold approximation, midfold bowing, and dysphonia. Subtle changes of pitch variation required in normal talking and singing will also be compromised with lack of TA innervation.

Posterior Cricoarytenoid (PCA).   The paired PCA is the lone abductor muscle of the vocal folds. Originating on the posterior surface of the cricoid cartilage, the muscle rises laterally and obliquely to the posterior muscular process of the arytenoid. When the muscle contracts, it rocks and slides the arytenoid, parting the arytenoids and abducting the vocal folds. The primary symptom of PCA paralysis is the inability to open the glottis on the involved side, creating a unilateral abductor paralysis.

Lateral Cricoarytenoid (LCA). The paired LCA is the primary adductor muscle of the vocal folds. The LCA originates on the superior, lateral surface of the cricoid arch and rises to the lateral muscular process of the arytenoids. When the LCA contracts, it slides the arytenoids together, which adducts the vocal folds. The LCA is an antagonist to the PCA: LCA relaxation facilitates PCA action and, conversely, relaxation of the PCA makes LCA adductory action easier. The primary symptom of LCA paralysis is vocal fold paralysis in the fixed, abducted, paramedian position.

Transverse Arytenoids. The transverse arytenoid muscles are the only unpaired muscles among the laryngeal intrinsic muscles. They are bilaterally innervated, crossing over the surfaces and space between the two arytenoid cartilages. When they contract, they have the effect of sliding the arytenoid cartilages together, contributing to vocal fold adduction. An RLN lesion may produce weakness or paralysis not only in transverse arytenoid function but in other adductory muscles as well.

Oblique Arytenoids. The oblique arytenoids are paired muscles, originating from the base of one arytenoid cartilage and rising obliquely to the apex of the opposite arytenoid. When they contract, they assist in bringing the arytenoids together, contributing to vocal fold adduction. It appears that, among those few people who can, with intent, produce ventricular phonation, differential contraction of the oblique arytenoids enables the more superior–lateral surfaces (the insertion points of the false folds) to approximate, resulting in ventricular voice. If a unilateral oblique arytenoid is paralyzed from lack of RLN innervation, this further contributes to unilateral adductor paralysis.

Having had a quick but intense look at the central and peripheral nervous systems and the innervation of muscles responsible for voice, let us now consider various voice problems of a neurogenic origin using a dysarthria classification framework introduced by Darley, Aronson, and Brown (1975) and subsequently revised by others (Duffy, 2005; Dworkin and Culatta, 1996; Yorkston et al., 1999). This revised classification system includes seven dysarthria subtypes, the categories of which are primarily based on neuromuscular abnormalities unique to each form: flaccid, unilateral upper motor neuron, spastic, ataxic, hypokinetic, hyperkinetic, and mixed.

Dysarthria is a disturbance of muscular control over the speech mechanism due to damage to the central or peripheral nervous system. Therefore, it is reasonable to expect that irregularities in speed, strength, timing, and accuracy may be observed in the systems of respiration, voicing, resonance, articulation, and prosody, either singly or in combination. Because voice is so intimately associated with respiration, resonance, articulation, and prosody in all seven dysarthria types, each subtype will be addressed.

FLACCID DYSARTHRIA

Flaccid dysarthria is usually caused by unilateral or bilateral damage to specific cranial nerves, irrespective of whether the disturbances occur at their nuclei in the brain stem or somewhere along their extracranial route to the speech subsystem muscles that they innervate. Damage to the peripheral nervous system causes a flaccid paralysis with underlying involvement of weakness, reduced force of muscle contraction, and reduced range of motion.

Vocal Fold Paralysis

Flaccid dysarthric patients who suffer damage of the cranial nerve X anywhere along its path from the medulla to the larynx have voice difficulties as a result of vocal fold paralysis. The physician's and SLP's roles are to confirm the diagnosis and to be certain that the movement deficit is not caused by mechanical causes, such as arytenoid cartilage dislocation or subluxation, cricoarytenoid arthritis or ankylosis, or a neoplasm (Rubin and Sataloff, 2007). Furthermore, the type and extent of dysphonia largely depends on the lesion site and whether the damage is unilateral, bilateral, partial, or complete.

Cricothyroid Muscle Paralysis. The SLN branches first or higher than the RLN from the descending vagus nerve and soon branches again into its internal and external branches that insert directly into the larynx. Because of its relatively direct course after it has branched out of the vagus down to the larynx, the SLN is rarely injured by trauma. Although other etiologies may be considered, viral infection appears to be the most common cause of SLN involvement, unilateral or bilateral, causing paralysis of left or right (or both) cricothyroid muscles (Dursun et al., 1996). Cricothyroid function is primarily in the tensing of the vocal fold, essential for elevation of pitch as well as contributing to vocal fold adduction. On examination, the patient displays a slight rotation of the involved vocal fold to the normal side as well as a slight bowing of the vocal fold on the involved side (Tanaka, Hirano, and Umeno, 1994). The patient's primary voice symptoms are an inability to elevate or lower pitch and some breathiness (due to the bowing). The virally caused cricothyroid paralysis is usually temporary, with the patient responding well to corticosteroids and antiviral agents. For those with longer-lasting paralysis, El-Kashian and colleagues (2001) reported promising results with selective reinnervation of the cricothyroid muscle, and Nasseri and Maragos (2000) reported postoperative improvements with type IV and type I thyroplasty. In addition, voice therapy has been found helpful in correcting the effects of the anterior glottal rotation (Dursun et al., 1996).

Bilateral Vocal Fold Paralysis.　Bilateral paralysis of the vocal folds is usually the result of lesions high in the trunk of the vagus nerve or at the nuclei of origin in the medulla. If the lesion is above the nodose ganglion, other muscles innervated by the vagus, as well as muscles supplied by other cranial nerves, will be affected as well. These high lesions include tumors at the base of the skull, carcinoma, or trauma. In the case of children, bilateral vocal fold paralysis is a common cause of neonatal stridor (Baker, Sapienza, and Collins, 2003). Most cases are associated with intracranial pathology such as meningomyelocoele, hydrocephalus, or Arnold-Chiari malformation. Other reports of rare etiologies are motor axonal neuropathy (Marchant et al., 2003) and familial clustering with autosomal recessive mode of inheritance (Raza et al., 2002).

Bilateral vocal fold paralysis may be of the abductory or adductory type; both are life threatening. Voice per se is of secondary concern to respiratory survival and feeding. In bilateral adductor paralysis, neither vocal fold is capable of moving to the midline, thus making phonation impossible and placing the individual at risk for aspiration. In abductor paralysis, the vocal folds remain at the midline, causing serious respiratory problems for which most patients will need a tracheostomy. Andrews and Summers (2002), Hoffman, Bolton and Ferry (2008), and Harvey-Woodnorth (2004) offer specific procedures for the SLP to use in working with young children with bilateral vocal fold paralysis—that is, how to manage the tracheostomy, the use of tracheal valves, and the need for minimizing the negative effects of the vocal fold dysfunction on the child's expressive language and speech development.

Continued bilateral vocal fold paralyses may require surgery to improve greater airway competence in both children and adults. Surgical reinnervation of the muscles of the vocal folds has been successfully reported by Crumley and Izdebski (1986). Perhaps used more often is the unilateral removal of one arytenoid with cauterization of muscular attachments to stimulate eventual contracture, resulting in more anterior glottal closure with posterior airway dilation (Tucker and Lavertu, 1992).

Zealer and colleagues (2003) reported in a pilot study that electrical stimulation to the posterior cricoarytenoid muscle via an implant resulted in improved vocal fold movement for three patients. Laser surgery has been successful in decreasing open glottal space for bilateral adductor fold paralysis, and laser arytenoidectomy for bilateral abductor paralysis has successfully opened the glottis. An alternative to surgery for some patients with abductor vocal fold paralysis may be inspiratory pressure threshold training. Baker, Sapienza, and Collins (2003) reported reductions in dyspnea during speech and exercise for a six-year-old child with congenital bilateral abductor paralysis after eight months of respiratory muscle strength training.

Unilateral Vocal Fold Paralysis (UVFP).　Disease or trauma to the recurrent laryngeal nerve (RLN) on one side is the most common form of laryngeal paralysis

(Case, 2002; Rubin and Sataloff, 2007). Because of the extended course of the left RLN, traveling down the neck and looping around the aortic arch in the chest and then traveling up again to the larynx, the left RLN appears to be more prone to traumatic or surgical injury than the right RLN. Bhattacharyya, Kotz, and Shapiro (2002) reported that of 64 patients presenting with UVFP, 53 cases were left-sided. In a retrospective review of patient cases, researchers at Georgetown University reported that isolated right VFP comprised only 3.1% of 778 laryngeal evaluation cases (Hughes et al., 2000). Surgical trauma predominated as an etiology, followed by viral and ideopathic causes. The authors commented that an unexpectedly high number of cases of VFP were caused by anterior laminectomy, accounting for 36% of cases. Etiologies of UVFP, of course, may also be location specific. Researchers in Scotland found a high rate of vocal fold palsy secondary to bronchogenic carcinoma, likely, the authors speculate, associated with the high levels of smoking in Scotland (Loughran, Alves, and MacGregor, 2002).

When the RLN is compromised on one side, the laryngeal adductor muscles (particularly the lateral cricoarytenoid) are not able to perform their adductory role. This keeps the paralyzed fold fixed in the paramedian position; that is, neither fully abducted nor adducted. The vocal fold remains at the paramedian position for both inspiration and expiration (including attempts at phonation).

On endoscopy, we see the paralyzed fold remaining abducted as the normal vocal fold moves to midline. Because of the proximity of the folds at the anterior commissure, there is usually some anterior approximation, which helps to set the two folds into vibration during phonation attempts. Colton and Casper (1996) discount that there is any slight crossover of the normal fold to meet the paralyzed fold, and, generally, what we observe on phonation attempts is the vibration of the paralyzed fold set in motion by the outgoing airflow passing between the two folds, particularly at the anterior one-third. Also, the Bernoulli effect, described in Chapter 2, plays a role here in drawing the two folds together.

The voice in UVFP is markedly dysphonic or aphonic. Perceptual characteristics include breathy, hoarse vocal quality, reduced phonation time, decreased loudness, monoloudness, diplophonia, and pitch breaks. The breathy vocal quality, reduced loudness, and short phonation times can be attributed to air escape through an open glottis during phonation. Hoarseness, pitch breaks, and diplophonia can be associated with reduced ability to adjust the internal tension of the paralyzed vocal fold. Excessive supraglottal constriction (hyperfunction) may contribute to the perception of hoarseness.

Because many traumatic vocal fold paralyses have spontaneous recovery within the first 9 to 12 months postonset, permanent corrective procedures should be delayed until voice intervention has been tried. In many cases, strengthening the vocal muscles and improving speaking technique result in very good voice quality and surgery is unnecessary (Schindler et al., 2008). Behavioral voice therapy may be the only treatment required or it may suffice as a temporary measure until medical intervention is feasible. One study found that voice therapy reduced mean airflow rate in 16 patients with UVFP by nearly 50% (McFarlane, Watterson, et al.,

1998). The techniques we normally introduce in clinic are half-swallow boom, head positioning, tuck-chin, digital manipulation, focus, tongue protrusion /i/, yawn–sigh, pitch shift up, and inhalation phonation. Each technique affords an anatomical and physiological rationale for improving voice in individuals with UVFP, as demonstrated in the following case study.

Mr. S. was a Korean-born gentleman who underwent surgery and subsequent radiation therapy for thyroid cancer. Postsurgery and radiation, Mr. S. reported a deterioration of voice, and his surgeons reported that he had sustained a right vocal fold paralysis. He reported that, in addition to speaking difficulties, on occasion he experienced dysphagia, especially on thin liquids. Swallow dysfunction secondary to UVFP is not unusual; indeed, researchers at Harvard Medical School reported that, for 64 patients presenting with UVFP, radiographically significant penetration or aspiration occurred in approximately one-third (Bhattacharyya, Kotz, and Shapiro, 2002).

Perceptually, phonation was breathy and diplophonic at times. Phrases were brief and tended to decline in volume toward the ends. Head turned right with right digital manipulation of the thyroid cartilage increased vocal loudness while maintaining vocal quality. Mr. S. extended the chin and tensed the neck strap muscles, notably when beginning a phrase. New techniques of chin down with focus eliminated these maladaptive behaviors.

Acoustic measures using a sustained /a/ revealed an F_0 (fundamental frequency) of 104 Hz, with a relative average perturbation (RAP) of 2.98% and shimmer of 12.2% (see Chapter 6 for acoustic assessment of the voice). F_0 was within normal limits; however, RAP and shimmer were above normal limits. Head turn right and right digital pressure revealed reduced RAP of 1.7% at 121 Hz, which is not within normal limits, but improved from baseline. Shimmer was reduced to 4.37% employing these techniques. Transglottal airflow was reduced to 266 mL/s from 468 mL/s with head turned right and right digital manipulation.

Rigid videoendoscopy with stroboscopy revealed a right vocal fold at the paramedian position. Phonation revealed an immobile right vocal fold and longitudinal glottal gap, even though the left vocal fold adducted to the midline. Medial compression was observed, as was seen by the bulging of the left ventricular fold.

Mr. S. received six hours of intensive voice therapy focused on eliminating maladaptive behaviors and improving vocal quality and intensity. Yawn–sigh followed by vowel initial productions were successful for increasing amplitude and vocal quality. This was followed by focus with nasal glide stimuli. We were sensitive to the multicultural nature of this case, and the phonemes that comprise the Japanese and Korean languages were explored. Mr. S. was able to identify voiced and voiceless sounds and to make phonation and resonance adjustments for smooth voiced to voiceless transitions. The primary clinician was assisted by an undergraduate clinician who spoke Japanese.

When Mr. S. felt comfortable with the techniques, he was introduced to new speaking situations within the clinic. He lectured for 15 minutes before an undergraduate class. Students reported full intelligibility. Mr. S. observed that he is asked to speak in large rooms, often without a microphone. For these occasions we recommended that he use a personal voice amplifier. Personal voice amplifiers vary widely in features and corresponding costs. In a recent study involving voice amplification as a control condition, Roy and colleagues (2002) used the ChatterVox portable amplifier; however, many others are available over the Internet and at local electronics stores. Finally, Mr. S was provided with a video and written home program to help to maintain the gains made in the clinic.

Nonbehavioral Approaches to UVFP.   Since Arnold (1962) introduced the injection of Teflon as a surgical approach for promoting better medialization, there have been many advances in the treatment of unilateral vocal fold paralysis. Teflon injection is no longer the procedure of choice for unilateral vocal fold paralysis; rather, in greater use today are vocal fold injections using various soft tissue fillers and medialization thyroplasty. A review of the literature reveals soft tissue fillers of varying combinations, ranging from fat injections (Hsiung et al., 2000) to polyacrylamide hydrogel, a facial tissue filler (Lee, Son, et al., 2007). Readers are encouraged to explore the literature to learn of the long-term effects and voice outcomes of the various injection fillers and methods. Most researchers report that injections are a safe and largely durable treatment option of the management of glottal insufficiency, although there are reports that fat augmentation is reabsorbed, but can be repeated (Hsiung et al., 2000) and that in some cases the mucosal wave can be interrupted when the injection is to the superficial area of the vocal fold.

Thyroplasty I is a surgical approach to medialization of the paralyzed fold, using a free-moving wedge to move the paralyzed fold to midline (Dursun et al., 2008). The surgeon cuts a rectangular window out of the thyroid cartilage on the side of the paralyzed vocal fold. The patient is conscious during the procedure and produces voice when the surgeon places the wedge at various sites against the paralyzed fold. When it is confirmed that a certain site produces the best phonation, the wedge is fixed surgically at that point. Thyroplasty in the hands of a competent surgeon produces excellent results, and patients should expect "voice improvement as early as 1 month postoperatively and should remain stable with slight fluctuations for at least 6 months" (p. 576). Dean and colleagues (2001) introduced a modification of the thyroplasty technique by introducing a titanium implant with a micrometric screw that allows for secondary adjustment of medialization, if necessary. Titanium is MRI safe.

There are numerous reports on the long-term results of both injection and medialization thyroplasties. One notable study by Morgan, Zraick, Griffin, Bowen, and Johnson (2007) reported a retrospective study of 19 patients with UVFP who received either vocal fold injection or thyroplasty. Outcome measures were videostrobolaryngoscopy, perceptual analysis, and patients' subjective voice assessments. Results revealed that both approaches were comparable in their improvements of subjective and objective voice outcomes. Another procedure for unilateral paralysis involves reinnervating the paralyzed muscles by nerve grafts from the phrenic nerve, or by grafting a section of the superior laryngeal nerve with a portion of the hypoglossus nerve into the vocal fold adductor muscles. A more recent reinnervation technique described by Lorenz and colleagues (2008) is ansa cervicalis-to-recurrent laryngeal nerve anastomosis. Other approaches involve arytenoid adduction (Su, Tsai, Chuang, and Chiu, 2005).

Some patients, after injection or surgery, continue to display the hyperfunctional vocal behaviors they were using before treatment. Direct symptom modification can usually reduce such problems as squeezing the words out, using pushing behaviors, and using excessive glottal attack. Following injection or surgical forms of medialization, the SLP may help the patient reestablish a normal voice, giving some attention to adequate breath support, phonation free of effort, with some attention given to voice focus and adequate loudness.

Myasthenia Gravis

Although vocal paralysis is the most common voice problem associated with flaccid dysarthria, myasthenia gravis (MG) is not an uncommon dysarthria, with an incidence of 1 in 10,000. Some patients with myasthenia gravis experience problems of severe voice fatigue with associated problems in adequate breath support. MG is an autoimmune disease in which the neuromuscular junction becomes impaired as the patient uses that particular muscle or muscle group, resulting in extreme muscle fatigue. Muscles innervated by the cranial nerves in the head and neck are particularly vulnerable to the disease. In MG, the immune system (for reasons unknown) produces antibodies that attack the receptors that lie on the muscle side of the neuromuscular junction (Duffy, 2005). Symptoms occur because there is damage to the receptors at the neuromuscular junction, preventing the normal transfer of impulse from the nerve into the particular muscle. The disease occurs twice as often in women over men with females reporting the onset in their thirties and men reporting onsets in their sixties.

Typically, sustained repetitive performance of a particular muscle group will lead to complete performance fatigue: Tapping two alternate notes repeatedly on a piano will result in a progressively slower tapping rate with eventually an inability to continue the task. For the mysathenia gravis patient with voice problems, the patient experiences a vocal change with voice usage from a normal voice to a breathy, weak, barely audible voice. With a few minutes of complete voice rest, the voice will be restored, but after a few minutes of usage, the weak voice will return. In severe cases, the patient will report difficulty swallowing, with occasional nasal regurgitation (Llabrés et al., 2005).

The diagnosis of myasthenia gravis should always be suspected in patients who experience weakness after usage of the muscles of the eye, face, and throat, but with some recovery after rest. Because acetylcholine receptors are blocked, drugs that increase the presence of acetylcholine in the neuromuscular junction are useful in helping to confirm the diagnosis. "Edrophonium (Tensilon™) is most commonly used as the test drug; when injected intravenously, it temporarily improves muscle strength in people with myasthenia gravis" (Berkow et al., 1997, p. 333).

Accordingly, the treatment of MG is primarily medical, giving anticholinesterase medications, immunosuppressants, antimetabolite agents, and corticosteroids. Other options available to the patient are plasmapheresis, which removes AchR antibodies from the circulating plasma of patients with MG, intravenous immunoglobulin, and thymectomy (Armstrong and Schumann, 2003).

The speech–language pathologist often plays the primary role in discovering the disease. Patient complaints of deteriorating voice after usage, particularly when coupled with other visual symptoms, such as a drooping eyelid (ptosis) or new problems in swallowing, should be referred through the patient's primary care physician to a neurologist. At the evaluation, the SLP should give the patient sustained oral reading tasks; a determination should be made of how long oral reading must continue before vocal-speech deterioration is heard. From the onset of voice change, time measurements should be made of continued oral reading until further voicing is almost impossible. Then determine the amount of time required before there is some restoration of vocal strength. Beyond oral reading, the SLP might take measures of airflow and pressure, spirometric determination of air volumes, test diadochokinetic rates for various oral tasks, make glottographic determinations of vocal fold approximation, and administer articulation tests. Once the patient is receiving treatment with some form of drug regimen, the SLP should select any of these measures for comparison over time, giving objective evidence of medication effectiveness. The SLP's role is discovery and comparison of motor response data over time—not providing voice therapy. With appropriate acetylcholine levels achieved through medication, MG patients in early stages of the disease process will usually experience the levels of speech and voice competence they had before the onset of symptoms.

Guillain–Barré

A brief mention of Guillain–Barré (GB) is warranted at this point, because the onset of the disease is often expressed in dysphonia and dysphagia. GB is a disorder of unknown cause, but is frequently preceded by viral infection. It involves the focal demyelinization of spinal and cranial nerves. The disease process usually begins symmetrically in the lower extremities and advances superiorly, but other researchers have suggested that facial, oral–pharyngeal, and occular muscles occasionally are affected first. The patient often requires a tracheostomy and ventilatory support. Often the patient receives plasmapheresis and intravenous immunoglobulin (IVIg) as part of medical intervention. Approximately 65% of individuals recover from GB while the remainder are left with residual dysarthria and altered function in psychosocial situations (Bernsen et al., 2002).

UNILATERAL UPPER MOTOR NEURON DYSARTHRIA (UUMND)

UUMND is caused by a unilateral lesion to the CNS, involving both the pyramidal and extrapyramidal tracts. It is often observed in patients who have experienced a cerebrovascular accident (CVA), but it could be caused by other etiologies, such as tumor or trauma. A CVA, known more commonly as a *stroke,* is a temporary impairment of blood flow to the brain. Three types of CVA are generally recognized: thrombosis (the most common obstruction, a clot that forms within an artery obstructing the flow of blood); embolus (a traveling blood clot that lodges within an artery preventing the flow of blood); or hemorrhage (blood flows out of a break in an arterial wall). Because the distribution of blood for most of the higher areas of the brain (cortex through thalamus–basal ganglia) is distributed superior to the circle of Willis, the blood supply to each of the two cerebral hemispheres is unilateral. That is, each hemisphere has its own blood supply, which is why most strokes appear to involve motor and sensory function on one side of the body. A CVA in the left hemisphere will produce a right-sided weakness or paralysis; a right hemisphere stroke will involve the left side of the body.

Voice was once thought to be seldom affected by a single, unilateral cerebral lesion, because of the bilateral nature of corticobulbar innervation of the vagus nerve. Rather, imprecise articulation due to unilateral facial and lingual weakness is a primary deviant characteristic of UUMND. Nevertheless, Duffy and Folger (1986) reported a high percentage of dysphonia occurring in 56 cases of individuals with UUMND. Thirty-nine percent of patients had a moderate dysphonia, which was described as harsh or strained-harshness and 9% had reduced loudness. Duffy suggests that the dysphonia could reflect the effect of subtle vocal cord weakness, mild spasticity from the lesion, or possible spasticity from an *undetected* lesion in the contralateral hemisphere. UUMND is also associated with dysphagia, due to lip, buccal, and lingual involvement. These sensory–motor disturbances are normally mild and transient (Darley, Aronson, and Brown, 1975; Logemann, 1998; Metter, 1985).

SPASTIC DYSARTHRIA

Two or more neurogenic events (acquired or congenital) that result in bilateral cerebral lesions may produce severe voice symptoms from lesions to the pyramidal and extrapyramidal tracts bilaterally. Common neuromuscular symptoms include hypertonicity, exaggerated reflexes, paresis, and bilateral weakness of various speech and voice muscle groups. The voice symptoms are characteristic of a spastic dysarthria, also known as pseudobulbar palsy. Voice may be strained and strangled, brief in phonation time, low in pitch, and monopitch with variable loudness. Hypernasality may be present in some patients due to the slow and weak range of movement of the velum. Symptomatic of patients with bilateral pyramidal and extrapyramidal tract damage is emotional lability, which may severely influence voice quality and resonance. The patient will laugh or cry easily, inappropriately to the intensity of the stimulus. For example, we remember a 55-year-old patient with pseudobulbar palsy who, when meeting an old friend, would appear to be crying on inhalation and laughing on exhalation. His lability-influenced voice would have severe posterior focus with extreme hypernasality. He had so much massive escape of airflow through his nasal passages that his oral articulation was severely compromised. When he cried or laughed, his speech was unintelligible. Management of his voice was best helped by attempting to reduce his lability.

Voice therapy for patients with spastic dysarthria is highly individualized, depending on the speech subsystems that are compromised. Some of these approaches are illustrated on the accompanying DVD. Dworkin and Culatta (1996), Duffy (2005), and Yorkston and colleagues (2004) have discussed hierarchical approaches to voice and speech therapy, based on the compromised subsystem(s).

HYPOKINETIC DYSARTHRIA

Hypokinetic dysarthria is associated with a depletion of or functional reduction in the effect of the neurotransmitter dopamine on the activities of the basal ganglia. As described earlier, the basal ganglia are associated with providing proper background and tone for quick, discrete movements. The clinical features underlying basal ganglia pathology are rigidity, slow movement (bradykinesia), limited range of motion, and a resting tremor that is normally ameliorated through intentional movement. Although a number of etiologies may cause hypokinetic dysarthria, idiopathic Parkinson's disease (PD) is known as the prototypical hypokinetic dysarthria, as 98% of hypokinetic dysarthrias are of the Parkinson's type (Berry, 1983).

Parkinson's Disease

The Parkinson patient exhibits a hypokinetic dysarthria characterized by reduced loudness, breathy voice, monotony of pitch, intermittent rapid rushes of speech, and soft production of consonants. Some investigators of PD have found diminished function in one or more components of speech–voice; for example, Solomon and Hixon (1993) found significant respiratory difficulties as possibly contributing to the PD patient's voice symptoms; Ramig and others (1994) found that 35 of 40 PD subjects had bowed vocal folds. Duffy (2005) and Yorkston and colleagues (2004) write that many of these abnormalities can be related to the underlying neuromuscular deficits of rigidity, reduced range of movement, and slowness of movement in the laryngeal muscles. See Fahr, Elton, and UPDRS Development Committee (1987) for the Unified Parkinson Disease Rating Scale, a comprehensive and widely used rating scale to document levels of motor behavior and activities of daily living for individuals with Parkinson's disease.

It would appear that isolation of any one speech component for study in the PD patient will find a deficit in function. Fortunately, the most effective voice therapy approach is a holistic one, finding that to exaggerate one component helps improve function in all other components.

When patients attempt to speak in a quick conversational pattern, speech is often unintelligible due to the rapid and accelerated movement of the articulators.

When they speak with intent, however, their speech can be slower, louder, have better voice quality, and better articulation. Following the model of intention used in physical therapy for gait training (thinking where you are going to place each foot as you walk makes walking easier), the same model of intent works to improve speech. Using intention with these patients, the writers have asked PD patients to speak with an accent, or use a different pitch, or speak slower, or speak louder (Boone and Plante, 1993). Taking the automatic motor-set out of speaking by speaking intentionally different seems to help the patient's speech in all parameters: loudness, voice quality, appropriate pitch, and rate. More recent in-clinic trials have found that instructing patients to deliberately pronounce the final sound of each word has yielded increases in vocal loudness and intelligibility.

Ramig and colleagues (2001) and others (Spielman, Ramig, and Mahler, 2007) have studied the model of intention in a formal voice and speech improvement program that is driven by a number of perceptual features of phonation in Parkinson's disease. The main goal of the Lee Silverman Voice Treatment (LSVT) program is to increase vocal fold adduction and respiratory effort, which, in turn, is intended to increase loudness, vocal quality, and, subsequently, intelligibility.

One study of LSVT effectiveness had 40 PD patients receive one hour of voice therapy four times a week for one month, receiving 13 to 16 hours of individual voice therapy. There were three general therapy tasks: increasing vocal fold adduction, increasing respiratory support, and increasing maximum fundamental frequency range. Of all the therapy tasks, speaking "louder shout" seemed to be the most unique and beneficial part of the Silverman therapy approach. There was significant improvement in all variables studied between pre- and posttherapy treatment.

Sapir and others (2002) investigated whether increased loudness is maintained over several months after conclusion of the LSVT program. Judges listened to reading samples produced by two groups: one that had undergone LSVT and one that had undergone a high-effort respiratory treatment program. Of the two groups, the speech samples in the LSVT group were significantly more likely to be perceived as louder and of better quality at follow-up.

Researchers in the Netherlands suggested that increased respiratory–phonatory effort raises vocal pitch and laryngeal muscle tension (de Swart et al., 2003). These researchers generated an intervention program called Pitch Limiting Voice Treatment (PLVT), which instructs patients to increase respiratory support, but to phonate at a low pitch. A study comparing LSVT and PLVT revealed the same increases in loudness for both groups, but the authors suggested that PLVT limited increases in vocal pitch, thus preventing strained and pressed voicing.

For those patients who are initially stimulable for behavioral voice programs, but who experience difficulty generalizing the gains beyond the clinic, we have offered delayed auditory feedback (DAF), with mixed results. DAF is an instrumental procedure that feeds an individual's speech trace back to the individual's auditory system via earphones at a delayed rate. The effect of the delay is to slow speech rate, increase vocal loudness, and increase articulatory accuracy. Several case studies at this clinic and reports in the literature have suggested improved speech using DAF for individuals presenting with hypokinetic dysarthria (Downie, Low, and Lindsay, 1981; Hanson and Metter, 1983; Yorkston et al., 2004). These authors suggest that the benefits included marked reduction in speech rate, increased loudness, reduced phonetic errors, and increased acoustic distinctiveness.

DAF intervention produced remarkable results in the vocal intensity, rate, and intelligibility of an individual seen at our clinic with PD. This patient, a former physician, had received a thalamic (deep brain) stimulator four years earlier to reduce tremors and was taking Sinemet (combined levadopa and carbidopa). Nevertheless, speech was rapid and blurred and the voice was hypophonic. Various clinic probes of speaking with intent, to a metronome, pacing, respiratory–phonatory training, and hyperarticulation were not effective. He was fitted with the Kay Facilitator (KayPENTAX) set at the 170 ms feedback mode and the effect was dramatic. He increased vocal intensity, extended the vowels, and increased articulatory contacts, thus increasing intelligibility. He subsequently purchased a pocket-sized DAF unit that he wore at all times. He said the system was so innocuous that people thought he was listening to the ball game. Even though he did not return to his former practice, he did begin to deliver lectures at the medical school and spoke at Parkinson's disease support group meetings.

The diagnosis of PD and its medical management belongs to the neurologist, although we and many other voice clinicians have been instrumental in alerting health professionals to patients who present to our clinics with hypokinetic features that may have previously gone undetected. We have found that an interdisciplinary health care team, consisting of the SLP, physician, nurse, nutritionist, and various rehabilitation experts, comprises the best medical care for patients with this complex disorder. Over time, the period of relief from continued dopaminergic administration becomes shorter, requiring new medication protocols and possible neurosurgical approaches to reduce tremor, such as anterior thalamotomies (Stacy and Jankovic, 1992), pallidotomies (Schulz, Greer, and Friedman, 2000), and stereotactic surgery deep-brain stimulation. In deep-brain stimulation, a thin stimulator is surgically placed in the thalamus, the part of the brain that is believed to activate tremors. The stimulator is powered by a tiny generator implanted in the patient's chest. Different researchers have identified different areas of the thalamus that are most receptive to stimulation, resulting in reduced tremors. Hamel and colleagues (2003) suggest that stimulation of the subthalamic nucleus results in marked improvement in levadopa-sensitive Parkinsonian symptoms and levadopa-induced dyskinesias.

HYPERKINETIC DYSARTHRIA

Hyperkinetic dysarthria is difficult to define because of its many different clinical presentations, but it is generally associated with damage to the basal ganglia or an imbalance of neurotransmitters therein, specifically acetylcholine and dopamine.

Hyperkinetic means involuntary and uncontrolled movements, and it may be manifest in any or all of the subsystems of speech. Unlike most CNS-based dysarthrias, hyperkinetic dysarthria can manifest itself at only one level of speech production, sometimes only a few muscles at that level (Duffy, 2005).

Spasmodic Dysphonia

Spasmodic dysphonia is a relatively rare voice disorder that can be classified as a focal dystonia (Case, 2002), which falls under the cluster of hyperkinetic dysarthria. The patient exhibits a strangled harsh voice with observable effort in pushing the air out during most voicing attempts. Patients' voices sound strained, choked off with the attempts to voice, as if they are trying to push the outgoing airstream through a tightly adducted laryngeal opening. Endoscopic examination shows that the tight voice is indeed produced by hyperadduction (severe approximation) of the true folds, often accompanied by tight closure of the false vocal folds (ventricular folds) with supraglottal constriction of the aryepiglottic folds and contraction of the lower pharyngeal constrictors. The total laryngeal and lower pharyngeal airway appears to close down. No wonder we hear a strained, strangled voice in such patients. Nevertheless, Hirano and Bless (1993) caution that the voice clinician should not anticipate seeing one particular laryngeal pattern. They suggest that spasmodic dysphonia can be very heterogeneous, with presentation ranging from spasmodic hyperfunction to hypofunction to irregular twitching of the vocal folds.

In addition to the problem of voicing, patients with spasmodic dysphonia complain about the difficulties they experience trying to force expiratory air out whenever they desire to phonate. Aronson (1990) comments that the tight voice during adductor spasmodic dysphonia "occurs only during voluntary phonation for communication purposes and not during singing, vowel prolongation, laughing, or crying" (p. 161). However, in patients who have carried the diagnosis of spasmodic dysphonia for some period of time and who are more severe, we see symptoms of this disorder in prolonged vowels as well. The patients soon learn to expect phonation difficulties whenever they attempt to speak. In this sense, spasmodic dysphonia resembles stuttering. In European writings, in fact, the condition is sometimes called the *laryngeal stutter*. McFarlane and Shipley (1979) make a case for spasmodic dysphonia *not* being considered as laryngeal stuttering based on the greater number of important dissimilarities than important similarities between the two disorders. Most patients with spasmodic dysphonia experience some normal voice in certain situations. Case histories of these patients reveal that, in such situations as "talking to my cat" or "speaking to others in a pool while I tread water," patients have experienced normal voice.

The most common type of spasmodic dysphonia appears to be related to tight laryngeal adduction, known as adductor spasmodic dysphonia (ADSD). Aronson (1990), however, also described a second form of the disorder, known as abductor spastic dysphonia (ABSD), in which patients exhibit normal or dysphonic voices that are suddenly interrupted by temporary abduction of the vocal folds, resulting in fleeting aphonia. After such momentary aphonia, the patients' voice patterns are restored again (until the next aphonic break). Endoscopy shows that the vocal folds of such patients abduct suddenly, "exposing an extremely wide glottic chink" (Aronson, 1990, p. 185). More often than not, the abductor spasms appear to be triggered by unvoiced consonant sounds. The abductor-type disorder is a much rarer form of spasmodic dysphonia. For example, Davis and others (1988) reported that of 25 successive cases of spasmodic dysphonia observed in a Sydney, Australia, hospital, 24 were adductor type and one was an abductor type. The abductor spasm can often be treated successfully as a phonation break. Because the symptoms and the treatment of adductor and abductor spasmodic dysphonia are so different, the authors of this text will confine further comments about spasmodic dysphonia to the adductor type. Symptoms and treatment for the sudden abductory spasms described by Aronson (1990) are discussed as phonation breaks in this text.

Spasmodic dysphonia (SD) is classified as a form of focal dystonia. Dystonia is a neurological dysfunction of motor movements, either more generalized to major body movements or seen in focal disorders, such as in the eyelids (blepharospasm), in the neck (torticollis), or in the larynx (spasmodic dysphonia). The site in the brain where a lesion might occur that would cause spasmodic dysphonia is still not definitively known. One of the first studies using MRI, SPECT, or brain electrical activity mapping (BEAM) for identifying possible SD lesion sites was reported by Finitzo and Freeman (1989) who concluded that "SD is a supranuclear movement disorder primarily, but not exclusively, affecting the larynx. Fully half of our subjects evidence isolated functional cortical lesions" (p. 553). While there is increasing consensus among medical and voice pathologists that SD is a neurological problem (Chhetri et al., 2003), the treatment of SD has not embraced symptom-modifying medication or intracerebral neurosurgery treatments. Of all the intrinsic laryngeal muscles (except the important adductor, the lateral cricoarytenoid, which was not studied), it has been clearly demonstrated using simultaneous EMG recordings that only the thyroarytenoid (the vocal fold) has abnormal muscle activation during SD-voicing (Nash and Ludlow, 1996).

Exploring beyond the suspected site of lesion, Schweinfurth, Billante, and Courey (2002) attempted to identify risk factors and demographics in patients with adductor spasmodic dysphonia (ADSD). Results of a retrospective survey of 168 patients revealed that there "appears to be no significant environmental or hereditary patterns in the etiology of spasmodic dysphonia" (p. 220). The authors did identify some trends, however. The majority of patients were females (79%). A significantly higher incidence of childhood viral illness was found in the patients with SD (65%). Patients with SD had a significant incidence of both essential tremor (26%) and writer's cramp (11%), but no history of major illness or other neurological disorder.

Judgment Scales for Spasmodic Dysphonia. The description and quantification of the symptoms of spasmodic dysphonia require administration of perceptual judgment scales and instrumental measures. Because SD is a rare disorder, patients with SD may not be easily identified by clinicians who do not have extensive experience in its symptomology. Barkmeier, Case, and Ludlow (2001) point out that SD can easily be misinterpreted as an essential tremor or vocal hyperfunction, behaviors whose distinguishing features and etiologies we will attempt to isolate later in this section (Table 4.1). Barkmeier and colleagues (2001) investigated whether voice clinicians with infrequent exposure to SD patients could learn to identify speech symptoms of ADSD and ABSD compared to voice clinicians having extensive experience with these disorders. Results revealed that while the nonexpert judges tended toward false positive judgments for the speech symptoms of interest, the overall speech symptom profiles for each type of voice disorder appeared comparable to those obtained from the expert judges. Readers are encouraged to review this study to become familiar with the identification scale used.

Another excellent judgment scale developed (Stewart et al., 1997) for assessing the SD patient is known as the Unified Spasmodic Dysphonia Rating Scale (USDRS). The scale offers the SLP a standardized way of asking for speech–voice responses and a seven-point rating scale for evaluating such SD-voice parameters as overall severity, aspects of voice quality, abrupt voice initiation, voice arrests, loudness variations, tremor, expiratory effort, speech rate, speech intelligibility, and related movements and grimaces (Stewart et al., 1997, p. 100). The administration of the perceptual rating scale should precede such instrumental assessments as airflow and pressure data, fundamental frequency values, perturbation measures, and intensity documentation (see Chapter 6).

What treatment options are available today for reducing the hypertonic approximation of the vocal folds during SD voicing attempts? Let us consider separately several treatment options that can be offered to the SD patient: voice therapy, surgical resection of the recurrent laryngeal nerve, botulinum toxin (BTX) injection, and surgical modification of the vocal folds.

Voice Therapy for SD.   For a clinical lifetime, this writer (DB) has encountered each new SD patient with the optimism that the strangled-sounding, harsh voice could be modified by voice therapy, only to find repeatedly with each new patient that apparent success in producing an easy normal voice temporarily in the voice clinic seemed to have no carryover out of the clinic.

Case (2002) wrote of similar poor outcomes of traditional voice therapy, noting that many patients made slight improvements when speech was produced in small units, such as monosyllabic utterances, but rarely in contextual speech. "Historically, the poor prognosis is one of the most significant symptoms of this disorder and has been pathognomonic and diagnostic to it" (p. 189). There have been few reported positive outcomes for SD patients receiving voice therapy, such as Cooper's (1990) "direct voice rehabilitation" and the more conventional voice therapy. For the typical speech–language pathologist, our role with the SD patient is careful, meticulous assessment to permit evaluation of treatment outcomes and to combine voice therapy efforts with pharmacological or surgical treatment, before and after intervention.

Some trial voice therapy should follow assessment, used at least as diagnostic probes. Many SD patients experience an easier voice with less effort "pushing voice out" through working on an easy breath cycle, employing yawn–sigh relaxation methods coupled with hierarchy analysis. Boone (1998) has found both real-time amplification, auditory feedback, and masking (so patients cannot hear their own voicing) to be facilitative for some SD patients. Speaking on inhalation is reported as less likely to reduce the symptoms of long-standing adductor spasmodic dysphonia (Harrison et al., 1992). Roy, Ford, and Bless (1996) have employed the musculoskeletal tension reduction techniques recommended by Aronson (1990) with over 150 cases of muscle tension dysphonia, described under Laryngeal Massage in Chapter 7 of this text. Included in the group of muscle tension dysphonia patients were some SD patients (the number was not specified in the article) who received the manual lowering of their larynx but experienced only "transient improvements in voice that could not be stabilized or generalized" (Roy et al., 1996, p. 855).

In summary, from long clinical experience and in reviewing the literature, there are scarce efficacy data to show that the struggling of SD patients to get air out while producing harsh, strangled voice is resolved solely with voice therapy. Rather, those patients who do respond positively to voice therapy may likely have originally presented with a vocal hyperfunction, which often masquerades as SD. It would appear that voice therapy coupled with surgery or Botox injections offers the best therapeutic management of spasmodic dysphonia. These interventions are described in the following sections.

Recurrent Laryngeal Nerve (RLN) Sectioning.   Introduced by Dedo (1976), the RLN section (Izdebski, Dedo, and Boles, 1984) was the first widely used surgical procedure for SD. Patients are selected for RLN section after a thorough diagnostic evaluation by both the surgeon and the SLP, which includes an injection of Xylocaine into the RLN to produce a temporary unilateral adductor paralysis. The patient's airflow, relative ease of phonation, and change of voice quality are assessed. If there is marked improvement in airflow (greater flow rates with less glottal resistance) and in both ease and quality of phonation, the decision may be made to cut the RLN permanently. Postoperatively, then, the patient usually has an easily produced but breathy voice, similar in sound to the patient with unilateral adductor paralysis. Voice therapy focusing on a slight elevation of pitch, some ear training, head positioning, and digital manipulation have all been effective in developing a better-sounding voice.

The long-term results of RLN resection have been mixed. Wilson, Oldring, and Mueller (1980) reported a woman who had received RLN cut 13 months previously and then experienced a regeneration of the severed RLN and a return of spasmodic dysphonia; a second RLN resection again produced immediate relief from her phonatory struggle. Over three years Aronson and DeSanto (1983) followed 33 patients with spasmodic dysphonia who had each received RLN cut. Although all experienced improved voice and ease of airflow immediately after surgery, three years later 21 of them, or 64%, had failed to maintain their gains and were considered failures. Much different results were reported by Dedo and Izdebski (1983) on over 306 patients who had received RLN cut for spasmodic dysphonia; they reported that 92% of the patients maintained voice improvement and required less effort to phonate.

The arguments over the long-term effectiveness of RLN section as posed by Aronson and DeSanto (1983) versus Dedo and Izdebski (1983) contributed to a significant reduction in the use of RLN sectioning as a treatment for SD. Regeneration of the severed RLN appears to be the primary factor in symptoms of tight voice coming back a few months or years after RLN section. To meet this regeneration problem, Weed and others (1996) recommended the use of avulsion (tearing out or entire removal) of as much of the recurrent laryngeal nerve as is surgically possible. In the Weed study, long-term follow-up of RLN avulsion patients revealed that "72 to 78 percent of patients retained clear benefit from the procedure beyond 3 years" (p. 600).

Berke and colleagues (1999) described a surgical technique for ADSD that paralyzes the thryroarytenoid and lateral cricoarytenoid muscles bilaterally by denervating the recurrent laryngeal nerve branches to these muscles. To prevent unwanted reinnervation and to preserve muscle tone, the TA nerve branch is reinnervated with a branch of the ansa cervicalis. The procedure, the authors note, obviates the breathy voice and other typical sequelae of unilateral vocal fold paralysis. The long-term results of 21 sequential cases were reported, with 19 patients judged to have an "absent to mild" dysphonia following the procedure and one patient requiring further Botox treatments. The opposite vocal behaviors were reported by one patient presenting to our clinic for voice therapy. Twenty months earlier he underwent bilateral laryngeal adductor denervation with ansa cervicalis reinnervation. He reported that although he no longer had to worry about strained and strangled phonation, he now had to worry about a soft voice that was insufficient for many social and professional activities of daily living. This patient responded well to intervention for unilateral vocal fold paralysis (digital manipulation, focus, head positioning).

Even though higher airflow rates and lower pressures are noted after RLN surgery, many patients persist in maladaptive hyperfunctional postures, such as pushing and working hard to produce outgoing expiration, grimacing, and continuing to experience a marked reduction in normal prosody. Most of these hyperfunctional postures are unlearned with voice therapy, allowing us to agree with Dedo and Izdebski (1983) that the vast majority (92% in their study) of patients continue for years to enjoy improved voices with ease of airflow after RLN section.

Botulinum Toxin (BTX) Injections.   The primary approach today for treating SD appears to be the injection of botulinum toxin (BTX) in one or both vocal folds. For many years, injection of Botox into muscles in spasm has been found effective for eyelid spasms (blepharospasm) and for severe neck muscle spasms (torticollis).

More recently Botox is being used to treat limb contractures secondary to stroke (O'Brien, 2002) and chronic headaches (Loder and Biondi, 2002), not to mention the smoothing of hyperfunctional lines (read *wrinkles*).

One early report of successful use of Botox injections for SD patients (Blitzer and Brin, 1991) found that Botox injection into the thyroarytenoid (TA) experienced by 210 SD patients was "a relatively safe and effective mode of therapy for laryngeal dystonia" (p. 88). Botox is injected into the TA, unilaterally or bilaterally in very low dosages (1 to 3 U). While the typical site of injection for SD is on the vocalis section of the TA, there is strong research (Inagi et al., 1996) that found the best postinjection voice and the voice that lasted the longest was the result of unilateral injection toward the posterior end of the TA with some absorption occurring in the lateral cricoarytenoid (LCA). These authors concluded that Botox appears to have the best effect with a single "unilateral injection placed strategically at the posterior portion of the TA and directed toward the LCA so that both muscle groups are affected" (p. 306). Other Botox teams continue to use bilateral injections with slightly lower Botox dosages injected into each TA. The amount of Botox required and the site(s) of injection vary according to the experience of the individual team members and the patient's response to the drug. Holden, Vokes, Taylor, Till, and Crumley (2007) reported that a dose of 1.5 units per side appears to improve dose stability with no tachyphylaxis (rapidly decreasing response to a drug following administration of the initial dose) or increasing sensitivity to Botox over time. These researchers arrived at these conclusions in a retrospective study from 1991 to 2005 that included 13 patients who had received at least six Botox injections.

It is commonly observed in patients who have received Botox injection in the TA that they experience for a short time (two to three weeks) some mild symptoms of aspiration, coughing, and breathiness. Instead of tight phonation with low airflow rates and high subglottal pressures, the SD patient now displays temporarily the symptoms of a patient with unilateral vocal fold paralysis, that is, high flow rate, low pressure, and a breathy voice. The patient at this time requires counsel from the SLP that the aspiration and breathiness are temporary. About three weeks after injection, the patient should return to the SLP for voice therapy. Murry and Woodson (1995) found in 27 patients that those who received both injection plus voice therapy had significantly better flow rates and acoustic improvement than patients who received only Botox without follow-up voice therapy. Typically, those patients who received both Botox and follow-up voice therapy will maintain good, functional voice from four to six months. As the patient experiences increasing adductory tightness while phonating, reinjection of Botox will be required.

Murry and Woodson (1995) usually begin with "five voice-therapy sessions planned for each patient" (p. 462). Some patients may require less therapy and some may need more. Beginning therapy is designed to reduce continued vocal hyperfunction. The typical SD patient has used for many years hyperfunctional behaviors in an attempt to push voice out. Even though such excessive effort is no longer needed after injection, the patient's habit set of vocal hyperfunction continues. Counseling, showing the patient differential airflow rates, and listening to pre- and postinjection recordings can be used to help the patient cognitively recognize that effort for voicing is no longer required. A useful task is to model in front of a mirror or on videotape the saying of "ah" with no discernible effort, no visible neck muscle activity, resulting in a slightly easy, breathy voice. Stay with this task until the patient can demonstrate taking the work out of voicing. Therapy then follows with learning to find the optimal breath for saying a series of syllables on one expiration, perhaps reducing voice production in the beginning to saying only six to eight syllables per breath. If the patient is observed to squeeze out the last syllable or two, the syllable target per breath should be reduced further. Practice should be given to developing the number of syllables that can be comfortably voiced on one expiration. When breath volume gets low, the patient should pause; during the pause breath will renew without the patient doing anything consciously but pausing (Boone, 1997).

We have established a voice therapy practice plan that monitors the patient's vocal behaviors post-Botox injection. This program is individualized for each patient and normally begins with several follow-up telephone calls. We ask the patient whether the postinjection aspiration has resolved; we can hear any latent vocal hyperfunction, which would necessitate a follow-up visit to the clinic. Several weeks after injection, we listen for spasmodic vocal behaviors, which would also necessitate a return to the clinic. If we detect the return of the dystonia, we ask the patient to return for acoustic and airflow assessment and possible reinjection.

Essential Tremor

Organic or essential voice tremor is often viewed as a disorder separate from the other dysarthrias, yet it can be classified as a hyperkinetic dysarthria of tremor (Duffy, 2005). Essential tremor is the most common of the movement disorders and is considered a benign autosomal dominant condition with variable penetrance (Jankovic, 1986). The tremor may appear present in tongue, velar, pharyngeal, and laryngeal structures, producing a vocal tremor in the 4 to 7 per second range. Other patients with voice tremor may show similar tremorous movements in the hands, arms, neck, and face. Familial tremor is a common form of essential tremor (approximately 50% of all cases) often beginning in early adulthood. The patient shows exaggerated tremorous behavior, more than the normal tremor that may be observed in people who are overworking particular muscles, such as may be felt or seen while carrying a heavy weight, "like carrying a case of twenty-four quarts of milk." Another form of essential tremor appears to be related to aging (Benito-Leon, Bermejo-Pareja, and Louis, 2005).

Vocal tremor may also be heard in other neurogenic voice disorders, such as in spasmodic dysphonia and in Parkinson's disease. Such tremors must be differentiated from a diagnosis of essential tremor, which is basically intention tremor that appears to exist independently of other neurogenic conditions. The diagnosis of essential tremor is best made by eliminating contextual speech, asking the patient to sustain the production of vowels in isolation. The longer duration of the vowel, the more severe the tremor. On prolonged vowel production, the tremor is well isolated, permitting a frequency count and an acoustic evaluation of the tremorous voice. Endoscopic examination of the vocal folds while prolonging the vowel will show a structurally normal larynx with the vocal folds producing the alternate tension changes that are part of the overall tremor production. Flexible endoscopy can also reveal velar, pharyngeal, and tongue movements in absolute tremorous synchrony with one another, all contributing to the acoustic observation of voice tremor.

There is little in the literature to suggest adequate management of essential tremor, either medically or by voice therapy. The speech–language pathologist who first encounters an essential tremor patient, either of the familial or aging type, should make a referral to a consulting neurologist who might offer some medication control, reducing the severity (amplitude) of the tremor (but not its frequency). Professional meeting papers and anecdotal reports by voice clinicians offer three therapy approaches that seem to minimize voice symptoms: (1) reducing voice intensity levels appears to minimize tremor identification; (2) elevating voice pitch a half note seems to change the tension level of the vocal folds sufficiently to reduce severity of the tremor; and (3) attempting to shorten vowel duration while speaking minimizes the identification of voice tremor (we are less likely to hear it).

When clients understand the nature of voiced versus nonvoiced phonemes, they discover that by abbreviating the vowels and overarticulating the nonvoiced phonemes the tremor is less noticeable. In addition, we encourage the client to produce an "easy" /h/ at the beginnings of vowel initial words, such as /h/apples, to reduce the amplitude of tremor. This technique worked well for a young client who worked as a telephone receptionist at Andressen Towing. Prior to intervention, when announcing her company's name on the telephone, she produced the initial /a/ with extended vowel duration, which only served to announce the tremor. With intervention, she softened and abbreviated the /a/ by making the voice breathy, devoiced the /d/, and anticipated the production of the nonvoiced /ss/. Using these strategies, the perceptual features of the tremor were not eliminated but certainly attenuated.

Differences among Spasmodic Dysphonia, Essential Tremor, and Vocal Hyperfunction

Spasmodic dysphonia can easily be misinterpreted as an essential tremor or vocal hyperfunction. This comes as no surprise as the three conditions may present very similarly (Barkmeier, Case, and Ludlow, 2001). In Table 4.1 we have attempted to identify some of the differences of the disorders, although it should be noted that the disorders may, and do, overlap. For example, a patient with severe ADSD may attempt to control the capricious vocal fold movements by squeezing down on the supraglottal structures. SD is only differentially identified when the individual undergoes trial voice therapy that eliminates the hyperfunctional posturing.

TABLE **4.1**	Differences among Essential Tremor, Vocal Hyperfunction, and Spasmodic Dysphonia				
Disorder	**Age of Onset**	**Gender**	**Suspected Etiology**	**Presentation**	**Intervention**
Essential tremor	Any age	Predominantly females	CNS neurogenic	Regular rhythmic vocal arrest; may involve supraglottal structures	Behavioral; Botox not recommended due to numerous supraglottal structures involved
Vocal hyperfunction	Any age	Predominantly male children and adolescent and adult females	Functional	Various: anteroposterior and medial squeezing of supraglottal structures	Behavioral
Adductor SD	Two-thirds of onset between 40 and 60	Predominantly adult females	CNS neurogenic	Irregular vocal arrests involving TA muscle	Botox injection, surgery, behavioral

Huntington's Disease

Up to this point, we have described hyperkinetic dysarthrias whose symptomologies are progressive in severity, yet not life threatening. Huntington's disease (HD), in contrast, is an inherited autosomal dominant degenerative, neurological disease in which the first symptoms begin to emerge in middle age (40 to 50 years). Each child of an affected parent has an even 50% chance of inheriting the disease, with the onset of symptoms delayed until middle age. The disease is an extrapyramidal disorder of the basal ganglia, characterized by an overabundance of dopamine. This results in the onset of the disease beginning with occasional jerks or spasms in either the extremities or more centrally in speech and voice, progressing rapidly into chorea, athetosis, and mental deterioration. The typical voice symptoms include strained or strangled voice quality, monopitch, excessive loudness variations, equal stress on ordinarily unstressed words, with sudden forced changes in breath control (Yorkston et al., 2004). Among the most prominent symptoms are the jerky, irregular bursts of loud voice (Colton, Casper, and Leonard, 2005) and obvious interruptions of prosody. See Zraick, Davenport, and colleagues (2004) for a report on the nature of speech deficits in HD.

In the early stages of HD, the SLP can guide the patient into maintaining better speech and voice, permitting good, functional communication. Voice seems to remain more normal when the patient works on easy, forward prosody, maintaining a rate near 150 syllables per minute. Both the DAF and metronomic pacer of the Facilitator can help the patient develop and maintain a slower controlled speaking rate, which seems to smooth out some of the unacceptable jerkiness. The yawn–sigh has been found to be a useful technique for opening up the vocal tract and developing ease of voice production. Similar to the patient with Parkinson's disease (another disease of the extrapyramidal tract), speaking with greater intention often enhances the patient's speech and voice behavior (Boone and Plante, 1993).

As HD progresses, with death occurring 15 to 20 years after onset (Yorkston et al., 2004), the patient usually begins experiencing some cognitive decline. At about this time, attempts at modification of speech and voice are no longer successful. Extreme choreic interruptions of airflow and flailing athetoid movements make speech intelligibility impossible. Because of both cognitive decline and severe motor control limitations, "there are no reports in the literature of successful application of augmentative communication technology in Huntington's disease" (Yorkston et al., 2004, p. 158). Therefore, improving speech, voice, and functional communication in the HD patient is usually possible only in the first few years after onset of the disease.

The hyperkinetic movements that interrupt respiration, voice, and articulation in Huntington's disease are the same that underlie the severe dysphagia that patients experience in the moderate and severe stages of the disease process. Yorkston and colleagues (2004) identify notable swallowing disruptions, such as tachyphagia, respiratory chorea, and eructation, and recommend positioning, dietary, and assistive feeding strategies to maximize oral intake success and safety (p. 167).

ATAXIC DYSARTHRIA

Ataxic dysarthria is a CNS disturbance caused by damage to the cerebellum or the cerebellar control circuit, with resultant respiratory, phonatory, and articulatory dyscoordination that may make the patient sound inebriated. Common etiologies for ataxic dysarthria are degenerative disease (see MS later in this chapter), vascular disorders, tumors, and trauma.

In some patients, phonation is hoarse with a mildly tremorous overlay and respiratory function is interrupted by dyscoordinated inhalatory and exhalatory exchanges. Intervention for patients presenting with voice disturbances as a function of ataxia addresses those subsystems of speech that are most compromised. Intervention is similar to that described in the section for multiple sclerosis, which often presents with ataxic or ataxic–spastic symptoms. For patients presenting with reduced respiratory–phonatory coordination, we introduce Linebaugh's (1983) concept of optimal breath groups, that is, the number of syllables that a patient can produce comfortably on one breath. The patient is encouraged to experiment with breath support and keep utterances within the optimal breath group. One companion technique that has been particularly successful in clinic is to have the patient produce the word "boom" at the end of each breath group. This ensures that the patient has sufficient expiratory support for the entire phrase ("Take me to your summer home: *boom*"). Eventually, the "*boom*" is phased out. To regulate vocal amplitude and pitch, we introduce pacing, both tactile (Chapey, 2001) and auditory (KayPENTAX Facilitator), along with visual and auditory biofeedback on the Visi-Pitch or auditory only, using a digital or analog tape recorder.

MIXED DYSARTHRIA

This condition is a mixture of dysarthrias characterized by two or more of the aforementioned primary types. Mixed dysarthria is caused by multiple lesion sites within the nervous system, which may involve both the central and peripheral nervous systems.

Amyotrophic Lateral Sclerosis (ALS)

ALS is a progressive degenerative disease of unknown etiology involving the motor neurons of the cortex and the gray bodies within the brain stem and spinal cord. Involving both upper and lower motor neurons, the disease is often called *motor neuron disease*. It is also known as Lou Gehrig's disease. The speech–language pathologist often sees these patients initially relative to their early complaints of difficulty in articulating rapid speech, experiencing occasional hoarseness, and complaining of occasional swallowing problems. On peripheral oral examination, on extension of the tongue, fasciculations (wavelike muscle tremors) on the surface of the tongue may be observed. The diagnosis of ALS often requires nerve conduction velocity studies and perhaps a muscle biopsy to identify lack of or reduced innervation to particular muscle groups. The diagnosis is often related to exclusion of other identifiable etiologies. As ALS progresses, the patient often experiences proximal atrophy of extremities rather than distal (for example, shoulder atrophy before hand involvement or back tongue impairment more than anterior involvement). The ALS patient may develop voice harshness, hypernasality, back-pharyngeal resonance focus, breathiness, and monopitch. In addition to these voice symptoms, these patients report articulatory deterioration and increasing dysphagia.

Of life-threatening concern is the patient's growing inability to clear the throat and to cough. Because most ALS patients are experiencing continuing bulbar involvement, more clinical focus needs to be given to swallowing and coughing, rather than to speech and voice per se. Yorkston and colleagues (2004) present the speech scale from their amyotrophic lateral sclerosis severity scale, which rates the patient's speech–voice function.

In the early stages of the disease, we attempt to address respiratory, phonatory, and resonance support for speech, which may involve building a palatal lift for patients who present with weak or spastic velar function. A palatal lift consists of a palatal portion that is attached to the teeth and a lift portion that extends posteriorly to lift the palate in the direction of velopharyngeal closure. Fitting the lift requires adequate dentition to retain the device; however, lifts have been successfully built into upper denture plates. Working with the prosthodontist, we view the velopharyngeal port at rest and during speech activities using flexible endoscopy. We identify the points of air escape and fashion the lift so that velopharyngeal closure is adequate for voice, speech, and swallow, while still allowing for nasal breathing. A palatal lift is shown in Figure 9.6. It should be noted that palatal lifts are difficult to fit for patients with hyperactive gag reflexes that are unresponsive to desensitization; however, on occasion we have successfully reshaped a lift to accommodate sensitive patients. Lifts are also not appropriate for patients who are not cooperative and patients who respond to the presence of the lift with increased mucus production. This latter factor is a troublesome variable, especially in the area of dysphagia.

Whether a palatal lift is indicated, some voice improvements may occur by helping the patient to renew breath more often and to develop a high front voice focus, with some attention given to increasing speaking rate (we have found metronome pacing to be helpful).

As the disease progresses, the SLP must help the patient work on diet modification and swallowing (trying different head positions with good mouth closure). These patients normally have good cognitive function and follow suggestions well if the suggestions are within their motor ability to execute. As the Yorkston scale suggests, eventually the patient may require some kind of augmentative communication aid.

Before a communication aid is selected, the SLP must determine the patient's literacy and cognitive level, specifically when selecting icon- versus text-based systems, communication needs, and hand function and mobility. A number of text-to-speech devices are available that offer scanning options as the disease progresses (DynaWrite and the LightWRITER by DynaVox).

Multiple Sclerosis (MS)

Among various demyelinating diseases, multiple sclerosis is the most common. The three most popular theories of causation include an autoimmune basis, viral, and a genetic predisposition (Boyden, 2000). This progressive disease attacks the myelin sheath covering of nerves; and, it is believed, the nerves themselves, literally causing breaks in transmitting axons, within the white matter of the CNS. The symptoms of the disease depend on the site of involvement. The patient may experience either sensory deficits (tingling, numbness, visual changes) or motor deficits (weakness, spasms, lack of coordination); more commonly both sensory and motor systems are involved. Citing the early work of Darley, Aronson, and Brown (1975), nearly 60% of 168 patients studied were judged to be normal in speech adequacy (Yorkston et al., 2004).

The increasing presence of dysarthria with problems of voice in MS is generally related to multiple neural system involvement associated with cerebral, brain stem, and cerebellar factors. The voice problems experienced by MS patients were earlier described (Darley, Aronson, and Brown, 1975) and listed here from most common to least common: impaired loudness control, harsh voice quality, sameness of prosody and voice pitch control, decreased breath control, and hypernasality. If the MS patient is experiencing some or all of these symptoms, direct voice therapy can often minimize symptom effects, improving the patient's communicative effectiveness. Considering the progressive nature of the disease, communication between caregiver and patient is increasingly necessary over time.

Changing the patient's speaking rate (slightly slower or faster) will often have positive effects on loudness and harshness. The patient learns to pace speech or uses the metronome pacing program developed for use with the Facilitator. Improving rate control is also consistent with developing better coordinated breath support. MS patients may profit from reducing the number of words they say on one expiratory breath. Baseline measures of expiratory breath control can serve as a starting place. The SLP then instructs the patient to cut in half the number of words he or she has been saying. This reduces vocal fold tension, the tendency to squeeze out the last words of an utterance. Developing good vertical postural habits with the patient, keeping the chin down, and minimizing mouth opening (while at rest) all seem to afford the MS patient a neutral postural set before initiating speech–voice responses. This postural control and attempt to pace an even spoken response seems to inhibit the sudden jerkiness and loud voice excesses that interfere with effective communication.

In the advanced stages of the disease, natural speech–voice may not be possible. Setting up alternative means of communication, also, may have many obstacles, as the patient's hand control for using keyboards, pointing, or pressing switches may be seriously compromised by ataxia, spasticity, and excessive tremor. Also, in advanced stages of multiple sclerosis, the patient may have severe visual problems and even blindness. Many of these obstacles can be successfully identified and addressed by performing a comprehensive augmentative and alternative communication assessment, as described by Beukelman and Mirenda (2005, p. 448).

Traumatic Brain Injury

Traumatic brain injuries are caused by external forces acting on the head. Most TBIs are caused by motor vehicle accidents, falls, assaults, and, more recently, explosion injuries experienced by service members. These injuries can cause focal or diffuse lesions, axonal shearing, and hypoxia, secondary to vascular or tissue damage.

Dysarthria associated with TBI may be temporary or chronic, mild or severe, and accompanied or not by other language and cognitive disorders. Most dysarthrias are of the mixed type, and variability in the nature and severity of the physiological impairment calls for custom treatment programs based on a clear appreciation for the subsystems of respiration, phonation, resonance, articulation, and prosody. Studies of speech breathing, for example, reveal that individuals with TBI have lower vital capacities than nondisabled speakers (Murdoch et al., 1994). Kinematics of the same group revealed that the speakers with TBI had problems coordinating the actions of the rib cage and abdomen during speech. This incoordination is apparent in patients with TBI, many of whom take replenishing breaths at inappropriate phrase junctures during conversational speaking and oral reading tasks.

Victor was a 21-year-old male who experienced a TBI with bilateral basilar skull fractures, left-sided cerebral edema, and subarachnoid and subdural hemorrhages. He came to our clinic after spending 30 days in the intensive care unit on ventilatory support and one year in full-time rehabilitation. Victor presented with a mixed spastic–ataxic dysarthria; speech was characterized as slow at 82 words per minute, with reduced articulatory accuracy, reduced respiratory–phonatory coordination, and strained and strangled phonation, notably on the vowels. Voice ground to a glottal fry at the ends of phrases.

The first step in the voice and speech rehabilitation program was to familiarize Victor with the anatomical and physiological bases for voice and speech production. He learned that he indeed had sufficient breath support for speech; however, respiratory–phonatory coordination needed some adjustments. He also learned that he could produce more words at a more rapid rate when he increased pitch and abbreviated vowel duration times. Improved voice, speech, and prosody were targeted through a variety of tasks. Using the Visi-Pitch for audio and visual feedback, Victor generated novel sentences ranging from five to eight words. He viewed the pitch traces on the screen and immediately heard his productions using the digitized feedback option. The productions were judged using a $\pm$ rating scale for articulation, breath support, vocal quality, and overall presentation of the sentence. If Victor was dissatisfied with a production, he was reminded to modify breath support, increase pitch, and reduce vowel durations. At the end of the semester, respiratory–phonatory coordination for conversational speech had increased from 57% accuracy to 85% accuracy, speaking pitch increased from 94 Hz to an average 110 Hz, words per minute had increased from 82 to 89, and intelligibility had increased from 74% to 80%, as measured by listener transcripts. He began speaking over the telephone again and soon found employment at a youth league.

Summary

At the beginning of the chapter we looked at the neurological bases of human laryngeal function. We then reviewed abnormal neurological functions in the motor speech system and subdivided those abnormalities by site of lesion, with particular emphasis on laryngeal neurological dysfunction. We reviewed vocal pathologies associated with lower motor neuron dysfunction, notably vocal fold paralysis.

We then discussed the upper motor neurons system and explored numerous pathologies that serve to interrupt normal laryngeal function—primarily, spastic, hyperkinetic, hypokinetic, and mixed dysarthrias. We reviewed the latest research in behavioral, pharmacological, and surgical management of neurogenic voice disorders and explored voice programs from the perspective of the SLP.

Thought Questions

1. Describe vocal characteristics of a unilateral vocal fold paralysis. Describe the physiological underpinnings of the characteristics.
2. Describe similarities and differences among muscle tension dysphonia, essential tremor, and adductor spasmodic dysphonia.
3. Describe the vocal and resonance characteristics that may be observed in an individual with TBI.
4. Describe the vocal characteristics of hypokinetic dysarthria and some evidence-based intervention approaches.

5

Functional Voice Disorders

LEARNING OBJECTIVES

- Define the term "functional voice disorder"
- Differentiate primary from secondary muscle tension dysphonia
- List the changes that can occur in the larynx as a result of functional dysphonia
- Explain the causes of diplophonia
- Explain the causes of pitch and phonation breaks

In Chapters 3 and 4, we have considered voice disorders related to organic changes and/or neurological impairment of structures and function of the vocal tract. A large number of voice disorders have no organic or neurogenic causative origin and appear to be wholly functional in origin. Although the mechanisms of respiration, phonation, and resonance appear physically capable of normal voicing function, they lack the proper functional balance, resulting in a voice disorder. Although no organic or physical cause of the voice disorder is identified, the resulting physiologic imbalance may produce a voicing problem, classified as a functional voice disorder. Some continued functional behaviors, such as excessive yelling in children or continued throat clearing, may eventually cause laryngeal tissue changes (Lee and Son, 2005), such as nodules or polyps.

In order to promote the study of therapy outcome, we find that under the "functional voice disorder" label, there appear to be two different causes: psychogenic or excessive muscle tension. To evaluate the effectiveness of a particular voice therapy technique, such as changing voice loudness, the same technique could produce different outcomes, depending on which of the two functional disorder causes exist. For example, encouraging a louder or softer voice in the patient with psychogenic voice disorder might result in the rejection of the technique because the change of loudness might be in direct conflict with the patient's emotional needs. For the patient with a muscle tension dysphonia, speaking softer may be an excellent technique for reducing excessive muscular tension. Or conversely, using a louder voice might be an inappropriate therapy technique for a young schoolboy who is already observed to be the loudest talker in his classroom.

The cause of the functional voice disorder will dictate the kinds of therapy techniques required to reach a favorable therapy outcome. Accordingly, we will consider psychogenic voice disorders (PVD) separately from the typical voice disorder related to excessive muscle function, known as muscle tension dysphonia (MTD).

PSYCHOGENIC VOICE DISORDERS

In the classic definition of psychogenic voice disorders, the voice problem is typically resistant to change from various symptomatic voice therapy approaches. The patient's psychological trauma or conflicts may be strong enough to preserve the vocal symptoms. In some cases, psychological counseling or therapy may have to play a primary role in the total voice rehabilitation process. However, psychological factors sometimes are reactive to the emergence of a voice problem and are not the cause of the disorder; for these cases, voice therapy can play a primary and successful role.

The SLP working with patients with any of the four psychogenic voice disorders (falsetto, functional aphonia, functional dysphonia, and somatization, or Briquet's dysphonia) should be aware of possible psychological or psychiatric factors that may contribute to the disorder. The SLP trained in counseling or clinical psychology may well combine needed psychological support with voice therapy for these psychogenic patients. Or appropriate psychological or psychiatric referral may be indicated. The first three disorders listed may well have psychogenic causation. Somatization dysphonia is primarily a psychiatric conversion problem and requires close psychiatric management.

Falsetto

Other names for falsetto are puberphonia, juvenile voice, mutational falsetto, and incomplete voice mutation. From a singing point of view, some men and women can extend the singing voice well beyond the chest register, producing the falsetto or loft register. Some classical singing includes the counter-tenor voice where the singing voice extends well above middle-C (260 Hz). The high lyric soprano sings several octaves higher. Our concern with the falsetto voice is not in singing but in the speaking voice. Puberphonia or the mutational falsetto is the high-register voice produced primarily by the adolescent or adult male who has completed the physical maturational changes from prepubertal to postpubertal male. Falsetto may also occur in females; Verdolini, Rosen, and Branski (2006) cite a form of puberphonia ("juvenile resonance disorder") in postpubescent females.

Some young men with falsetto voices have found the transition from boy to manhood to be difficult. The rapid physical changes they have experienced may have been complicated by increased adultlike feelings and responsibilities. As an overall coping mechanism, these young men may continue to use their prepubescent voices. For this occasional puberphonic patient, some psychological counseling or therapy would be a required part of overall voice management. Most young men with puberphonia, however, uncover a normal speaking voice with only minimal voice therapy. These young men with mutational falsetto (we deliberately use the words *falsetto, puberphonia,* and *mutational falsetto* interchangeably as synonyms) are very accepting of voice therapy that helps them find and establish an appropriate lower voice pitch, and the vast majority achieve normal pitch levels and vocal quality after only brief exposure to voice therapy.

Voice therapy for puberphonia first requires a thorough review of the medical chart and perhaps medical evaluation confirming that the client has reached postpuberty status. When asked to cough, the cough usually sounds like that of an adult (both male and female patients will present a much lower pitch level than children when asked to cough). The SLP generally begins therapy for the puberphonic falsetto patient by demonstrating a cough and then extending phonation beyond the cough for a few seconds. Following the SLP cough demonstration, the patient is asked to do the same thing, cough and then extend the phonation after the cough on the same outgoing breath. In most cases, it is best to record the patient's cough response and then provide the patient with an auditory feedback model. The SLP then explains that the vocal folds are able to produce the lower phonation, and a brief word list can then be presented with each word said on the extended phonation following the cough.

If the cough is not successful in uncovering the patient's natural pitch, light digital pressure against the thyroid cartilage often "uncovers" the lower pitch. The patient is asked to say and prolong an "ah" for more than five or six seconds. During this extended phonation, the SLP applies light finger pressure on the patient's anterior thyroid cartilage, usually producing an immediate lowering of voice pitch. After several finger pressure productions, the patient is then asked to see if he or she can match the lower voice pitch. The therapy session should be recorded for immediate playback and discussion. Other therapy techniques presented in Chapter 7, masking and using glottal fry, have been found useful in eliminating the falsetto speaking voice.

Positive commentary about the appropriateness of using the newly found lower pitch should be supplemented with some counseling (Aronson, 1990). The majority of puberphonic patients present an excellent therapy outcome in one or two clinical sessions and seemingly rejoice in finding a voice that sounds like their peers. There are only a few anecdotal reports of occasional puberphonic patients requiring counseling or psychotherapy before releasing the need for continuing the falsetto voice. Following successful elimination of the high-pitched voice, the SLP should schedule all puberphonic patients for a three- or four-week follow-up to determine how he or she is doing, both from a voice and an emotional perspective.

Functional Aphonia

The unique aspect of functional aphonia is that the patient speaks in a whisper but continues speaking with the same rhythm and prosody of normal speech. Only voice is lacking. In order to rule out some form of organic involvement of the vocal folds, such as vocal fold paralysis as described in Chapter 4, these patients need a videoendoscopic examination to visualize vocal fold movement. When the aphonic patient is asked to say "ah," the normal vocal folds remain too far apart to permit phonation and often develop the open position used for a whisper production (Case, 2002). The visual examination will usually confirm normal function for both the cough and throat clearing. When swallowing, the aphonic patient exhibits both normal laryngeal elevation and vocal fold closure, both required to prevent aspiration into the airway below the larynx. When these patients are asked to speak, the larynx often appears to elevate excessively near the hyoid bone and is difficult to move manually in any direction.

In his classic text, *Clinical Voice Disorders,* Aronson (1990) describes a persistent functional aphonia as a possible "conversion aphonia." Aronson goes on to write that a conversion disorder is the "somatization" of an emotional disorder and can be "created by anxiety, stress, depression, or interpersonal conflict" (Aronson, 1990, p. 142). In somatization, it is believed that an unresolved psychological conflict results in a dysfunction of some bodily system (Starcevic and Lipsitt, 2001). We will consider the somatization of laryngeal function in greater detail later in this section. It appears clinically, however, that the majority of patients with aphonia do not seem to have a conversion causation, as they respond favorably to symptomatic voice therapy in one or very few therapy sessions. While normal phonation is usually restored by the SLP using only minimal exposure to voice therapy, emotional conflicts may require psychological or psychiatric therapy over a longer period of time (Gerritsma, 1991).

The onset of functional aphonia varies. Many aphonic patients say that their "voicelessness" came on gradually or only sporadically. Under tight emotional situations, they might "lose" their voices in a particular situation but recover normal voice after subsequent stress reduction. Sometimes aphonia occurs after patients have experienced some kind of laryngeal pathology or severe systemic disease; perhaps laryngeal edema during an acute infection may render voice impossible. Days or weeks later, after the initial infection that caused the voice loss is gone, the aphonia continues. Two aphonic patients who developed aphonia originally from an acute infectious disease seemed to subsequently incorporate the lack of voice into their lives (Boone, 1966b). Months after the onset of their aphonias, both patients were referred for voice therapy and made complete voice recoveries. For some patients, communication without voicing seems to help them temporarily meet their emotional needs.

A young boy, age 7, was found to have bilateral vocal nodules by his laryngologist, who told him to stop using his voice for a few weeks. The parents enforced the "voice rest" for four weeks, and the boy was never heard to use voice during that time. When the parents brought him back for a recheck, the nodules were gone but his voice was totally absent. Despite the physician's urgings and parental requests, the aphonia persisted for a month more. At a voice team conference, the child was presented as the "boy who had forgotten how to talk." He was subsequently scheduled for voice therapy and happily "found" his voice during the first therapy session. Over a four-year follow-up, he continued to have a normal prepubescent voice in all situations.

Patients with functional aphonia communicate well by gesture and whisper or by a high-pitched, shrill-sounding weak voice. Typical aphonic patients whisper with clarity and sharpness and rarely avoid communication situations; they communicate effectively by using facial expressions, hands, and highly intelligible whispered speech. What they lack in communication is voice. Embarrassed and frustrated by lack of voice, aphonic patients generally self-refer to a physician or speech–language pathologist. Despite Greene's (1980) warning that many patients with functional aphonia may require psychological counseling, most aphonic patients, in our experience, completely recover their normal voice with voice therapy alone (usually in the first session of therapy). Aphonic patients as a group, in fact, have an excellent prognosis. It is almost as if, for whatever reason, the patient has lost the set for phonation. The voice clinician's task is to help the patient find his or her voice primarily by helping the patient use nonspeech phonations, such as coughing and throat clearing, or by inhalation phonation or sometimes using masking noise (Chapter 7).

In Chapters 7 and 8, we consider in more detail some of the therapy facilitating techniques commonly used by the SLP for reestablishing voice in the functional aphonic patient. Therapy approaches include extending the cough and throat clearing, redirecting phonation achieved while singing or humming on a kazoo, and reading aloud with auditory masking. The patient's various responses to selected voicing tasks should be audiorecorded, affording immediate playback of any phonations the patient is able to produce.

FA.16

The voice therapy provided for a nine-year-old girl who had "lost" her voice following a severe influenza provides a good example of successful therapy for functional aphonia. For six weeks following a severe flulike infection, she communicated entirely by whisper with good facial animation and normal interactive communication with her listeners. In the therapy session, we had her read aloud. Using the Lombard effect (Newby, 1972), which is used to detect a hearing loss of the malingering type, the patient is asked to read aloud in a whisper and continue reading aloud as about 75 dB of speech-range masking is introduced. Like the patient who is falsifying hearing loss, the patient's oral reading immediately is influenced with the onset of the masking. As this girl read aloud in her whisper, masking was introduced, and she then started reading in a light voice. This voice was recorded and played back as the SLP commented, "Now your vocal folds seem to be coming together well." The girl was overjoyed with the discovery of her lost voice. Once voice is established, the SLP moves slowly to increase loudness as a drill activity and then works gently to produce voice interactively.

After voice is reestablished, the aphonic patient should be offered some psychological support with strong SLP assurance that the voice is "back for good." It usually is.

Functional Dysphonia

Some of the most abnormal or disturbed voices we hear have no organic or structural causes. The voice patient may be using the normal respiration system in an incorrect balance between initiating the airstream with the beginning of phonation, such as beginning voice after much expiratory air has been expelled. The patient may take in too small a breath or too large a breath for producing a normal voice. Or the patient with functional dysphonia may bring the vocal folds together in a lax manner, producing breathiness, or in a tight manner producing symptoms of harshness or tightness. Or patients may be speaking at inappropriate pitch levels, with voices too low or too high for their age and sex. Excesses of mouth opening, head position, or jaw positioning may alter the quality of the voice. Or the sound of the voice can be altered by tongue positioning within the mouth, either excessively back or too far forward. Excessive nasality can be added to voice production by a slight alteration in velopharyngeal closure. In using the label "functional dysphonia," we are suggesting that these components for producing voice are in a physiologic imbalance produced in part by the psychological needs of the patient.

The diagnosis of functional dysphonia implies that the voice problem has no physical or organic cause. This means in our evaluation and testing that normal structure and capability for normal function should be demonstrated. One approach is to include a number of diagnostic probes (see Chapters 6 and 7) to determine if the patient can imitate SLP modeling of pitch, loudness, or quality change, demonstrating capability for producing some normal voice behaviors. If the patient can demonstrate a normal voicing function, this is often a good place for the SLP to begin voice therapy intervention.

The patient often reports other problems associated with functional dysphonia, such as weight loss, difficulty swallowing, throat and neck pain, excessive coughing, or other somatic abnormalities. The SLP may uncover psychological complaints of worry, avoiding responsibility, shyness, excessive fears, and so on. Aronson (1990) states:

> A psychogenic voice disorder is broadly synonymous with a functional one but has the advantage of stating positively, based on exploration of its causes, that the voice disorder is a manifestation of one or more types of psychologic disequilibrium—such as anxiety, depression, conversion, or personality disorder—which interferes with normal volitional control over phonation. (p. 131)

Even though the patient may be capable of producing normal voice when requested to do so in the voice evaluation, the SLP must consider the relative weight of emotional factors possibly preventing the use of a normal voice in everyday living.

In functional dysphonia, there is often a mixture of emotional problems and faulty voice usage. The patient may exhibit vocal hypofunction, a weak, soft voice, or vocal hyperfunction, a loud, harsh voice. While the patient may demonstrate some emotional issues deserving of counseling or therapy, he or she may also have the capability of using a normal voice after voice therapy intervention. In Chapter 7, we will consider a few therapy approaches that are particularly effective with this functional dysphonia group of patients, such as counseling, hierarchy analysis, relaxation, respiration training, and vocal hygiene. Stemple's vocal function exercises were designed to strengthen and "balance the laryngeal musculature" and have been found to have a positive "holistic" effect for general voice improvement (Stemple, 2005). Faulty voice physiology may not necessarily have a strong emotional component.

Emotionality may play a minimal role in some children and adults with faulty voices who live with their voicing difference (mild hoarseness, inappropriate voice pitch, etc.) and do not think of this difference as being a "voice disorder." Listeners perceive their voices as different and perhaps unique but not as "disordered."

In their classic look at efficacy of voice therapy, Ramig and Verdolini (1998) describe most voice disorders as caused by "habits of vocal misuse and hyperfunction," medical/physical conditions, and/or psychological factors. We include voice misuse and vocal hyperfunction in the MTD section of this chapter as representing most of what the SLP sees in patients with functional voice problems. Many published studies that have considered the outcome of voice therapy for voice disorders have targeted the "misuse–hyperfunctional" type of disorders. The range of voice therapy methods for vocal hyperfunction include the accent method (Kotby, El-Sedy, Baslany, Abou-Rass, and Hegazi, 1991), resonant therapy (Verdolini, 2000), symptomatic therapy (Boone, McFarlane, and Von Berg, 2005), manual circumlaryngeal therapy (Roy, Gray, Simon, Dove, Corbin-Lewis, and Stemple, 2001), and physiologic therapy (Colton and Casper, 1996; Stemple, 2005). Vocal hyperfunctional behaviors over time often lead to tissue changes within the larynx, creating glottal margin disorders such as vocal fold thickening, nodules, and polyps (as we will see in our discussion of muscle tension dysphonia).

When functional dysphonia is classified as a psychogenic voice disorder, priority is given both to the emotional support of the patient and the concomitant voice differences. Sometimes the voice client does not have a voice disorder but only a voice difference, such as poor breathing influencing a soft voice or using a pitch level that is not appropriate. While vocal differences can be treated by the SLP using voice therapy techniques, there are other disciplinary approaches (NATS, 2008; VASTA, 2008) that can be helpful in learning to optimize vocal function. The client with a "different" voice might on occasion be better served by a member of the National Association of Teachers of Singing (NATS) or the Voice and Speech Trainers Association (VASTA) rather than by an SLP. NATS members have long recognized the connection between emotions and the optimal production of both speech and singing. Similarly, members of VASTA have developed voice improvement methods that help the actor and speaker minimize speech differences that might negate performance. In the treatment of psychogenic dysphonias, there needs to be greater future interaction between the psychologist or psychiatrist, the SLP, and the teachers/coaches of the singing and speaking voice.

Somatization Dysphonia (Briquet's Dysphonia)

In reviewing the clinical files of hospital and university voice clinics, we find rare clinical occurrences of voice patients who may be classified as having somatization dysphonia or showing symptoms of Briquet's dysphonia. In somatization dysphonia, the voice patient shows beyond dysphonia an array of possible conversion symptoms, such as laryngeal pain, neck and shoulder pain with stiffness, shortness of breath, depression, and extreme vocal fatigue (Verdolini, Rosen, and Branski, 2006). Historically, these patients might have carried the diagnosis of Briquet's syndrome but in recent years would fit under the diagnostic label of somatoform or somatization disorders (APA, 1987). The SLP may be overwhelmed by the severity of patient symptoms, soon realizing that the presenting dysphonia is but a small part of the patient's overall problem. Such a patient should be referred for an extensive medical workup and psychiatric evaluation–treatment.

The voice evaluation of such patients may typically reveal an elevated voice pitch and increased hoarseness with a reduced signal-to-noise ratio. Vegetative laryngeal functions (coughing, prevention of aspiration, etc.) may remain normal. The voice symptoms often begin in late adolescence extending into young adulthood, and from the beginning are surrounded by many other symptoms, the severity of which may present greater problems to the patient than the presenting dysphonia. The prevalence of somatization dysphonia is much greater in women than men by a ratio estimated to be as high as 10 to 1 (Verdolini, Rosen, and Branski, 2006). Critical to the diagnosis is the absence of any physical evidence that can support the cause of the dysphonia and the other related symptoms. Somatization dysphonia is a true conversion disorder, and management appears possible only with successful identification and reduction of emotional and psychological factors.

EXCESSIVE MUSCLE TENSION DISORDERS

Muscle Tension Dysphonia

Muscle tension dysphonia is a persistent dysphonia resulting from excessive laryngeal musculoskeletal tension and associated hyperfunctional true and/or false vocal fold vibratory patterns (Dworkin, Meleca, and Abkarian, 2000). Morrison and colleagues first described muscle tension dysphonia as the occurrence of vocal dysfunction in the absence of laryngeal structural abnormalities (Morrison, Rammage, Belisle, Pullan, and Nichol, 1983). MTD can also be categorized as primary or secondary based on whether organic pathologic conditions contribute to trigger the dysphonia behavior (Rosen and Murry, 2000a). Primary muscle tension dysphonia occurs *in the absence* of current organic pathology, without obvious psychogenic or neurologic etiology. Secondary muscle tension dysphonia occurs *in the presence* of current organic pathology or psychogenic or neurologic etiology. Secondary MTD is believed to originate as a compensatory response to the primary etiology. Muscle tension dysphonia can be seen in both adults and children (Lee and Son, 2005).

A number of laryngeal and supralaryngeal configurations can be observed in muscle tension dysphonia. These include anterior–posterior compression, medial compression and a sphincterlike combination of these two (Koufman and Blalock, 1991). Excessive vocal fold tension resulting in an underapproximation of the vocal folds may also be observed (Hillman and Verdolini, 1999). In some patients medial compression may be a normal configuration, however, and must be interpreted in light of other laryngoscopic findings (Behrman, Dahl, Abramson, and Schutte, 2003).

Numerous factors may contribute to the development of muscle tension dysphonia, including deviant body posture and misuse of neck and shoulder muscles, high stress levels, excessive voice use, persistently loud voice use, and laryngopharyngeal reflux disease (Altman, Atkinson, and Lazarus, 2005). Patients frequently demonstrate significant emotional stress and they may also suffer from depression (Dietrich, Verdolini-Abbott, Gartner-Schmidt, and Rosen, 2008; Seifert and Kollbrunner, 2005). Understandably, voice-related quality of life is diminished in persons with muscle tension dysphonia (Kooijman, de Jong, Oudes, Huinck, van Acht, and Graamans, 2005).

For the inexperienced and experienced voice clinician alike, muscle tension dysphonia can sometimes be difficult to differentiate from other forms of dysphonia. This is because some patients with adductor spasmodic dysphonia, vocal tremor, or muscle tension dysphonia present with symptoms that overlap to such a degree that a correct diagnosis is not easy. Findings from a number of recent studies examining diagnostic elements such as patient interview, visualization of the larynx, acoustic and aerodynamic evaluation, and perceptual judgments may help the clinician arrive at the correct diagnosis in a timely manner (see Barkmeier and Case, 2000, and Dworkin, Meleca, and Abkarian, 2000, for reviews). For example, comparison of laryngeal behaviors during quiet breathing, counting from 1 to 10 in usual voice compared with falsetto and whispered speech, comparison of all-voiced versus all-voiceless utterances, variation of pitch and loudness during sustained phonation versus connected speech, and singing or crying may elicit differing patterns between adductor spasmodic dysphonia and muscle tension dysphonia. The key difference between laryngeal behaviors in individuals with adductor spasmodic dysphonia and muscle tension dysphonia is the consistency of laryngeal postures across and within each of the examination tasks. Patients with muscle tension dysphonia maintain hyperadduction of the involved laryngeal structures across all tasks, whereas those with adductor spasmodic dysphonia tend to demonstrate more intermittent hyperadduction (Leonard and Kendall, 1999). In patients with adductor spasmodic dysphonia voice severity is perceived to be worse for connected speech than sustained vowels; this is not the case in patients with muscle tension dysphonia, where no difference is usually heard (Roy, Gouse, Mauszycki, Merrill, and Smith, 2005). Furthermore, in patients with MTD voice severity is generally perceived to be the same on connected speech regardless of whether the sentences are all-voiced or all-voiceless; this is not the case for patients with adductor spasmodic dysphonia (Roy, Mauszycki, Merrill, Gouse, and Smith, 2007). See the previous discussion in Chapter 4 to read more on the differences among essential tremor, muscle tension dysphonia, and adductor spasmodic dysphonia.

Reinke's Edema

Chronic diffuse swelling of the superficial lamina propria of the vocal fold is known as Reinke's edema (Thibeault, 2005), also referred to as polypoid corditis, polypoid laryngitis, or polypoid degeneration of the vocal fold. In Reinke's edema, a gelatinous material develops in Reinke's space, usually seen bilaterally. It is associated strongly with smoking, frequently with chronic vocal hyperfunction, and occasionally with laryngopharyngeal reflux (Koufman, 1991; Marcotullio, Magliulo, and Pezone, 2002). A localized area of unilateral Reinke's edema may be seen and is sometimes referred to as a pseudocyst. Frequently occurring on the middle of the free edge of the vocal fold and usually unilateral, it is associated with vocal fold paresis, not inflammation (Koufman and Belafsky, 2001).

Reinke's edema and related forms of vocal fold thickening often affect the anterior two-thirds of the glottal margin (the vibrating portion of the vocal folds) or the membrane covering the muscular portion of the vocal fold. This is in contrast to vocal nodules and polyps, which usually affect a localized area of the vocal fold. The more extensive the condition, the more likely it is that the voice will be affected.

Dysphonia resulting from Reinke's edema and related conditions is often responsive to voice therapy. A behavioral program that promotes easy and proper use of the vocal mechanism (vocal reeducation), along with reducing the source of the irritation (such as eliminating an allergy, reducing smoking, eliminating laryngopharyngeal reflux, or curbing vocal abuse) is probably the best management of the problem. Many of the voice therapy facilitating approaches presented in Chapter 7 have been effective in reducing Reinke's edema and related conditions. Surgical treatment of vocal fold thickening, without removing the cause of the problem, will not usually be a permanent solution to the dysphonia. Our strong preference is to have a serious course of voice therapy first, which will generally eliminate the need for phonosurgery (surgery to improve the voice).

If Reinke's edema is extensive and a first course of voice therapy is not effective, then medical–surgical intervention may be warranted (supplemented still by voice therapy). In a study by Dursun, Ozgursoy, Kemal, and Coruh (2007) 15 patients with Reinke's edema who underwent microlaryngoscopic surgery were reported to have experienced significant positive changes in voice quality and laryngeal status. These researchers further reported no recurrence of Reinke's edema one year following surgery, speculating that the removal of redundant mucosa of the vocal fold reduced the risk of recurrence and provided better quality of voice (p. 1027).

Vocal Fold Nodules

Vocal fold nodules are the most common benign lesions of the vocal folds in both children and adults. They are caused by continuous abuse of the larynx and misuse of the voice. Nodules are generally bilateral, whitish protuberances on the glottal margin of each vocal fold, located at the anterior–middle third junction. However, McFarlane and Watterson (1990) demonstrate in their study of 44 cases of vocal nodules that there can be considerable variation in the size, number, and location of vocal nodules in both children and adults. Of the observed and documented variations, perhaps the most striking is that nodules can range from singular to two, three, and even four (quad nodules) in number. While these variations are interesting, two important facts remain: First, nodules are responsive to voice therapy, and second, the classic description of number and location on the vocal folds (juncture of anterior and middle third) is generally accurate. Vocal nodules are typically characterized as bilateral, midmembranous vocal fold lesions of the basement membrane zone and the superficial layer of the lamina propria (McFarlane and Von Berg, 1998; Rosen and Murry, 2000a). In the early stages of development, the nodule is soft and pliable. With continuous phonotrauma, the nodule becomes more fibrotic and may become either slightly larger or more focused, smaller, and harder.

As the bilateral nodules approximate one another on phonation, there is usually an open glottal chink anterior and posterior to the nodule contact point, which results in a glottal hourglass figure. This open glottal chink (produced by the nodules coming together in exact opposition to one another) results in a lack of complete vocal fold adduction. This faulty approximation leads to breathiness in the voice and air wastage. Also, the increased mass of the nodules added to the vocal folds contributes to a lower voice pitch and increased aperiodicity (usually judged as hoarseness), leading to a breathy, flat kind of voice that often seems to lack appropriate resonance. Patients complain that they need to clear their throat continually and often that they have excessive mucus or something on the vocal folds. Excessive throat clearing often becomes an identified vocal abuse, which may lead to further enlargement or further organization and consolidation of the nodules. Typical patients with vocal nodules complain that their voices seem to deteriorate with continuous voicing; they may start the day with fairly good voices that become increasingly dysphonic with continuous use. Following prolonged speaking or singing, perhaps coupled with vocal abuse and misuse, phonation rapidly deteriorates.

Small nodules and recently acquired ones can be successfully treated with voice therapy (Ruotsalainen, Sellman, Lehto, Jauhiainen, and Verbeek, 2007). Holmberg, Hillman, Hammarberg, Södersten, and Doyle (2001), reporting on voice therapy success for 11 adult females with vocal nodules, found a significant decrease in severity of dysphonia following behavioral voice therapy. In addition, video-laryngostroboscopy at the end of therapy showed that the nodules had decreased in size and that edema was reduced for nearly all clients. McFarlane and Watterson (1990) reported success in 44 cases presenting both large and small nodules in children and adults, in both singers and nonsingers. They also document with pictures the before and after therapy conditions of the larynx of a child and an adult singer. The nodules were completely resolved via voice therapy. Boone (1982) developed a four-point program for adults with vocal nodules that focuses on identifying abuse–misuse; reducing the occurrence of such abuse–misuse; searching with the patient for various voice therapy facilitating approaches that seem to produce an easy, optimal vocal production; and using the facilitating approach that works best as a practice method. Although we strongly recommend voice therapy as the primary treatment for nodules, we also acknowledge that larger or long-established nodules may be treated by surgery, followed by a brief period of complete voice rest and then voice therapy (Pedersen and McGlashan, 2001). However, a trial period of voice therapy is an appropriate conservative course of treatment prior to surgery for nodules in nearly all cases (Pedersen, Beranova, and Moller, 2004). If voice therapy must follow surgical treatment, then why not begin with a period of voice therapy? It is not unusual clinically for new nodules to reappear several weeks after surgical removal of nodules in both children and adults. Unless the underlying hyperfunctional vocal behaviors are identified and reduced, vocal nodules have a stubborn way of reappearing.

Vocal nodules in children before puberty are more common in boys. In their review of 254 cases of children with vocal nodules, Shah, Woodnorth, Glynn, and Nuss (2005) reported that nodules were more commonly observed in males between the ages of 3 to 10 years. Laryngopharyngeal reflux disease was present in one-fourth of the cases reviewed by Shah and colleagues, and in three-fourths of the cases there was evidence of vocal hyperfunction (p. 903). As boys get older, there is less evidence of nodules, and adolescent and adult females show a higher prevalence of nodules (Herrington-Hall, Lee, Stemple, Niemi, and McHone, 1988; Nagata, Kurita, Yasumoto, Maeda, Kawaski, and Hirano, 1983). However, in discussing the fact that vocal fold lesions are more common in women than men, Koufman and Belafsky (2001) suggest that differences in incidence may be multifactorial and related to hormonal, anatomic, inflammatory, and aerodynamic factors. Shah, Feldman, and Nuss (2007) have developed a reliable scale for grading the size of vocal nodules in children, which should facilitate objective analysis of outcomes when studying and following pediatric patients with vocal nodules.

It is generally accepted that nodules result from vocal hyperfunction and are therefore often observed in individuals who exhibit hyperfunctional vocal behaviors. Some could be referred to as vocal overachievers. Green (1989) found that children with vocal nodules demonstrated more aggressive behaviors, acting out, and disturbed relationships with peers, compared to children with normal voices. This was not supported, though, in a study by Roy, Holt, Redmond, and Muntz (2007), who reported no evidence of amplified aggressiveness or immature behavior in children with vocal nodules compared to children with normal voices. Roy and colleagues did report, however, that children with nodules use their voice for socializing more than children with normal voices.

Although symptomatic voice therapy has been effective in reducing or eliminating vocal nodules, young patients with vocal nodules often require strong psychological support by the voice clinician (Andrews and Summers, 2002; Toohill, 1975). Merati, Keppel, Braun, Blumin, and Kerschner (2008) studied voice-related quality of life of children with voice disorders and reported significant impairment in those with vocal nodules, particularly in the social–emotional and physical–functional domains. The effect of vocal nodules on children may depend on the age of the child. Connor, Cohen, Theis, Thibeault, Heatley, and Bless (2008) assessed the attitudes of children with dysphonia across four age groups (toddler, ages 2–4; preschool, ages 5–7; school age, ages 8–12; and adolescent, ages 13–18) and found that as children got older, social and emotional handicap became greater from having vocal nodules and other forms of dysphonia. Providing therapy to children with vocal nodules is important, as they do not simply "outgrow" the problem. De Bodt and colleagues (2007) questioned 91 adolescents in whom nodules were diagnosed in childhood and found that 21% had voice complaints persisting into postpubescence, with a statistically significant difference between boys and girls. Nodules were still present in 47% of the girls and 7% of the boys, with significant higher long-term risks for dysphonic girls with allergy.

Vocal Fold Polyps

A vocal fold polyp is a focal abnormality of the superficial lamina propria, usually at the same site where vocal fold nodules occur. This lesion, however, is thought to be slightly deeper within the superficial lamina propria. Vocal fold polyps are usually unilateral, but a reactive lesion is often found on the vocal fold immediately across from the polyp. Unlike vocal nodules, which result from continuous or chronic vocal fold irritation, polyps are often precipitated by a single vocal event. For example, a patient may have indulged in excessive vocalization, such as screaming for much of an evening, which produced some hemorrhaging on the membrane at the point of maximum glottal contact. Such hemorrhagic irritation eventually results in formation of either a translucent, fibrotic, hyaline, hemorrhagic, or mixed polyp that adds mass to the vocal fold. Once a small polyp begins, any continued phonotrauma will irritate the area, contributing to its continued growth.

An excellent description of vocal fold polyps, their formation, and their treatment was developed by Kleinsasser (1982), who reviewed 900 cases of polyps. Three-fourths of patients were male and one-fourth female, with the mean age of both being around 40 years. In 90% of the cases polyps were unilateral, in 5% they were bilateral, and in 5% they were both multiple and unilateral. Over 80% of patients smoked and other contributing factors included inhaled allergens and irritants. As described by Rubin and Yanigisawa (2003, p. 74), the gross appearance of vocal fold polyps varies: They may be reddish or white, large or small, and sessile (broad-based) or pedunculated (narrow-necked on a stem). Most are small and sessile, however. As polyps become more advanced, they become increasingly more pedunculated. Polyps are associated with other vocal fold pathologies in 15% of cases (Bouchayer and Cornut, 1991).

Kleinsasser (1982) described vocal fold polyps as being responsive to surgery. Sometimes, surgery can be performed in the office as opposed to the hospital (Woo, 2006). The goal of modern vocal fold surgery is to preserve as much superficial lamina propria as possible and to disrupt the glottal margin as little as possible. Thus microflap surgery designed to raise a flap of mucosa, remove a benign lesion via suction, and then lay the flap back down on the vocal fold is common (Courey, Garrett, and Ossoff, 1997; Hirano, Yamashita, Ohno, Hitamura, Kanemasu, and Ito, 2008). Another technique, epithelial cordotomy, involves microdissection between the polyp and the residual normal superior lamina propria while disturbing as little of the epithelium as possible (Benninger, 2000; Hochman and Zeitels, 2000). Cohen and Garrett (2007) examined the utility of voice therapy alone for patients with vocal fold polyps and cysts. In their study of 57 patients, almost half experienced an improved voice. Factors such as length of dysphonia, smoking status, allergy, and gastroesophageal reflux treatment, were not associated with treatment outcome. They also found that the type of polyp was associated with voice improvement. Specifically, patients with translucent polyps were more likely to experience an improved voice than those with fibrotic, hyaline, or hemorrhagic polyps. Finally, disappearance of the polyp was not observed in most of the cases where voice improvement was noted.

Unless the causative behaviors are identified and ameliorated, polyps often recur after surgery. With voice therapy and attempts to use the laryngeal mechanisms more optimally, polyps can be significantly reduced in size or permanently eliminated. We have seen even professional singers return to a singing career with an improved vocal hygiene and improved singing technique after surgery and voice therapy (Lavorato and McFarlane, 1983). We prefer voice therapy as the first approach to treatment of a sessile polyp and surgery followed by voice therapy when initial voice therapy fails to achieve the desired response. This opinion is supported by the research of Zeitels, Hillman, Desloge, Mauri, and Doyle (2002), who suggest that successful management of vocal fold lesions depends on prudent patient selection and counseling, ultraprecise surgical technique, and vigorous vocal rehabilitation using various voice facilitating approaches (see Chapter 7).

Traumatic Laryngitis

In mechanical or traumatic laryngitis patients experience swelling of the vocal folds as a result of excessive and strained vocalization. Phonotrauma such as yelling, screaming, abrupt and strained voice usage, chronic coughing, habitual throat clearing, and forceful singing are common causes of traumatic laryngitis. Typical traumatic laryngitis may be heard in the voices of excited spectators after a sporting event or rock music concert. In the excitement of the event, with their own voices masked by the noise of the crowd, fans scream at pitch levels and intensities they normally do not use. Under these speaking conditions the surface tissues of the true (and possibly, false) vocal folds experience intense friction, thermal agitation, and molecular breakdown (Dworkin, 2008). The vocal fold edema is accompanied by irritation (erythema) and increased blood accumulation.

The acute stage of functional laryngitis is at its peak during the actual yelling or traumatic vocal behavior, with the vocal folds much increased in size and mass. In general, the greater the irregularity, size, and consistency of the gap between the vocal fold free edges during the closed phases of vibration, the more severe the dysphonia. Variably hoarse–breathy, harsh, strained, and low-pitched voice abnormalities result from the underlying glottal incompetence. In the case of functional laryngitis secondary to yelling or a similar form of vocal abuse, eliminating the abuse usually permits the vocal mechanism to return to its natural state. The temporary laryngitis experienced toward the end of a sporting event or concert is usually relieved by a return to normal vocal activity, and most of the edema and irritation vanish after a good night's sleep.

Chronic laryngitis may typically produce more serious vocal problems if the speaker attempts to speak above the laryngitis. Because the temporary edema of the vocal folds alters the quality and loudness of the phonation, the speaker increases vocal efforts, which only increases the irritation of the folds, thereby compounding the problem. Finally, if such hyperfunctional behavior continues over time, what was once a temporary edema may become a more permanent polypoid thickening, sometimes developing into vocal fold polyps, vocal fold nodules, hyperkeratosis, or scarring. For this reason, functional laryngitis should be promptly treated by eliminating the causative abuse and, if possible, by enforcing a short period (less than one week) of complete voice rest. Although voice rest in itself is not a cure for most voice disorders, this is not true for traumatic laryngitis. Complete or absolute voice rest, which means no phonation or whispering for several days, is usually enough for irritated vocal fold margins to lose their swelling and return to their normal shape. It is important that voice rest designed to promote healing of irritated vocal fold surfaces *not* include whispering; whispering (as most people do it) still causes too much vocal fold movement, and irritation from the rubbing together of the approximating surfaces of each fold is still possible. Studies have shown that during forced whisper there are increases in expiratory muscle activity and airflow, and the ventricular folds often may be brought into function (Pearl and McCall, 1986). The events that cause traumatic laryngitis must be identified and curbed.

Ventricular Dysphonia

Ventricular dysphonia, sometimes known as *dysphonia plicae ventricularis* or false fold phonation, occurs more often than previously indicated (Boone, 1983). While ventricular dysphonia may be produced by the vibration of the approximating ventricular folds, it more often is produced by the true vocal folds vibrating in an abnormal fashion due to the false folds (ventricular folds) riding (or loading) the true folds.

Sometimes the ventricular voice becomes the substitute voice of patients who have had resection due to severe disease of the true folds (such as cancer, severe recurrent respiratory papilloma, or large polyps). The ventricular voice is usually low-pitched because of the large mass of vibrating tissue of the ventricular bands (as compared to the smaller mass of vibrating tissue of the true folds) or from the combined mass of the true and false vocal folds. In addition, the voice has little pitch variability and is therefore monotone. Finally, because the ventricular folds have difficulty in making a good, firm approximation for their entire length, the voice is usually quite hoarse and may also be breathy. This combination of low pitch, monopitch, and hoarseness makes most ventricular voices sound very unpleasant. If no persistent true cord pathology continues to force patients to use their ventricular voices, this disorder usually responds well to voice therapy. Sometimes, however, hypertrophy (enlargement) of the ventricular folds is present, which makes their normal full retraction somewhat difficult. Ventricular phonation is impossible to diagnose by the sound of the voice alone (Maryn, De Bodt, and Van Cauwenberge, 2003). Laryngoscopic examination during phonation shows the ventricular folds coming together, covering (partially or completely) from view the true folds that lie below (Nemetz, Pontes, and Vieira, 2005).

Some ventricular dysphonias display a special form of diplophonia (double voice), in which the true folds vibrate and also drive the ventricular folds to vibrate because the false folds are sitting on the true folds (loading the true cords with ventricular folds). In our experience, more often than not, the ventricular folds do not vibrate as a sole source of sound but load the true vocal folds. The true vocal folds are dampened by the false folds. Identification and confirmation of what vibrating structures the patient is using for phonation can best be made by frontal tomographic x-ray (coronal) of the sites of vibration. Ventricular phonation can also be diagnosed sometimes by nasoendoscopy and endoscopic stroboscopy (McFarlane, Watterson, and Brophy, 1990). In ventricular phonation, the true vocal folds will be slightly abducted, with the ventricular bands above in relative approximation and very possibly resting on the true vocal folds. In normal phonation, the opposite relationship between the true folds and the ventricular bands occurs; that is, the true folds are adducted and the ventricular bands are positioned laterally from the midline position. Once ventricular phonation is confirmed by laryngoscopy or x-ray, any physical problem of the true cords that might make normal phonation impossible should be eliminated. We consider both the elimination of ventricular phonation and its occasional need to be taught when we present voice therapy for special problems in Chapter 8.

In many ways ventricular phonation is a symptom of other conditions. For example, when one true fold is paralyzed or too stiff (due to postsurgical scarring) to vibrate, the false fold is brought into the phonatory act. Figures 5.1 and 5.2

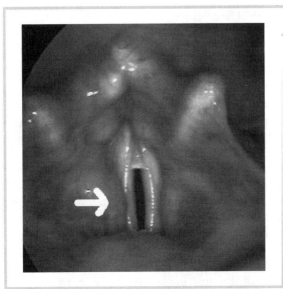

FIGURE **5.1**

Ventricular Fold Phonation

Prolapsed right ventricle in a 75-year-old trumpet player. Voice is low in pitch, hoarse, and breathy, due to the false vocal fold impinging on the true vocal fold.

show ventricular fold vibration compensating for a prolapsed right ventricle. Note how the facilitation approach of inhalation phonation decreases the impingement.

We have known ventricular phonation to become habituated after a bout of flu when the true vocal folds were too swollen to vibrate. Ventricular fold phonation in such cases is a compensation used by the patient. It is usually not the best

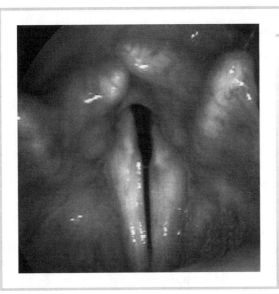

FIGURE **5.2**

Intervention Using Inhalation Phonation

Note that with the facilitating approach of inhalation phonation, the false vocal fold impinges less on the true vocal fold.

compensation for the problem and is generally responsive to voice therapy such as inhalation phonation or pitch elevation of breathy voice onset, as discussed in Chapter 7.

Diplophonia

The term *diplophonia* means "double voice." A diplophonic voice is produced with two distinct frequencies occurring simultaneously. Diplophonia is the consequence of irregular vocal fold vibration. It may be produced by some normal speakers voluntarily, but is more likely to be heard in patients with mass lesions, vocal fold paralysis, vocal fold scarring, laryngitis and other inflammatory conditions, muscle tension dysphonia, puberphonia, or paradoxical vocal fold movement (Ishi, Ishiguro, and Hagita, 2006; Vertigan, Theodoros, Winkworth, and Gibson, 2007). Auditory–perceptual and acoustic analyses usually form the basis for a diagnosis of diplophonia. Laryngostroboscopy is of limited diagnostic value because the tracking of the frequency of vocal fold vibration is dependent on a single frequency (Kendall, Browning, and Skovlund, 2005).

The treatment of diplophonia is aimed at eliminating the source of the second voice. Sometimes, surgical removal of a mass lesion or surgical repositioning and tensing of a paralyzed vocal fold will eliminate diplophonia (Tsukahara, Tokashiki, Hiramatsu, and Suzuki, 2005). More often, though, diplophonia is corrected by voice therapy (discussed in Chapters 4 and 7), accomplished by reducing any laryngeal hypertension that may be contributing to production of a second sound source. Videoendoscopy is helpful in identifying the source of the undesired vibration and guiding voice therapy in reestablishment of normal voice production.

Phonation Breaks

A phonation break is a temporary loss of voice that may occur for only part of a word, a whole word, a phrase, or a sentence. The individual is phonating with no apparent difficulty when suddenly a complete cessation of voice occurs. Such a fleeting voice loss is usually situational and it usually happens after prolonged hyperfunction. Typical patients with this problem work too hard to talk, often speaking with great effort, and suddenly experience a complete voice break. Such patients usually struggle to find their voice by coughing, clearing their throat, or taking a drink of water. In most cases, phonation is restored and remains adequate until the next phonation break, which may occur in only a few moments or not for days. Other than continued vocal hyperfunction, no physical condition seems to cause these phonatory interruptions. They may result from a variety of physiological sources, ranging from reduced subglottal air pressure near the end of a phrase to the loading of the true vocal fold by the ventricular fold or mucus on the true fold. Many times these breaks result from excessive laryngeal muscle tension and inappropriate adjustments of the otherwise normal mechanism.

Voice patients who experience phonation breaks rarely show them during voice evaluation sessions. In their histories, however, such patients report the occurrence of phonation breaks, often with much embarrassment when they occur. Occasionally patients have been told by their employers that they must learn to use their voices correctly (without voice breaks) or they would lose their jobs. Fortunately, the treatment of phonation breaks is relatively simple: taking the work out of phonation and eliminating inappropriate vocal behaviors such as excessive coughing and violent throat clearing. Some of the voice therapy techniques described in Chapter 7 that are designed to reduce vocal hyperfunction (tongue protrusion /i/, chant–talk, nasal–glide stimulation, warble), are most effective in eliminating the phonation break problem. Specific therapy procedures for phonation breaks or more severe abductor spasms are discussed in Chapter 7.

Pitch Breaks

There are two kinds of pitch breaks. One is a developmental phenomenon seen primarily in boys experiencing marked pubertal growth of the larynx, and the other is caused by prolonged vocal hyperfunction, particularly while speaking at an inappropriate (usually too low) pitch level.

The rapid changes in the size of the vocal folds and other laryngeal structures produce varying vocal effects during the pubertal years. Boys experience a lowering of their fundamental frequency of about one octave; girls, a lowering of only about two or three semitones (Wilson, 1987). This change does not happen in a day or two. For several years, as this laryngeal growth is taking place, boys will experience temporary hoarseness and occasional pitch breaks. Wise parents or voice clinicians witness these vocal changes with little comment or concern. These mass–size increases of puberty tend to thwart any serious attempts at singing or other vocal arts. Luchsinger and Arnold (1965) point out that much of the European literature on singing makes a valid plea that the formal study of singing be deferred until well after puberty. Until a male child experiences some stability of laryngeal growth, the demands of singing might be inappropriate for his rapidly changing mechanism. Laryngeal strain is a real concern when serious singing is attempted during this period. One of the authors was told by Beverly Sills, the most famous of recent sopranos, that she stopped singing altogether for three years during puberty. Interestingly, Beverly Sills, unlike any other opera singer we know, had only a single voice teacher for her entire child and adult career.

The age and rate of pubertal development varies markedly. From the pediatric literature we find that the main thrust of puberty for any one child seems to take place in a total time period of about four years six months. The most rapid and dramatic changes occur toward the last six months of puberty (this is when pitch breaks, if they occur, may be observed in some boys). Most pubertal changes begin at age 12 in boys, a little earlier in girls, and are completed by age 16.

Younger children and adults might experience a different kind of pitch break, related to the voice breaking an octave (sometimes two octaves) up or an octave down when speaking at an inappropriate pitch level. When individuals speak at an inappropriately low frequency, their voice tends to break one octave higher; if they speak too high in the frequency range, their voice may break one octave down.

Pitch breaks can also result from overall vocal fatigue. Heavy users of voice, such as actors after prolonged rehearsals or during long-running performances, may begin to experience pitch breaks after hours of prolonged voicing. Vocal hyperfunction—speaking with too much effort—will sometimes result in either pitch or phonation breaks. Such pitch breaks are usually warnings that the vocal mechanisms are being overworked and being held at an inappropriate pitch level for a prolonged period of time. We refer to such pitch or phonation breaks as *vocal limping*, just as one limps when walking with an injured foot. With a little temporary voice rest (two or three days) and initiation of techniques of easy phonation (such as glottal fry or yawn–sigh), fatigue-induced pitch and phonation breaks usually disappear.

SUMMARY

The majority of voice disorders are related to vocal hyperfunction. Vocal excesses, such as voicing too loud and too long and excessive throat clearing, are examples of causal factors of symptoms of aphonia or dysphonia. These we classify as functional disorders, perhaps resulting in vocal fold thickening, nodules, or polyps. Psychogenic voice disorders, on the other hand, often manifest themselves in a hoarse voice with no physical cause, or complete loss of voice due to emotional trauma or conflict. In the cases of both psychogenic and MTD voice disorders, an element of counseling is recommended along with intervention so that the client recognizes the underlying antecedent events. Once these events are identified, the client is better prepared to eliminate or reduce those events before, or as, they occur.

Thought Questions

1. Discuss the differences between psychogenic voice disorders and muscle tension dysphonia. Describe treatment approaches to each.
2. List causes of vocal fold thickening.
3. Cite published research reporting successful treatment for vocal nodules.
4. What are two types of pitch breaks?

Voice Evaluation

LEARNING OBJECTIVES

- Define the terms *assessment, evaluation,* and *diagnosis*
- Describe the screening process for voice disorders
- List the major elements of the voice assessment
- Describe the noninstrumental assessment of voice
- Describe the instrumental assessment of voice

When encountering a patient presenting with a voice disorder, the clinician begins a systematic process of assessment, evaluation, and diagnosis. *Assessment* is the process of collecting relevant data for clinical decision making. *Evaluation* is an appraisal of the implications and significance of the assessment. *Diagnosis* calls for the clinician to make a decision as to whether a problem exists, and if so, differentiating it from other similar problems. In a medical model, diagnostic emphasis is also put on identification of possible causes and maintaining factors (Paul, 2002).

The results of the voice evaluation serve as the foundation for a sound treatment plan. As such, the voice evaluation must be a carefully and scientifically validated procedure performed by a competent clinician. Ideally, the voice assessment should follow examination of the patient by a laryngologist, who is an ear, nose, and throat (ENT) physician with special knowledge of the larynx and voice. In instances where a patient is assessed prior to examination by the laryngologist, the clinician should reserve diagnosis and treatment planning until results of the medical assessment can be evaluated. While it is the province of the laryngologist to make a laryngeal diagnosis and establish and oversee a medical management plan, it is the province of the speech–language pathologist to make a voice diagnosis and to establish and carry out a voice therapy plan.

Although we present the comprehensive voice evaluation here in a separate chapter, it is important for the reader to appreciate that effective voice therapy requires continuous assessment and evaluation. Many of the assessment instruments and procedures described in this chapter are also used in voice therapy. Finally, while we believe in the value of using appropriate instrumentation for assessment, it is the knowledgeable and skilled clinician who is of ultimate value in the evaluation, diagnosis, and treatment of the patient with a disordered voice.

SCREENING FOR VOICE DISORDERS

The prevalence of voice disorders in school-age children is usually reported as between approximately 5 and 9% (Oates, 2004), but some studies place the prevalence rate in the double digits (Lee, Stemple, Glaze, and Kelchner, 2004). In one large study of preschool children (Duff, Proctor, and Yairi, 2004), voice disorders were identified in nearly 4% of the students examined. Kahane and Mayo (1989) suggest that the vast majority of children with voice disorders are never seen by a speech–language pathologist. This is supported by reports from Davis and Harris (1992) and Broomfield and Dodd (2004) estimating that children with voice disorders make up less than 5% of a clinician's caseload.

Individuals other than the school clinician often identify the majority of children with voice problems (Davis and Harris, 1992). A vocal feature such as abnormal voice quality is noticed by the child's teacher, nurse, or family member, and subsequent contact is made with the clinician. The ability of such individuals to make accurate judgments about the normalcy of voice is not quite as good, however, as that of an experienced clinician (McFarlane, Holt-Romeo, Lavorato, and Warner, 1991). Therefore, rather than relying on other well-meaning individuals to refer children for therapy, the clinician should develop screening procedures for the early identification of children with voice problems.

Most public and private schools have screening programs to identify speech and language disorders in new students and those in certain grades at specified times of the year. By using some kind of voice screening form, clinicians are better able to identify and document those children in need of voice assessment and potential treatment. With very little additional testing time per child (five minutes or so) a voice screening can be added to existing speech and language screening protocols. The importance of identifying and managing voice disorders in children cannot be overemphasized, because dysphonia can impact a child's educational and psychosocial development, as well as his or her physical and emotional health.

Clinicians in various settings have developed different screening forms. The items on the screening form usually represent the aspects of voice that the clinician considers important for identifying children who may be having voice problems. The screening form helps the clinician focus, organize, and report listening observations. Two easy-to-administer screening protocols are the voice screening form in the *Boone Voice Program for Children* (Boone, 1993) and the Quick Screen for Voice (Lee, Stemple, and Glaze, 2005).

The Quick Screen for Voice, which addresses respiration, phonation, and resonance, is designed to be administered in about 10 minutes and may be used with students from preschool through high school. The clinician responds to a checklist of observations made during spontaneous conversation, picture description, imitated sentences, recited passages, counting, and other natural samples of voice and speech. The student fails the screening if one or more disorders in production are found in any section. Lee and colleagues report in the manual accompanying this instrument that approximately 10% of preschool students in a field test failed the voice screening, a prevalence rate in line with that reported in the literature by others (Boyle, 2000).

The Boone Voice Program for Children Voice Screening Form (see Figure 6.1), which also addresses respiration, phonation, and resonance, can be administered relatively quickly and is appropriate for students in all grades. The clinician listens to natural samples of voice and speech, and for each of the scale judgments (pitch, loudness, quality, nasal resonance, oral resonance) notes whether the child's voice sounds like the voices of peers of the same age, gender, and race. To facilitate ease of scoring, a simple three-point system is used to record perceptual judgments. Specifically, if a child's voice appears lower in pitch than that of his or her peers, the minus sign (−) is circled; if pitch appears normal, the neutral symbol (N) is circled; if the pitch level is higher than the child's peers, the plus sign (+) is circled. Inadequate loudness is specified as minus (−); normal loudness as neutral (N); and excessive loudness as (+). A breathy, hoarse voice is marked as (−); normal voice quality as neutral (N); and a tight, harsh voice as (+). If hyponasality (insufficient nasal resonance) is noted, the form is checked with a (−); normal nasal resonance is marked (N); and hypernasality (too much nasal resonance) is marked with a (+). Oral resonance deviations do not occur as often as other problems; however, excessive posterior tongue carriage that produces inadequate oral resonance is marked as (−), normal oral resonance is marked as (N), and excessive front-of-the-mouth resonance characterized by a baby-thin voice is marked as (+). If the child receives either a (−) or (+) on any of the five clinical parameters, he or she should be rechecked within a few weeks. Arrangements should be made for full medical and voice evaluations for those individuals who on follow-up continue to demonstrate some departures in voice from their peers (Boone, 1993).

MEDICAL EVALUATION FOR VOICE DISORDERS

The American Speech-Language-Hearing Association (ASHA) *Preferred Practice Patterns for the Profession of Speech–Language Pathology* (2004d) states:

> All patients/clients with voice disorders must be examined by a physician, preferably in a discipline appropriate to the presenting complaint. The physician's examination may occur before or after the voice evaluation by the clinician. (p. 99)

FIGURE **6.1**

A Voice Screening Form

VOICE SCREENING FORM
The Boone Voice Program for Children

Name _____ Sex M F Grade _____
School _____ Teacher _____
Examiner _____ Date _____

VOICE RATING SCALE

Circle the appropriate symbol(s)

Pitch	− N +	Describe:
Loudness	− N +	Describe:
Quality	− N +	Describe:
Nasal Resonance	− N +	Describe:
Oral Resonance	− N +	Describe:

S/Z RATIO

Record 2 trials of [s] and 2 trials of [z] expirations

s = _____ seconds
s = _____ seconds

                                 Longest s ÷ by Longest z = S/Z Ratio: _____

z = _____ seconds
z = _____ seconds

DISPOSITION:

❑ Complete voice evaluation required (one or more rating of + or − or an S/Z ratio of greater than 1.2)
❑ No further evaluation required
❑ Second screening required _____
                          (Date)

Comments:

Source: From Boone, D. R. (1993). *The Boone Voice Program for Children* (2nd ed.). Austin, TX: Pro-Ed.

If, for whatever reason, a patient arrives to be treated for some form of dysphonia but has not had a previous medical examination, the clinician should wait to make treatment recommendations until the medical information is obtained. The voice evaluation by the speech–language pathologist may begin, however, even in the absence of the medical information. A case history can be taken, and assessment of respiration, phonation, and resonance can be conducted; only the decision about whether to begin voice therapy need be deferred until all medical information is obtained. This is because a patient's voice may sound a particular way for a number of reasons, some more serious and complicated than others. For example, a particular patient's vocal symptoms may include decreased speaking pitch, pitch variability, and pitch range; decreased loudness, loudness variability, and loudness range; increased breathiness; voice breaks; and vocal fatigue. Such complaints are common when there is an additive vocal fold mass. However, such a mass lesion may take the form of a nodule, for example, which is benign, or it may take the form of an invasive malignant tumor. Without a complete medical examination, the clinician does not know the etiology of the voice disorder.

The roles of the laryngologist and speech–language pathologist differ in regard to evaluation of the voice disordered patient, though the assessments conducted by each may overlap. In general, the laryngologist's primary role is to identify and manage those conditions or diseases that interfere with normal voice production, while the speech–language pathologist's primary role is to evaluate and facilitate voice production given the patient's known medical status. Optimally, the laryngologist and the clinician work together in evaluating and managing the patient. McFarlane, Fujiki, and Brinton (1984) have discussed this team relationship from the view of the speech–language pathologist:

> The most desired goal is to be regarded by these professional practitioners as peer professionals. This means that we must be able to talk intelligently about their field (be "bilingual," using our jargon and theirs) and their clients, provide a valuable and effective treatment service to their patients, and possess a knowledge and skill base somewhat unique from these other specialties. (pp. 133–134)

In larger urban cities, patients may have ready access to a voice care team in settings such as local hospitals and clinics, private otolaryngology practices, or academic medical centers. However, in smaller or rural cities, access may be quite limited. In such cases, patients may have to travel sometimes a considerable distance to see a laryngologist. In such cases, it is important that the patient understand why he or she being asked to see the laryngologist. A brief written note from the referring clinician can often help facilitate communication between the patient and laryngologist. If the patient is a child who failed a voice screening, for example, inclusion of the voice screening record form may help the parents to discuss their child with the laryngologist and help focus the child's examination. On completion of the medical examination, it is equally important for the laryngologist to communicate the findings to both the patient (or parent, where applicable) and the referring clinician. Depending on the nature of the medical examination, a variety of written forms may be used, including a narrative/descriptive note stating the medical diagnosis and findings, record forms for specific types of assessment (such as laryngoscopy), and copies of photos or videos of the larynx and related structures.

Sataloff, Spiegel, and Hawkshaw (2003) have written extensively about the history taking and physical examination of patients with voice disorders. They suggest the use of a history questionnaire (often completed in advance) to help the patient document all the necessary information, sort out and articulate any problems, and save office time in recording information (p. 138). Figure 6.2 lists the essential items covered in such a questionnaire. Depending on the nature of the patient's chief complaint and symptoms, additional areas of questioning may be pursued.

The cause of a voice disorder can often be suggested from a detailed history and interview. Nevertheless, a comprehensive physical examination is necessary to confirm or rule out certain medical conditions, which may require the laryngologist to consult with specialists such as neurologists, pulmonologists, endocrinologists, psychiatrists, internists, physiatrists, and others with special knowledge of and interest in voice disorders. Physical examination should include an assessment of general physical condition and a thorough ear, nose, and throat evaluation. Depending on the patient's age and observed signs, additional areas of examination may be pursued (McMurray, 2003; Pontes, Yamasaki, and Behlau, 2006).

Visual inspection of the larynx is perhaps the most important procedure for understanding the cause of a voice disorder and its potential for treatment. Research has documented the importance of laryngoscopy for improved diagnosis of voice disorders (Galli et al., 2007; Grillone and Chan, 2006; Hirano and Bless, 1993; McFarlane, 1990; Noyes and Kemp, 2007; Sanli, Celebi, Eken, Oktay, Aydin, and Ayduran, 2008). Office-based visual examination of the larynx traditionally takes one of two forms: mirror laryngoscopy or endoscopic laryngoscopy (more commonly referred to as laryngeal endoscopy). In mirror laryngoscopy, a small laryngeal mirror is placed at the back of the patient's mouth and light is shined on the mirror from the physician's headset. If the mirror is angled properly, a reflected view of the hypopharynx can be seen. In laryngeal endoscopy, either a rigid fiberoptic scope is placed in the mouth or a flexible fiberoptic scope is passed through the nasal passages. The rigid laryngoscope has a prism at the end that directs light and receives images at an angle of either 70° or 90°, permitting optimum visualization of the normal inverted-V position of the vocal folds. Figure 6.3 lists the advantages and disadvantages of these indirect laryngeal examination methods.

Assessment, Evaluation, and Diagnosis of Voice Disorders by the Clinician

In an interview with Thibeault (2007), Bless describes the clinician's role in the evaluation of voice disorders as follows:

> The clinician's role is to describe the structure and function of the larynx and make recommendations regarding further testing needed to understand the etiology or maintenance of the voice problem and to make recommendations for treatment. (p. 4)

FIGURE **6.2**

Sample Medical History Questions

How old are you?

What is your voice problem?

Do you have any pressing voice commitments?

How much voice training have you had?

Under what kinds of conditions do you use your voice?

Are you aware of misusing or abusing your voice during singing?

Are you aware of misusing or abusing your voice during speaking?

Do you have pain when you talk or sing?

What kind of physical condition are you in?

Have you noted voice or bodily weakness, tremor, fatigue, or loss of control?

Do you have allergy or cold symptoms?

Do you have any breathing problems, especially after exercise?

Have you been exposed to environmental irritants?

Do you smoke, live with a smoker, or work around smoke?

Do any foods seem to affect your voice?

Do you have morning hoarseness, bad breath, excessive phlegm, a lump in your throat, or heartburn?

Do you have trouble with your bowels or your belly?

Are you under particular stress or in therapy?

Do you have problems controlling your weight; are you excessively tired; are you cold when other people are warm?

Do you have menstrual irregularity, cyclical voice changes associated with menses, recent menopause, or other hormonal changes or problems?

Do you have jaw joint or other dental problems?

Do you or others living with you have hearing loss?

Have you suffered whiplash or other bodily injury?

Did you undergo any surgery prior to the onset of your voice problems?

What medications and other substances do you use?

FIGURE **6.3**

Advantages and Disadvantages of Laryngeal Examination Methods

I. Mirror laryngoscopy
  A. Advantages
    1. Quick overview of laryngeal anatomy and physiology
    2. Prognostic for either rigid or flexible laryngoscopy
  B. Disadvantages
    1. Poorly tolerated by some patients
    2. Can only assess sustained vowels and not connected speech or singing
    3. Alters typical laryngeal behavior
II. Rigid (oral) laryngoscopy
  A. Advantages
    1. Excellent lighting, contributing to good photography
    2. Excellent magnification, contributing to good videography
  B. Disadvantages
    1. Poorly tolerated by some patients
    2. Can only assess sustained vowels and not connected speech or singing
    3. Cannot assess the entire vocal tract
    4. Alters typical laryngeal behavior
III. Flexible (nasal) laryngoscopy
  A. Advantages
    1. Well-tolerated by almost all patients
    2. Minimal alteration of typical laryngeal behavior
    3. Can assess connected speech and singing across the vocal range
    4. Can assess the entire vocal tract
  B. Disadvantages
    1. Optics and magnification inferior to that of rigid (oral) laryngoscopy
IV. Stroboscopy (coupled to rigid or flexible laryngoscopy)
  A. Advantages
    1. Allows for examination of vocal fold vibratory behavior
  B. Disadvantages
    1. Requires that patient produce a steady fundamental frequency
    2. Requires additional technical skills of the examiner

Source: Modified from Koufman (2003).

The American Speech-Language-Hearing Association (ASHA) has published a comprehensive document titled *Preferred Practice Patterns for Speech-Language Pathology* (ASHA, 2004d), in which preferred practice patterns for voice assessment and treatment are described, stating in part that voice assessment is provided to identify and describe

- Underlying strengths and deficits related to a voice disorder or a laryngeal disorder affecting respiration and communication performance
- Effects of the voice disorder on the individual's activities (capacity and performance in everyday communication contexts) and participation
- Contextual factors that serve as barriers to or facilitators of successful communication
- Participation restrictions for individuals with voice disorders or laryngeal disorders affecting respiration

The document also describes the voice assessment clinical process as including

- Review of auditory and visual status
- Relevant case history, including vocal use history, medical status, education, vocation, and cultural and linguistic background
- Standardized and nonstandardized methods:
  - Perceptual aspects of vocal production/behavior
  - Acoustic parameters of vocal production/behavior
  - Physiological aspects of phonatory behavior
  - Patient's/client's ability to modify vocal behavior (e.g., stimulation probes)
  - Emotional/psychological status
  - Medical history and associated conditions
  - Observation or review of articulation, fluency, and language
  - Functional consequences of the voice disorder
  - Use of perceptual and/or instrumental measures, including
    - perceptual ratings
    - acoustic analyses
    - aerodynamic measures
    - electroglottography
    - imaging techniques such as endoscopy and stroboscopy (these procedures may be conducted and interpreted in collaboration with other professionals)
- Selection of standardized measures for voice assessment with consideration for documented ecological validity
- Follow-up services to monitor voice status and ensure appropriate intervention and support for individuals with identified voice disorders

The remainder of this chapter will describe in detail much of the voice assessment clinical process outlined above. We recognize that not every patient will need to undergo all the assessments listed, and we recognize that not every clinician will have access to, and comfort with, the equipment needed to conduct all the assessments. It is our intent here to provide sufficient breadth and depth, knowing that the individual clinician will have the final "voice" in evaluating what is needed for any given patient.

Review of Auditory and Visual Status

Hearing acuity is important in monitoring and regulating one's own voice production (Lee, Hsiao, Yang, and Kuo, 2007). Thus, hearing loss has the potential to alter respiration, phonation, resonance, and prosody (Boone, 1966a; Higgins, McCleary, Ide-Helvie, and Carney, 2005; Horga and Liker, 2006). For example, an elderly patient may have a hearing loss and/or his or her spouse may have a hearing loss. In this clinical scenario, the patient may potentially develop a functional dysphonia characterized by inappropriate pitch and/or loudness and/or glottal attack. Other clinical scenarios include a child with a congenital hearing loss or a teen or adult with noise-induced hearing loss. About 8% of persons in the United States have hearing loss, which may vary from mild loss of sensitivity to total loss of hearing (Liu and Yan, 2007). The prevalence of hearing loss accelerates dramatically with age. It is estimated that hearing loss is found in 5% of children under the age of 17, 23% of those 18 to 44, 29% of those 45 to 60, and 43% of those 65 or older (Davis, Stephens, Rayment, and Thomas, 1997; National Academy on an Aging Society, 1999). Self-reported hearing loss can be identified in half of those aged 85 years and older (Mulrow and Lichtenstein, 1991). These numbers are expected to rise with the rapidly increasing number of elderly people (Hobbs and Stoops, 2002). When evaluating the patient with a voice disorder, a hearing screening should be conducted by the clinician when hearing difficulty is suspected, either from patient self-report or behavioral observation of others (Bogardus, Yueh, and Shekelle, 2003). Conducting hearing screenings in such a situation is within the ASHA (2007) *Scope of Practice for Clinicians* and is addressed in the ASHA (2004d) *Preferred Practice Patterns for Speech-Language Pathology.* It is unknown from review of the literature to date whether persons with voice disorders have a higher incidence of hearing loss than peers without a voice disorder.

Visual acuity is also an important consideration when assessing the person with a voice disorder. Decreased visual acuity may lead a patient to misjudge distance from the listener and alter his or her voice in ways that are detrimental. If visual feedback is provided by a mirror reflecting the patient's head and body posture, or a computer monitor showing a voice tracing, it is important that the patient be able to see well. In the case of the alaryngeal speaker who is learning to use an electrolarynx, visual acuity is important in learning to place the electrolarynx in the right location. More than 38 million Americans age 40 and older are estimated to experience blindness, low vision, or an age-related eye disease, with persons older than age 65 being the most affected (Congdon, Friedman, and Lietman, 2004).

Case History

During the case history the clinician must establish rapport with the patient so that information will be freely and honestly shared, and so that he or she will ultimately feel empowered to change their behavior if called upon to do so. Behrman (2006) has written recently about the concept of motivational interviewing (MI), which centers on eliciting in a nonthreatening manner the patient's motivation to adhere to behavioral change. Behrman also describes certain clinical considerations for patients with voice disorders that may be expected to affect resistance, and therefore adherence, to voice therapy. Such considerations may include a history of controlling interactions with medical professionals, previous exposure to exaggerated vocal hygiene messages, confusion regarding vocal identity, failure of other treatment modalities such as voice rest and medical management, prior experience with nonadherence in voice therapy, and lack of support from individuals in the patient's life, including business colleagues, friends, and family members (p. 216). The clinically astute clinician will monitor his or her own verbal and nonverbal behaviors during the case history interview so as to elicit clinically relevant information from the patient in a supportive and motivating manner.

In the sections below we provide an overview of the key areas in the case history and interview. Other areas may be pursued, depending on the particular clinical scenario.

Description of the Problem and Cause.   It is valuable in understanding patients to ask directly what they feel are the problems and what might have caused them. It is often effective to ask the same questions of family members, a spouse, or teachers. The different views about what the problem may be and the various guesses about probable causation may offer tips for management. Patients' descriptions often reveal much about their own conceptualization of the problem. What a patient feels the problem is may not be consistent with the opinions of the referring physician or the clinician, a discrepancy that may be due to what we call "the patient's reality distance." This distance may be the result of the patient's lay background and inability to understand adequately what has been explained. Often we hear highly discrepant reports of "what the doctor said" as a patient recounts the diagnoses of previous clinicians. More often this distance is primarily the result of the patient's reluctance to accept and cope with the real problem. An individual's defenses may lead to a description of the problem that is not consistent with the perceptions of others. What a patient says about a problem may, however, provide the clinician with insights that no amount of observation or testing can match.

Onset and Duration of the Problem.   How long patients believe they have had the voice problem is important. Acute and sudden onset of a dysphonia usually poses a severe threat to a patient. That is, it keeps the patient from carrying out his or her customary activities (playing, singing, acting, selling, preaching, teaching, campaigning, or whatever). Sudden onset of aphonia or dysphonia deserves thorough exploration by both the laryngologist and the clinician. Some dysphonias develop very gradually. Such gradual, fluctuating dysphonias are often related to varying situations in which patients may find themselves; sometimes they only occur during moments of stress or after fatigue. A history of slow onset sometimes suggests a gradually developing pathology, such as the development of Reinke's edema or dysphonia that is an early developing symptom of some kind of progressive neurological disease. Voice therapy, like other forms of remedial therapy, is usually more successful with those patients who are motivated to overcome their problems. Patients with a long history of indifference toward their dysphonia usually present an additional challenge to the clinician and a more unfavorable prognosis than those who have recently acquired the disorder, depending, of course, on the type and etiology and relative extent of the pathology involved.

Variability of the Problem.   Most voice patients can provide rather accurate timetables of the consistency of their problem. If the severity of a voice problem is variable, a clinician may be able to identify those vocal situations in which the patient experiences the best voice and the worst voice. The typical patient with vocal hyperfunction reports a better voice earlier in the day, with increasing dysphonia later in the day as the voice is used more. For example, a high school social studies teacher reported a normal-sounding voice at the beginning of the day; toward the end of the day, after six hours of lecturing, he reported increasing hoarseness and a feeling of "fullness and dryness in the throat." Voice rest and then dinner at the end of the day usually restored his voice to its normal pitch and quality. Obviously, such fluctuation in the daily quality of the voice enables the clinician to identify easily the situations contributing to the patient's vocal abuse. Another patient, whose dysphonia was closely related to allergy and postnasal drip experienced during sleep, presented this variation in hoarseness: severity in the morning on awakening, decrease in severity with usage of the voice, complete disappearance by late afternoon, and severity again the next morning.

The variation of the voice problem can provide even more specific clues as to what situations most aggravate the disorder. A nightclub singer reported that she had no voice problem during the day in conversational situations or while practicing her repertoire. She developed hoarseness only at night and only on those nights she sang. Further investigation of her singing act revealed that the adverse factors were the cigarette smoke around her, to which she was unusually sensitive, and the noise of the crowd, above which she had to increase her volume to be heard. Her singing methods were found to be satisfactory. A change of jobs to a summer tent theater provided her with immediate relief. It was also recommended that she invest in a more sophisticated and powerful sound system.

Description of Vocal Use (Daily Use–Misuse).   Abuse, misuse, and overuse of the voice cause most functional voice problems. It is important for clinicians to determine how voice patients are using their larynges in most life situations. The voice a child or adult exhibits in the clinician's office may in no way represent the voice used on the playground, in the classroom, or in other settings. Sometimes patients can recreate some of their aversive laryngeal behaviors as a demonstration for the clinician, but more often a valid search for aversive vocal behaviors requires the clinician to visit the environment where the abuse–misuse occurs. Successful voice clinicians must thus build into their schedules actual visits to playgrounds, theaters, churches, courtrooms, or offices. Case (2002), for instance, has demonstrated the effects of cheerleading on the larynges of teenagers, comparing laryngoscopic examinations before and after two weeks of attendance at a cheerleading camp. His data strongly suggest that continued cheerleading has a direct adverse effect on the larynges of the majority of the adolescents studied. It is obviously important for the clinician to identify the vocal use pattern of the patient.

FA.20

Additional Case History Information.   It is important to determine at the time of the voice evaluation whether the patient has ever had previous voice therapy. If so, what type of past therapy would have obvious relevance to present management? When previous voice therapy attempts have failed to improve the vocal quality or have been unsuccessful in reducing a vocal pathology, the knowledge of previous therapy is important. We must, however, make every effort to present the appearance of a fresh and different approach to the patient who has experienced failure in previous voice therapy; even if we use the same goals of therapy as before, we must redirect the new approach to voice therapy in a manner that appears to the patient to be headed down a completely different road. Determining whether other members of the family have similar voice problems is helpful. We have had particular patients present a certain voice problem, only to interview members of the family and find that all or many of them have the same voicing patterns.

Once a patient is comfortable with an examiner, or perhaps after voice therapy has begun, a social history should be taken to provide the clinician with useful information about the patient as a person. One patient spoke with two completely different voices, constantly shifting between one voice and the other. When we asked why she used these two voices, she said her first voice was "my voice before I died." Further case history questioning revealed that she had been a patient in a mental hospital on two occasions. It became clear as the interview progressed that she was still having psychological problems and her voice disorder was a symptom of a more serious unresolved disorder. She was convinced that she had died and that she was now a channel for another person who had also died. The different voices represented different people.

On completing a thorough records review and patient interview, the next step for the clinician is to systematically assess each aspect of voice production, with an eye towards differential diagnosis, determining prognosis for change, and formulating a treatment plan. The clinician may use instrumental or noninstrumental approaches to assess the voice. The noninstrumental approach relies on behavioral observation of the patient, examination of the patient's oral–peripheral mechanisms, auditory–perceptual judgments about various aspects of the voice (e.g., pitch, loudness, quality, respiratory–phonatory control, resonance, effort, etc.), and patient self-assessment of voice impairment, disability, and handicap (voice disordered quality of life). In the instrumental approach the emphasis is on obtaining indirect measures of voice production (e.g., visualization of the larynx, acoustic measures of the voice signal, aerodynamic measures of pressure and flow, physiological measurement of laryngeal muscle function, etc.). Each approach has its advantages and limitations, and it is incumbent on the clinician to be skilled at using both approaches and to have a clear purpose in using each.

While it may seem that the instrumental approach is less subjective than the noninstrumental approach, it should be noted that a skilled voice clinician can conduct a valid assessment of voice with or without instrumentation. The use of instrumentation does not ensure more accurate results. In the hands of a well-trained clinician the use of instrumentation does add important elements of documentation and quantification, which may or may not be available without instrumentation. Be that as it may, one should not rely on instrumentation to strengthen weak powers of observation, modest clinical skills, or lack of knowledge about voice production. Instrumentation alone will not compensate for mediocre skills. The most important skills are to be able to listen critically and carefully and to analyze objectively.

Noninstrumental Assessment

Behavioral Observation.　Keep in mind that observation of patients often tells more about them than their histories and assessment data. Clinicians must become critical observers, attempting to describe behavior they see rather than merely labeling it. Writing observations about a patient is one of the few ways clinicians can note what they observe (audio and video recordings are two other means). Even here, however, it is important for clinicians to minimize any subjectivity by describing only what they see and hear and not adding interpretation to the observation.

Because voice difficulties are often symptomatic of the inability to have satisfactory interpersonal relationships, it is imperative that the clinician consider the patient's degree of adequacy as a social being. Patients who exhibit extremely sweaty palms, who avoid eye contact with people to whom they are speaking, who speak through clenched teeth, who use excessive postural changes or demonstrate facial tics, who sit with a masked, nonaffective facial expression, or who exhibit obvious shortness of breath may be displaying behaviors frequently considered as symptomatic of anxiety. Their struggle to maintain a conversational relationship may be accompanied by much struggle to phonate. Such observed behavior in the voice patient may be highly significant to the voice clinician planning a course of voice remediation. The decision about whether to treat a problem symptomatically (that is, by voice therapy) or by improving the patient's potential for interpersonal adjustment (perhaps by psychotherapy) is often aided by a review of the observations of the patient. A patient who demonstrates friendly, normal affect is telling the clinician, at least superficially, that he or she functions well in a two-person relationship; this information may well have clinical relevance. Such observations are extremely valuable to voice clinicians planning treatment approaches. Note, however, that in our experience very few voice patients require referral for psychotherapy.

The Oral–Peripheral Mechanism Examination.　Careful assessment of the oral–peripheral mechanism is part of the voice assessment. Although we focus on assessment of the larynx and respiratory systems, examination of the face, oral and nasal cavities, and pharynx is also required.

Beyond observing obvious problems in breathing, some attention should be given to the amount of neck tension. The accessory neck muscles and the supralaryngeal strap muscles in some patients literally stick out like bands as the patient speaks (this is also observed in untrained singers). Often, mandibular restriction is closely associated with neck tension; affected patients speak through clenched teeth, with little or no mandibular movement. Such restricted jaw movement places most of the burden of speech articulation on the tongue, which, to produce the various vowels and diphthongs in connected speech, must make fantastic adjustments if no cavity-shaping assistance from the mandible is forthcoming. Another externally observable hyperfunction of the vocal tract is unusual downward or upward excursion of the larynx during the production of various pitches. Any unusual movement upward while phonating higher pitches, or unusual movement downward while phonating lower ones, should be noted. The angle of the thyroid cartilage may be palpated externally by the fingers (digitally) as the patient sings a number of varying pitches; typically the fingertips will feel little discernible change in thyroid angle as the patient sings up and down the scale. Sometimes, however, the thyroid cartilage can be felt to rock forward slightly in the production of high pitches, as it sweeps upward to a higher position toward the hyoid bone. It is helpful to gently move the larynx manually from side to side to note the degree of tension with which the strap muscles of the neck hold the larynx in place. We also ask patients to move their larynx manually from side to side and to observe how fixed it appears compared with the clinician's own larynx.

Any really noticeable amount of lifting or lowering of the larynx, as well as the tipping forward of the thyroid cartilage in the production of high pitches, should be noted as possible hyperfunctional behavior. However, the majority of hyperfunctional behaviors associated with voice problems are probably not directly observable from examination of the oral–peripheral mechanism. For example, to determine the extent of the tongue's impinging on the oropharyngeal space we would need to rely on oral or nasal laryngoscopy.

Auditory–Perceptual Assessment. Clinicians appear to prefer auditory–perceptual measures over instrumental measures when assessing dysphonia and documenting therapy progress (Bassich and Ludlow, 1986; Carding, Carlson, Epstein, Mathieson, and Shewell, 2000). Behrman (2005) surveyed voice clinicians regarding common diagnostic practices in patients referred for therapy with the diagnosis of muscle tension dysphonia. Each respondent reported that perceptual assessment of voice quality was very important for therapy tasks, such as defining overall therapy goals, defining specific therapy session goals, helping the patient to achieve a target production, providing reinforcement to the patient, and measuring treatment outcome. Furthermore, the clinician's perceptual assessment of voice quality was reported to occur significantly more commonly than stroboscopic, acoustic, aerodynamic, and electroglottographic assessments. Behrman concluded: "Efforts to make voice quality assessment standard and strengthen perceptual scaling methods appear well justified, given its dominant role in voice evaluations" (p. 468).

When performing an auditory–perceptual evaluation of voice quality, the clinician should consider a number of factors that might influence their resulting judgments (Kent, 1996). These include the nature of the speaking task, listener experience and training, and the type of rating method used (Kreiman, Gerratt, Kempster, Erman, and Berke, 1993). A variety of voice perceptual scales are available for clinical use, including the GRBAS scale (Hirano, 1981), the Buffalo Voice Profile system (Wilson, 1987), the Hammarberg scheme (Hammarberg, Fritzell, Gauffin, Sundberg, and Wedin, 1980), the Vocal Profile Analysis scheme (Laver, Wirz, MacKenzie, and Hiller, 1981), and more recently, the Consensus Auditory Perceptual Evaluation of Voice (CAPE-V) (Kempster, Gerratt, Verdolini Abbott, Burkmeier-Kraemer, and Hillman, 2008). Of these, the GRBAS scale has been studied most extensively (Carding et al., 2000; Yamaguchi, Shrivastav, Andrews, and Niimi, 2003).

The GRBAS Scale was developed by The Committee for Phonatory Function Tests of the Japanese Society of Logopedics and Phoniatrics. Each parameter on the GRBAS scale represents a dimension of phonation: G (grade) represents the overall severity of voice abnormality; R represents roughness; B represents breathiness; A represents aesthenic (weakness); and S represents strain. The GRBAS uses a four-point, equal-appearing interval (EAI) rating scale of 0 (normal) to 3 (extreme) for all five parameters.

The CAPE-V was drafted following the Consensus Conference on Auditory-Perceptual Evaluation of Voice held at the University of Pittsburgh in June, 2002. The conference was sponsored by ASHA's Division 3 (Voice and Voice Disorders) and brought together scientists, researchers, and clinicians interested in the problem of measuring voice quality. The instrument known as the CAPE-V was drafted by a working group of five participants following the conference and it was designed with two specific psychometric properties in mind: (1) It uses visual analog scales for rating several characteristics of voice, and (2) it is unanchored. The CAPE-V shares several of the parameters of the GRBAS scale. Judges rate six aspects of voice (Overall Severity, Roughness, Breathiness, Strain, Pitch, and Loudness) by placing a tick mark on a 100 mm line. The instrument includes two unlabeled scales in the event a voice includes other significant features (e.g., tremor).

An ASHA-sponsored national multicenter CAPE-V validation study, completed by Zraick and colleagues (Zraick, Klaben, Connor, Thibeault, Kempster, Glaze, et al., 2007), examined agreement for expert clinicians' ratings of dysphonia using the CAPE-V and the GRBAS. Inter-rater and intra-rater reliability across both scales was also assessed. It was reported that expert clinicians' perceptions of dysphonia appeared to be reliable and unaffected by rating instrument and that the CAPE-V appeared to be more sensitive than the GRBAS to small differences within and among patients. These findings are consistent with those of Karnell, Melton, Childes, Coleman, Dailey, and Hoffman (2007).

Quality of Life in Persons with Voice Disorders. Two basic approaches to quality of life measurement in persons with voice disorders are available: generic assessments that provide a summary of overall health-related quality of life, and specific assessments that focus on specific communication-related quality of life. In a recent survey of diagnostic practices of experienced voice clinicians (Behrman, 2005) 94% responded that communication-related quality of life instruments are important for assessment of treatment outcomes, and 81% considered the data from such instruments important in defining overall therapy goals (p. 460).

In general, voice disordered patients report poor overall health-related quality of life and communication-related quality of life (Cohen, Dupont, and Courey, 2006). The clinician should be aware, however, that variables such as life events and experiences, personality factors, and the effects of adaptation may influence reported subjective well-being (O'Connor, 2004).

Zraick and Risner (2008) provide a comprehensive review of instruments for assessing communication-related quality of life in persons with voice disorders. Table 6.1 lists some of the instruments currently available to clinicians, most of which are pyschometrically sound (Agency for Healthcare Research and Quality, 2002; Franic, Bramlett, and Bothe, 2004).

TABLE **6.1**	Major Voice Disordered Quality of Life (VDQOL) Instruments
Instrument Name and Acronym	**Developers**
Voice Handicap Index (VHI)	Jacobson, Johnson, Grywalski, Silbergleit, Jacobson, and Benninger (1997)
Voice Handicap Index—10 (VHI-10)	Rosen, Lee, Osborne, Zullo, and Murry (2004)
Voice Handicap Index—Partner (VHI-P)	Zraick, Risner, Smith-Olinde, Gregg, Johnson, and McWeeny (2006)
Pediatric Voice Handicap Index (pVHI)	Zur, Cotton, Kelchner, Baker, Weinrich, and Lee (2007)
Singing Voice Handicap Index (SVHI)	Cohen, Jacobson, Garrett, Noordzij, Stewart, Attia, Ossoff, and Cleveland (2007)
Vocal Performance Questionnaire (VPQ)	Carding, Horsley, and Docherty (1999)
Voice Symptom Scale (VoiSS)	Deary, Wilson, Carding, and MacKenzie (2003)
Voice Activity and Participation Profile (VAPP)	Ma and Yiu (2001)
Voice-Related Quality of Life (V-RQOL)	Hogikyan and Sethuraman (1999)
Pediatric Voice-Related Quality of Life (PVRQOL)	Boseley, Cunningham, Volk, and Hartnick (2006)
Voice Outcomes Survey (VOS)	Glicklich, Glovsky, and Montgomery (1999)
Pediatric Voice Outcomes Survey (PVOS)	Hartnick (2002)

Source: Adapted from Zraick and Risner (2008).

Instrumental Assessment

Laryngoscopy.   It is worth noting that indirect laryngoscopy, as described earlier in this chapter, is not the sole province of the physician. Appropriately trained clinicians may employ indirect laryngoscopy (and other laryngeal visualization techniques) in accordance with ASHA's *Scope of Practice for Clinicians* (2007). A joint statement regarding the use of videolaryngoscopy has been developed by the American Academy of Otolaryngology Voice and Swallow Committee and ASHA's Special Interest Division 3 (Voice and Voice Disorders) and states in part, "Clinicians with expertise in voice disorders and with specialized training in videolaryngoscopy are professionals qualified to use this procedure for the purpose of assessing voice production and vocal function" (ASHA, 1998a). ASHA has also published a position statement regarding laryngeal videostroboscopy (2004e), a technical report on laryngeal videostroboscopy (2004f), and a knowledge and skills document for clinicians with respect to vocal tract visualization and imaging (2004c). Figure 6.4 lists some of the competencies expected of clinicians performing laryngeal videostroboscopy (ASHA, 1998b).

Many times the information gained from laryngeal videostroboscopic visualization of the larynx has been the most important information derived from the diagnostic assessment (McFarlane and Watterson, 1990; McFarlane, Watterson, and Brophy, 1990). When coupled with the other information, visualization of the larynx has greatly improved accuracy of diagnosis and has set the foundation for successful voice therapy plans.

Acoustic Analyses.   Due to advances in technology and greater affordability of equipment, acoustic analysis of the voice is becoming increasingly more common in clinical practice. For acoustic measurements to be valid, they must be able to (1) discriminate the normal from dysphonic voice, (2) correlate positively with the clinician's auditory–perceptual judgments of the voice, and (3) be sufficiently stable to assess change across time (Stemple, Glaze, and Klaben, 2000). The most routinely obtained measures assess the following five acoustic properties of the vocal signal: (1) fundamental frequency, (2) intensity, (3) perturbation, (4) sound spectrography, and (5) signal (or harmonics)-to-noise ratio.

Frequency.   Average fundamental frequency (average F_0) is the rate of vibration of the vocal folds and is expressed in Hertz (Hz), or the number of cycles of vocal fold vibration per second. Fundamental frequency correlates with the auditory perception of pitch. A number of fundamental frequency measures can be obtained, depending on the clinical scenario. Three aspects of frequency are commonly assessed: (1) speaking fundamental frequency (SFF), (2) frequency variability, and (3) phonational frequency range (PFR). A fourth frequency-related measure, the voice range profile (VRP), is also sometimes obtained in conjunction with measurement of intensity and will be discussed in that section.

Speaking fundamental frequency is the average F_0 in connected speech and is correlated with the perception of habitual pitch. Habitual pitch is defined by Case

FIGURE **6.4**

Competencies and Skills of Speech–Language Pathologists Performing Laryngeal Videoendoscopy/Stroboscopy (LVES)

1. Familiarity with the various roles of otolaryngologists, speech–language pathologists, nurses, and support staff involved in the provision of LVES
2. Ability to communicate well with otolaryngologists, nurses, and patients in an interdisciplinary patient care environment
3. Familiarity with normal and pathological laryngeal anatomy and physiology, medical terminology as it pertains to laryngeal disorders, and principles and techniques of voice treatment
4. Familiarity with the various approaches to becoming trained to perform LVES
5. Ability to identify, select, assemble, operate, and maintain the equipment necessary to perform LVES
6. Ability to recognize and identify patients who are appropriate for LVES
7. Ability to technically perform LVES using oral and flexible endoscopes in a manner that yields maximum quality recordings
8. Ability to interpret effects of vocal behavior and laryngeal anatomy on laryngeal physiology in coordination and cooperation with medical colleagues
9. Ability to concisely describe LVES findings and interpretations for professional communication purposes
10. Ability to organize, store, and retrieve LVES data for quality assurance and treatment efficacy purposes

Source: This excerpt from *Training Guidelines for Laryngeal Videoendoscopy/Stroboscopy* [Guidelines] (1988), published by the American Speech and Hearing Association (ASHA), is reprinted by permission. Readers are directed to the ASHA website (www.asha.org) to access the Guidelines (and any updates) in its entirety.

(2002) as "the modal or average pitch heard in a continuing sample of speech, the level around which normal pitch inflections occur." While there is no "optimal pitch" for a given speaker, there is usually a habitual pitch that is best for the patient during the initial period of voice therapy. We use the term "best pitch" to describe the pitch that best results in a slightly louder voice of clearer quality that can be produced with an economy of physical effort and energy. It is worth noting that we tend to use a relatively small range of frequencies toward the lower end of our range. An individual's habitual pitch is dependent on his or her age, gender, and race. There are published average F_0 and SFF norms for a variety of speaker groups, and it is incumbent on the clinician to use these norms when making a clinical judgment about the suitability of a particular patient's habitual pitch (Andrews and Summers, 2002; Zraick, Gregg, and Whitehouse, 2006).

Various methods have been proposed for eliciting SFF. Zraick, Skaggs, and Montague (2000) compared SFF across different speaking tasks (automatic speech, elicited speech, spontaneous speech, and reading aloud) and reported no significant differences. Zraick, Birdwell, and Smith-Olinde (2005) compared SFF across different speaking durations (1, 5, 15, 30, and 60 seconds) and reported significant differences between the 30- and 60-second samples. Zraick, Gentry, Smith-Olinde, and Gregg (2006) compared SFF across different social contexts (speaking during a voice evaluation, in public, to a peer, to a superior, to a subordinate, and to a parent or spouse) and reported that SFF differed depending on who was the patient's communication partner. Results of these studies (and others) indicate that SFF should probably be interpreted in light of how it was elicited. It is generally reported that the adult male voice is somewhere near 123 Hz, an adult female, 220 Hz, and a child's voice, between 264 and 294 Hz.

Frequency variability is the range of SFFs used in connected speech. Normal voices have some frequency variability, perceived by the listener as acceptable changes in prosody. In some dysphonic speakers, however, frequency can be either more or less variable than expected or tolerated by the listener. Increased frequency variability may be perceived as a childlike "sing-song" prosody, while decreased frequency variability may be perceived as monotone. Abnormal frequency variability may have a functional, organic, or neurological basis.

Frequency variability is measured in terms of the standard deviation (SD) from the average F_0. F_0SD reflects the range of frequencies around the average F_0, measured in Hertz. F_0SD in normal connected speech is around 20–30 Hz but can be greater depending on the speaker's mood. For steady-state sustained vowels F_0SD should be even lower (3–6 Hz); higher F_0SD values can indicate a patient's difficulty with control of frequency. When F_0SD is converted to semitones it is referred to as pitch sigma. Pitch sigma should be around 2–4 semitones for connected speech (there are 12 semitones in an octave).

Phonational frequency range, more commonly referred to as maximum phonational frequency range (MPFR) is defined by Hollien, Dew, and Philips (1971) as "that range of vocal frequencies encompassing both the modal and falsetto registers; its extent is from the lowest tone sustainable in the modal register to the highest in falsetto register, inclusive." MPFR is one of the most frequently obtained voice measures (Hirano, 1989) and can be measured in Hertz, semitones, or octaves. An MPFR of about three octaves (36 semitones) is expected for healthy young adults, with a smaller MPFR expected in older adults (Kent, 1994). The patient's MPFR should be determined as a prelude to identifying that person's best pitch level (the patient's easiest and most compatible voice pitch) at which to begin therapy probes.

Zraick, Nelson, Montague, and Monoson (2000) compared two methods for eliciting MPFR (stepping from lowest to highest note versus gliding from lowest to highest note) and reported that stair-step progression through the range resulted in a larger MPFR. Zraick, Keyes, Montague, and Keiser (2002) compared whether the lowest or highest pitch should be obtained first and reported that obtaining the lowest pitch followed by the highest pitch resulted in a larger MPFR. Results of these studies (and others) indicate that MPFR should probably be interpreted in light of how it was elicited.

Intensity.   Vocal intensity corresponds with the acoustic power of the speaker and correlates with the auditory perception of loudness. Intensity is typically reported in dB SPL (decibels sound-pressure level). A number of intensity measures can be obtained, depending on the clinical scenario. Three measures of intensity are commonly assessed: (1) habitual intensity, (2) intensity variability/stability, and (3) intensity (dynamic) range. A fourth intensity-related measure, the voice range profile (VRP), is also sometimes obtained in conjunction with measurement of frequency.

Habitual loudness is the average loudness level used by the speaker for the majority of their vocalizations. For most speakers, their habitual loudness should be loud enough to allow them to be heard over background noise but not so loud that it brings the listener discomfort or distraction (Awan, 2001). Normal conversational speech usually is in the range of 65–80 dB SPL, with an average for males and females (adults and children) of around 70 dB SPL (Baken, 1996). Older adults may exhibit a slightly less intense conversational voice. Various methods have been proposed for eliciting habitual intensity. Key considerations when measuring intensity are the mouth-to-microphone distance, the level of ambient or background noise, speaking task, and SFF. Although no standard exists, a common mouth-to-microphone distance is 12 inches (30 cm). One should document the distance and use this consistently when comparing intensity values across sessions. Zraick, Marshall, Smith-Olinde, and Montague (2004) suggest that clinicians use more than one task to determine habitual loudness. For example, values elicited by having the patient count from 1 to 10, speak spontaneously, and read aloud could be averaged before a determination is made about whether therapy to address loudness is necessary.

Intensity variability is the range of intensities used in connected speech. Normal voices have some intensity variability, perceived by the listener as acceptable changes in intonation. In some dysphonic speakers, however, intensity can be either more or less variable than expected or tolerated by the listener. In connected speech, decreased intensity variability may be perceived as monoloudness. Abnormal intensity variability may have either a physiological etiology (such as Parkinson's disease, vocal fold paralysis, or hearing loss) or may result from learned behavior.

Intensity variability is measured in terms of the standard deviation (SD) from the average intensity. This SD reflects the range of intensities around the average intensity, measured in dB SPL. Intensity SD for a neutral, unemotional sentence is around 10 dB, but can be higher depending on the speaker's mood.

Intensity (dynamic) range reflects the physiologic range of intensities, from softest nonwhisper to loudest shout, that the patient can produce without undue physical strain. People rarely speak at either end of their dynamic range (approximately 50–115 dB) for extended periods. Therefore, the clinician should focus his or her attention on the dynamic range available to the patient around the patient's habitual loudness. For example, if a patient's habitual loudness is 70 dB in most speaking environments and situations, then intentionally varying the intensity by

±15 dB should result in a voice (and speaker) perceived as more dynamic. The dynamic range depends on the F_0 produced and tends to be greatest for F_0 in the midrange and less for F_0 that is much lower or higher (Ferrand, 2007). The fact that F_0 and intensity covary leads some to propose the use of the voice range profile (VRP) to assess some patients.

The VRP from a phonetogram or phonogram (see Figure 6.5) is a graphic display of the relationship between intensity and F_0. The patient is asked to phonate the vowel /i/ or /a/ at select frequencies across his or her frequency range (modeled by a tone-generator such as a piano or pitch pipe or presented by computer software), both as softly and loudly as possible. The upper contour of the VRP represents the patient's maximum phonation threshold (maximum intensity at each frequency) and the lower contour represents the patient's minimum phonation threshold (minimum intensity at each frequency). A normal VRP should have an oblique-oval shape; at the physiologic extremes of vocal range, there is a minimal intensity difference between the soft and loud phonations (LeBorgne, 2007). A constricted (compressed) VRP indicates that the patient has difficulty achieving normal frequency and intensity ranges. Obtaining a complete VRP for some patients can be challenging, leading some to propose various customized VRP protocols for clinical use (Holmberg, Ihre, and Södersten, 2007; Ma, Roberston, Radford,

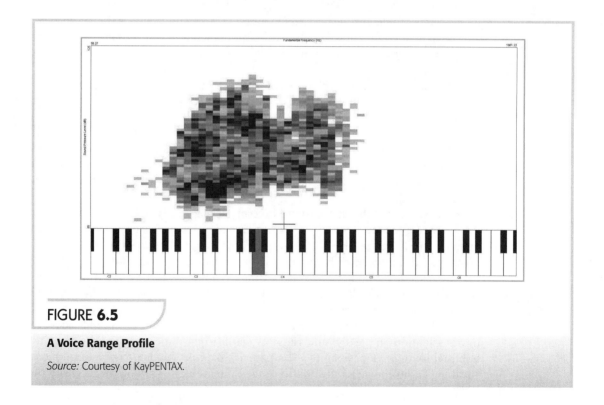

FIGURE **6.5**

A Voice Range Profile

Source: Courtesy of KayPENTAX.

Vagne, El-Halabi, and Yiu, 2007; Wingate, Brown, Shrivastav, Davenport, and Sapienza, 2007; Wingate and Collins, 2005).

Perturbation.   Perturbation is defined by Titze (1994) as the variability or irregularity in a system. Applied to voice, then, it is the cycle-to-cycle variability in the vocal signal. A small amount of cycle-to-cycle variability is expected in the normal voice, which results from aperiodic vibration of the vocal folds. Unlike the frequency/intensity variability previously discussed, perturbation is aimed at identifying the short-term cycle-to-cycle, nonvolitional variability, not the longer-term, volitional word or utterance (prosodic) trends. As such, perturbation measures can only be derived from vowels, most accurately, sustained vowels or steady-state portions of vowels extracted from connected speech. Two commonly obtained perturbation measures are jitter and shimmer.

Jitter is the short-term variability in fundamental frequency, while shimmer is the short-term variability in the amplitude of the acoustic waveform. There are a variety of perturbation measures from which to choose, making valid selection and interpretation difficult (see Behrman, 2007, and Ferrand, 2007, for descriptions of the most common perturbation measures). Standardization is almost nonexistent when it comes to perturbation measures, making them potentially less clinically useful, particularly when comparing research results across sites, clinicians, and equipment manufacturers. Further limiting the clinical utility of perturbation measures is the fact that a direct correlation between jitter and shimmer and voice impairment does not exist (Kreiman and Gerratt, 2005). Also, because a coherent database of normative perturbation values does not exist, perturbation cannot be used to reliably differentiate between normal and abnormal voices (Behrman, 2007). Generally, jitter of less than 1.0% and shimmer of less than 2.6% are considered normal clinically. Children demonstrate higher jitter and shimmer than adults, and older adults demonstrate higher jitter and shimmer than younger adults (Gorham-Rowan and Laures-Gore, 2006). Perturbation is best interpreted in combination with other instrumental assessment data and clinical impressions.

Sound Spectrography.   Sound spectrography is the graphic representation of the frequency and intensity of the sound wave as a function of time. The resulting graphic, known as a spectrogram, reflects the harmonic structure of the glottal sound source and the resonant characteristics of the vocal tract. Frequency is displayed on the vertical axis, time is represented on the horizontal axis, and intensity is represented by the darkness of the trace on the screen or paper (see Figure 6.6). The fundamental frequency is always represented by the lowest energy band, with energy in the higher frequencies in bands above. When grayscale is used, darker gray bands represent greater energy. When obtaining a spectrogram the clinician needs to decide how the spectrograph should filter and then display the sound signal. Two choices are possible—narrow-band filtering and wide-band filtering. The bandwidth refers to the analysis window around the fundamental frequency. With narrow-band filtering there is good frequency resolution but poor time resolution. In wide-band filtering, there is good time resolution

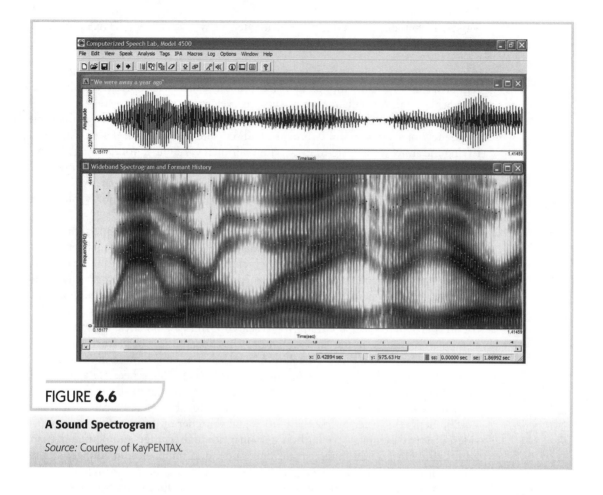

FIGURE 6.6

A Sound Spectrogram

Source: Courtesy of KayPENTAX.

but poor frequency resolution. That is, the narrow-band spectrogram displays individual harmonics well, while the wide-band spectrogram displays a number of harmonics at once.

Signal (or Harmonics)-to-Noise Ratio. The harmonics-to-noise ratio (HNR) is a measure of the ratio of energy in the fundamental and harmonics to the energy in the aperiodic (or noise) component of the voice signal (Yumoto, Gould, and Baer, 1982). It is typically reported in dB SPL. HNR quantifies the relative amount of additive noise (aperiodic vibration) in the voice signal (Murphy and Akande, 2007; Shama, Krishna, and Cholayya, 2007). In breathiness the excessive escape of air adds turbulent noise (aperiodic vibration); in harshness/hoarseness irregularity of vocal fold vibration adds noise. Thus, a higher HNR indicates that the harmonic components of the voice are more intense than the noise components. Stated another way, the lower the HNR, the more noise there is in the voice.

Generally, a HNR of approximately 12 dB or greater is indicative of a voice with normal quality (Yumoto et al., 1982), with higher normative HNRs commonly reported (Awan and Frenkel, 1994; Horii and Fuller, 1990). Ferrand (2000, 2002) has reported that HNRs for children and older adults are lower than HNRs for young and middle-aged adults. HNR correlates well with the perception of dysphonia (de Krom, 1995), making it a useful clinical measure.

Aerodynamic Measurements.   Just as with acoustic voice analysis, aerodynamic analysis of the voice is becoming increasingly more possible and common in clinical practice. Aerodynamic measures reveal indirect physiologic information about the valving activity of the larynx. Routinely obtained measures include (1) lung volumes and capacities, (2) air pressure, (3) airflow, (4) laryngeal resistance, and (5) durational measures such as maximum phonation duration and the s/z ratio. Each of these will be described following a brief discussion of respiratory patterns.

Prior to quantitatively assessing respiration, we suggest careful observation of the patient's breathing patterns. An inefficient breathing pattern or a lack of coordination between inspiratory and expiratory movements can contribute to dysphonia. For example, the patient may have to take more frequent breath groups, or they may adopt increased musculoskeletal tension resulting in vocal hyperfunction. Three basic types of breathing patterns have been described: clavicular, thoracic, and diaphragmatic–abdominal.

- *Clavicular breathing.* This inefficient type of breathing is probably the easiest to identify. The patient elevates the shoulders on inspiration, using the neck accessory muscles as the primary muscles of inspiration. This upper chest breathing, characterized by noticeable elevation of the clavicles, is unsatisfactory for good voice for two reasons. First, the resulting weak and shallow inspiration does not provide adequate respiratory support for speech and voice. Secondly, overuse of many of the neck accessory muscles for respiration (particularly the sternocleidomastoids) may effect an increase in laryngeal tension (Prater, Swift, Miller, and Deem, 1999).
- *Thoracic breathing.* This type of breathing is characterized by expansion of the thorax and contraction of the abdomen during inspiration, reversed during expiration. It is the normal breathing pattern for most people. In some cases, however, thoracic breathing can be characterized by shallow breathing punctuated by breath holding or gasping.
- *Diaphragmatic–abdominal breathing.* This may well be the preferred method of respiration, especially if the patient has heavy vocal demands, as in singing or acting. This breathing pattern is characterized by abdominal and lower thoracic expansion on inspiration, with little noticeable upper chest movement, and a gradual decrease in abdominal and lower thoracic prominence on expiration.

Hixon and Hoit (1998, 1999, 2000) have written extensively about the clinical evaluation of speech breathing and have also published a comprehensive text on the evaluation and management of speech breathing disorders (Hixon and Hoit,

2005). These authors emphasize the role of the speech breathing case history in evaluating patients. The speech breathing case history described by Hixon and Hoit (2005) includes the following sections: (1) alerting signs and symptoms; (2) airway risk factors; (3) medical evaluations, diagnoses, and treatments; (4) breathing and speaking experiences; and (5) client perceptions of speech breathing. Figure 6.7 lists some of the alerting signs and symptoms described (p. 196) and Figure 6.8 lists some of the abnormal client perceptions of speech breathing (pp. 200–201).

Lung Volumes and Capacities.   Part of evaluating respiratory adequacy is measuring the patient's lung volume. Lung volumes refer to the amount of air in the lungs at a given time and how much of that air is used for various purposes, including speech (Solomon and Charron, 1998). Lung volumes include *tidal volume* (amount of air that can be inspired and expired in a normal breathing cycle), *inspiratory reserve volume* (maximum amount of additional air that can be inspired after a tidal inhalation is completed), *expiratory reserve volume* (maximum volume of air that can be expired after a tidal expiration), and *residual volume* (air remaining in the lungs even after a maximum exhalation). Lung capacities combine various lung volumes and include *inspiratory capacity* (tidal volume + inspiratory reserve volume), *vital capacity* (tidal volume + inspiratory reserve volume + expiratory reserve volume), *functional residual capacity* (expiratory reserve volume + residual volume), and *total lung capacity* (tidal volume + inspiratory reserve volume + expiratory reserve volume + residual volume). Lung volumes and capacities vary depending on the patient's age, gender, level of physical exertion, and vocal training. Data reported by Hoit and Hixon (1987) and Hoit and colleagues (1989, 1990) indicate that, in general, lung volumes and capacities increase from infancy through puberty and then remain stable until advancing age, when they decrease slightly.

FIGURE **6.7**

Alerting Speech Breathing Signs and Symptoms

Frequent coughing

Persistent hoarse voice

Coughing up mucus

Coughing up blood

Wheezing

Difficulty breathing

Chest pain

Numbness, weakness, coordination problems, or involuntary movements

Source: From Hixon and Hoit (2005).

FIGURE **6.8**

Abnormal Client Perceptions of Speech Breathing

Frequent awareness of breathing

Hunger for air

Uncomfortable urge to breathe

Breathlessness

Shortness of breath

Hard work to breathe

High effort to breathe

Weak breathing muscles

Tired breathing muscles

Difficulty inhaling

Difficulty exhaling

Tightness in chest

Difficulty coordinating breathing movements

Need to think about breathing

Feelings of distress with breathing

Feelings of panic with breathing

Source: From Hixon and Hoit (2005).

Air Pressure. Various air pressures are necessary for speech. These include pressure inside the lungs, pressure below the vocal folds, and pressure inside the oral cavity. Air pressure is measured and expressed in units of cmH_2O. The total pressure that a person can generate may be as high as 50 cmH_2O or more, yet the pressure needed for conversational speech is only around 5–10 cmH_2O. Greater pressures than this may be required, however, depending on syllable stress and loudness demands (Stathopoulos and Sapienza, 1997). Pressure below the vocal folds is estimated indirectly by measuring oral pressure during production of the closed portion of a voiceless bilabial consonant such as /p/. When producing this consonant, the lips are closed and the velopharyngeal port is sealed and the glottis is open—thus, pressures throughout the system are equal. Oral pressure is measured by a pressure transducer connected to a small tube placed just inside the mouth (Smitheran and Hixon, 1981).

Airflow. Laryngeal airflow is the volume of air passing through the glottis in a fixed period of time. It is typically measured in cubic centimeters (cc) or milliliters (mL) per second. For example, the /a/ vowel produced with a normal voice quality is characterized by an approximate laryngeal airflow of 100 cc/sec (Baken, 1996). That same vowel produced with a breathy voice quality (perhaps by a patient with large bilateral nodules) would be characterized by a laryngeal airflow of higher than 100 cc/sec due to excessively decreased glottal resistance to airflow. At the opposite end of the continuum, that same vowel produced with a strained–strangled voice quality (perhaps by a patient with adductor spasmodic dysphonia) would be characterized by a laryngeal airflow of less than 100 cc/sec due to excessively increased glottal resistance to airflow. Peak airflow (i.e., greatest flow) can be considerably higher than 100 cc/sec and depends on articulatory demands. For example, peak airflow during production of fricatives and stop consonants may exceed 500 cc/sec (Stathopoulos and Weismer, 1985). Children and older adults tend to demonstrate higher laryngeal airflows than younger adults (Stathopoulos and Sapienza, 1997).

Laryngeal Resistance.   Laryngeal resistance is a measure derived from peak intraoral pressure and peak airflow during production of the /pi/ syllable repeated at a rate of approximately 1.5 syllables/second. Peak intraoral pressure is estimated from the /p/ portion of the syllable and peak airflow is measured from the /i/ portion of the syllable. A breathy voice would suggest decreased laryngeal resistance, while a strain–strangled voice would suggest increased laryngeal resistance. When interpreting laryngeal resistance values, the clinician must examine the relative contribution of pressure and flow to that value.

Maximum Phonation Duration (Time).   Maximum phonation duration (MPD) is an indirect index of laryngeal airflow. MPD is the greatest length of time over which the /a/ vowel can be sustained at the patient's most comfortable pitch and loudness following a maximal inhalation. Verbal encouragement and a clinician model are usually given, and the longest of three trials is usually reported. If airflow is high, MPD is shorter than normal; if airflow is low, MPD may be longer than normal. Normative data for MPD across the age span is found in a review by Kent, Kent, and Rosenbek (1987) of maximum performance tests of speech production. Average MPD is 10.5 seconds for six-year-olds, increasing to approximately 28 seconds for young adults, and declining to 13 seconds for the elderly. The authors point out, however, that variability is large. Perhaps one of the most efficient uses of MPD is as a baseline against which future comparisons can be made.

s/z Ratio.   The s/z ratio is also an indirect index of laryngeal airflow. To obtain the s/z ratio, the clinician asks the patient to first sustain the /s/ as long as possible, and then to sustain the /z/ as long as possible. Verbal encouragement is usually given, and the longest /s/ and longest /z/ from one of three alternating /s, z/ trials is used to calculate the ratio. The s/z ratio of normal subjects approximates 1.0, indicating that the voiceless exhalation time (the /s/) closely matches maximum phonation duration (the /z/) (Tait, Michel, and Carpenter, 1980). In 95% of their patients with glottal margin pathologies (nodules, polyps, thickening), Eckel and Boone (1981) found s/z ratios greater than 1.4, indicating marked reduction in voiced duration values.

Rastatter and Hyman (1982) reported in their prepubertal patients with vocal fold nodules that the presence of vocal nodules did not affect the s/z ratio, whereas the durations of /s/ and /z/ and the variance observed across multiple productions of /z/ are affected and should be considered as diagnostically significant. It should be cautioned that the s/z ratio is a crude, quick appraisal technique based on the possibility of air wastage due to a vocal fold lesion (Trudeau and Forrest, 1997). It may be helpful for those clinicians without the benefit of instrumentation. Elevated s/z ratios may be a red flag to check the glottal edge of the vocal folds for an additive lesion, or to suspect glottic insufficiency due to vocal fold paralysis (Miller, 2004).

Electroglottography.   Electroglottography (EGG) is a noninvasive technique for obtaining an estimate of vocal fold contact patterns during phonation. A gold electrode is placed on each side of the thyroid cartilage at a level corresponding to the position of the vocal folds. A small electrical current is passed between the electrodes. Vibrations of the vocal folds rhythmically change the contact area between them, which is registered as variable changes in the electrical resistance between the electrodes. Resistance increases when the glottis is opening or open and decreases when the glottis is closing or closed. The resulting waveform, called an electroglottogram or laryngogram (see Figure 6.9) reveals summary information about vocal fold contact over time, with peaks and troughs representing maximum points of open and closed phases. The EGG can be used to visualize various types of voice quality. For example, Figure 6.10 shows electroglottograms for a prolonged /i/ vowel produced with a normal voice quality, a breathy voice quality, and a hoarse voice quality.

THE CLINICAL VOICE LABORATORY

Instrumental analysis of voice, as described in this chapter, is common in many voice clinics and other settings where voice patients are evaluated. Due to advances in microprocessor technology, computer-based hardware and software systems are becoming more affordable and automated. Be this as it may, clinical instrumentation, no matter how sophisticated, cannot replace the mind, eyes, and ears of a well-trained clinician. That is, instrumental data must be paired with clinical impressions and auditory–perceptual judgments of voice to be used meaningfully.

When instrumentation is utilized, there are principles of calibration, standardization of measurement technique, data interpretation, reliability of measures, hygiene, and examiner training that are fundamental to valid outcomes (Brown, Vinson, and Crary, 1996; Klein, Piccirillo, and Painter, 2000). At a minimum, the clinician should be mindful of the following equipment considerations when obtaining voice recordings for clinical purposes: (1) sound isolation and ambient room noise, (2) microphone choice, (3) sound-level meter choice, (4) cable choice, (5) computer specifications, (6) recording software, and (7) choice of video recorder and monitor (Spielman, Starr, Popolo, and Hunter, 2007).

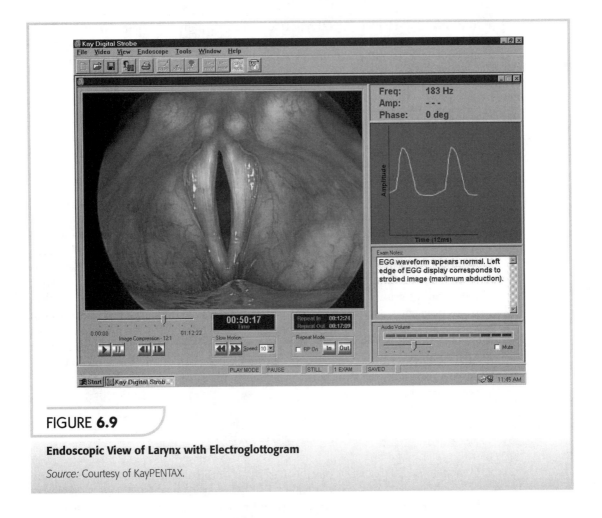

FIGURE **6.9**

Endoscopic View of Larynx with Electroglottogram

Source: Courtesy of KayPENTAX.

Stemple and colleagues (2000, p. 180) suggest that the clinical utility of in-strumental measures can be assessed on four levels of clinical application. Specif-ically, does the instrumentation: (1) identify the existence of a voice problem? (2) assess the severity or stage of progression of the voice problem? (3) identify the dif-ferential source of the voice problem? and (4) serve as a primary treatment tool for behavioral modification, biofeedback, or patient education? These questions often guide the choice of instruments used and the recording protocols that are followed.

Clinical Instrumentation for Acoustic Analysis

A relatively inexpensive clinical instrument for the measurement of pitch is the piano or electric keyboard. Isolated vowels or connected speech can be produced by the patient and pitch-matched on the keyboard by the clinician (see Figure 6.11). With

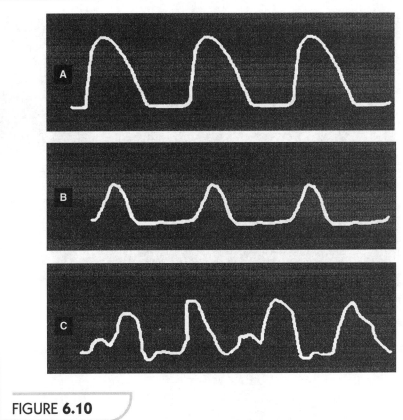

FIGURE **6.10**

Electroglottograms

These three electroglottograms are productions of the /i/ vowel with (A) normal vocal quality, (B) breathy quality, and (C) hoarse vocal quality. The normal trace (A) demonstrates a sharp vertical rise, a narrow peak, an even return to baseline, and a substantial closed phase. Trace (B), the breathy voice quality, is represented in the sloping voice onset, rather than the vertical rise seen in the normal trace and the long open phase. Trace (C), the hoarse voice, is indicated by the lack of a uniform wave form from one cycle to the next.

a piano or keyboard (or pitch pipe, for that matter), it is possible to estimate SFF, frequency variability, and MPFR because the tones produced by the human voice can be matched to the musical notes of these instruments. For example, in Hertz, the typical adult male voice is somewhere near B2 (123 Hz), an adult female voice is in the vicinity of A3 (220 Hz), and a child's voice is somewhere between C4 and D4 (262 to 294 Hz). Each octave on a musical instrument comprises eight whole tones, with each tone represented by an alphabetical letter. Sharps and flats

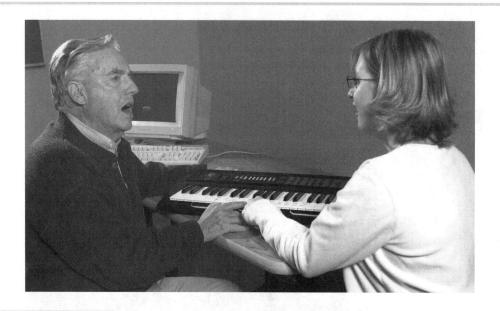

FIGURE **6.11**

A Typical Electronic Keyboard Used in Voice Evaluation and Therapy

represent semitones. There are 12 semitones in an octave. Each C begins a new octave. Each octave represents a doubling of frequency of vocal fold vibration. Therefore, an increase from C3 to C4 represents a doubling of frequency (131 Hz + 131 Hz = 262 Hz). See Table 6.2 for a musical note to frequency chart.

A relatively inexpensive clinical instrument for the measurement of loudness-related parameters is the Level II sound-level meter, such as can be commonly obtained from a vendor such as RadioShack. Analog and digital versions are available. Most consumer sound-level meters are sensitive from 40 to 130 dB SPL, with slow or fast response for checking peak and average signal levels. The sound-level meter should have the ability to employ different weighting filters, with a C or linear weighting being the most desirable for voice recordings. Typically, the sound-level meter is held by the clinician at a distance of 50 cm from the speaker.

The Visi-Pitch IV (Model 3950, KayPENTAX Corp.) is a widely-used clinical instrument for measuring habitual pitch and loudness, frequency and intensity variability, and MPFR and dynamic range, among other things (Figure 6.12). The Visi-Pitch IV extracts acoustic parameters during speech production and presents them in real time, providing clients with clear, intuitive visual displays. Target vocalizations provided by a clinician can be compared to client attempts, both graphically

TABLE **6.2**	Musical Note to Frequency Chart				
Note	**Freq. (Hz)**	**Note**	**Freq. (Hz)**	**Note**	**Freq. (Hz)**
A_1	55	A_3	220	A^5	880
B_1	62	B_3	245	B^5	988
C_2	65	C^4	262	C^6	1046
D_2	73	D^4	294	D^6	1175
E_2	82	E^4	330	E^6	1318
F_2	87	F^4	349	F^6	1397
G_2	98	G^4	392	G^6	1568
A_2	110	A^4	440	A^6	1760
B_2	123	B^4	494	B^6	1975
C_3	131	C^5	523	C^7	2093
D_3	147	D^5	587	D^7	2349
E_3	164	E^5	659	E^7	2637
F_3	175	F^5	698	F^7	7294
G_3	196	G^5	784	G^7	3136

Note: The notes are sequentially numbered, from left to right on the piano keyboard, starting with the first C-octave. All decimals are rounded off. The Visi-Pitch will only record between 0–1600 Hz.

Source: Reprinted courtesy of KayPENTAX.

and with auditory playback. Monitoring important speech–voice behaviors with concrete visual displays helps clients reach therapy goals more easily.

The Computerized Speech Lab (Model 4500, KayPENTAX Corp.) is a more comprehensive hardware system than the Visi-Pitch IV, with optional software and database options (Figure 6.13). Some of the more clinically useful Computerized Speech Lab (CSL) options for voice include: Auditory Feedback Tools (Model 3506), Disordered Voice Database (Model 4337), Games (Model 5167), Multi-Dimensional Voice Program (Model 5105), Real-Time EGG Analysis (Model 5138), Real-Time Pitch (Model 5121), Real-Time Spectrogram (Model 5129), and the Voice Range Profile (Model 4326). The Multidimensional Voice Program (MDVP), for example, analyzes and displays 33 different vocal parameters, including the more commonly reported jitter, shimmer, and harmonic-to-noise ratios.

The Nagashima Phonatory Function Analyzer (Model PS77E, Kelleher Medical, Inc.) measures habitual pitch and loudness. If a mask is used, then pitch and loudness can be measured in connected speech. With a disposable mouthpiece (as shown in Figure 6.14) only sustained vowels may be analyzed. Of particular value is the fact that this instrument is capable of five simultaneous acoustic and aerodynamic

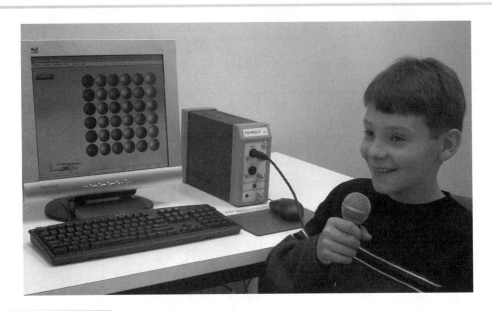

FIGURE **6.12**

A Visi-Pitch IV in Clinical Use

Source: Courtesy of KayPENTAX.

measures of voice: (1) average fundamental frequency, (2) sound pressure level, (3) mean flow rate, (4) expiratory lung pressure, and (5) airway resistance.

Many voice disorders are chronic or recurring conditions that result from faulty and/or abusive vocal behaviors. Such behaviorally based disorders are difficult to assess and rehabilitate because patient self-reporting and self-monitoring is subjective and often unreliable. Instrumentation has recently become available that gives clinicians and researchers quantitative data on a patient's voice use throughout the day. The Ambulatory Phonation Monitor (KayPENTAX) developed in conjunction with researchers at Sensimetrics Corporation and clinicians at Massachusetts General Hospital, is a portable device worn by clients (Figure 6.15) to capture important parameters of vocal behavior over an entire day of normal activity (Cheyne, Hanson, Genereux, Stevens, and Hillman, 2003). The Ambulatory Phonation Monitor (APM) works via an accelerometer that measures the vibration of the skin of the neck occuring during phonation. The accelerometer signal is analyzed to provide percentage phonation time, fundamental frequency, sound pressure level, and vocal dosage. The APM may facilitate carryover of behaviors that are established in voice therapy by providing vibrotactile biofeedback to the user when voice usage parameters exceed limits set by the therapist. The Denver Center for the Performing

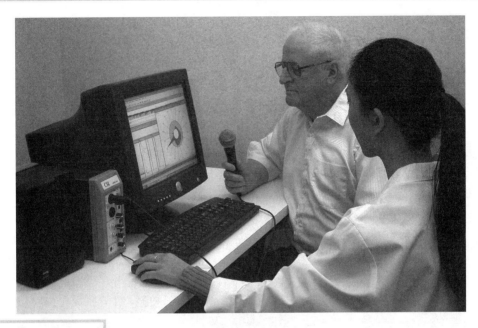

FIGURE **6.13**

Computerized Speech Lab

Source: Courtesy of KayPENTAX.

Arts has also developed a vocal dosimeter which provides similar measures for research purposes (Popolo, Svec, and Titze, 2005).

Recently, high-speed digital imaging (HSDI) of the larynx has been evaluated for clinical value compared to traditional laryngostroboscopy (Patel, Dailey, and Bless, 2008). Laryngostroboscopy works by synchronizing the flash of the stroboscopic light with the fundamental frequency of the vocal fold vibration, revealing an average pattern of vibration across multiple cycles. It requires a periodic voice signal and is of somewhat limited value with severely dysphonic patients. HSDI captures several thousand frames per second, providing a true view of vocal fold movement that does not require periodic phonation, and is able to visualize vocal fold vibration irrespective of the degree of aperiodicity and level of dysphonia. Patel and colleagues conclude that HSDI has value for evaluating grade II (moderate hoarseness) and grade IV (severe hoarseness) voice qualities and patients with neuromuscular conditions. In addition, HSDI provides valuable information on vocal fold movement that is not available via laryngostroboscopy, including the observation of phonatory onset, very short voicing segments, and spasms. Limitations of HSDI (compared to laryngostroboscopy) include the lack of audio, the

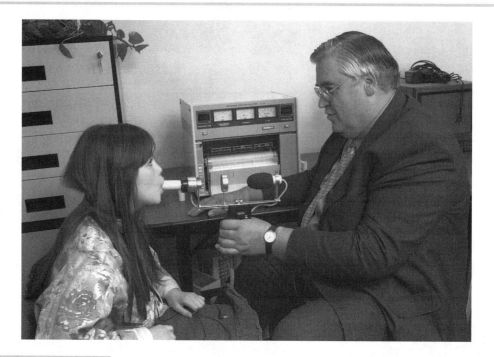

FIGURE **6.14**

Phonatory Function Analyzer

The phonatory function analyzer is used here to evaluate phonation time (in seconds), fundamental frequency (Hz), vocal intensity (dB SPL), airflow rate (mL/sec), and total volume of air (mL) during each phonation attempt.

inability to use a flexible endoscope with the procedure, and a limited sample of phonation (usually 2 seconds).

Clinical Instrumentation for Aerodynamic Analysis

The aerodynamic capacities and volumes we need to measure can be determined by using wet or dry spirometers. In the wet spirometer a container floats in water placed in a larger container. As air is introduced to the smaller floating container, it floats higher in proportion to the volume of air introduced. The distance or rise of displacement is measured in terms of cubic centimeters or liters. Some spirometers are of the dry type. A flexible container enlarges on inspiratory tasks and decreases in volume on expiratory tasks, in both instances measuring the volume of displacement. Recent advances in technology have resulted in miniaturization

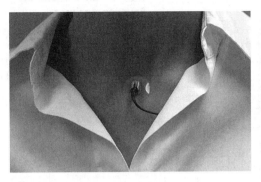 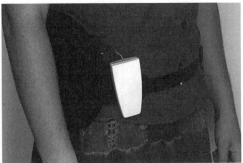

FIGURE **6.15**

An Ambulatory Phonation Monitor in Use

Source: Courtesy of KayPENTAX.

and digitization of dry spirometers, allowing for ease of use and reduced cost compared to wet spirometers.

Relatively inexpensive pressure measuring gauges and manometers are available to measure airflow pressures. For example, Hixon, Hawley, and Wilson (1982) described a simple water manometer test that can be used to estimate the ability to generate respiratory driving pressure sufficient for voice and speech. The test requires a drinking glass that is 12 cm deep or deeper, filled with water and calibrated in centimeters by a marker pen. A plastic straw is attached to the cup with a paper clip. The bottom tip of the straw is anchored at 10 cm below the rim. The patient is instructed to blow bubbles through the straw. If the patient maintains a stream of bubbles for 5 seconds with the straw at a depth of 10 cm (10 cm H_2O), the authors suggest that breath support is sufficient for most speech purposes.

The Nagashima Phonatory Function Analyzer, described previously in regard to acoustic voice analysis, is also quite beneficial when examining aerodynamic voice parameters and their interaction with acoustic voice parameters. For example, when one parameter, such as pitch, is altered during clinical stimulation, the effect on another parameter, such as airflow rate, is easily demonstrated. The tracing in Figure 6.16 demonstrates that a slight elevation in pitch during the production of a vowel can reduce the excessive airflow rate that gives rise to the perception of extreme breathiness in this adult patient with bowed vocal folds. An improved vocal quality, with reduced breathiness, is correlated with the tracing of reduced airflow.

The Phonatory Aerodynamic System (KayPENTAX Corp.) is the latest pneumotachograph-based system for aerodynamic analysis (Figure 6.17). The PAS allows the clinician to obtain measurements of average phonatory flow rate, sound

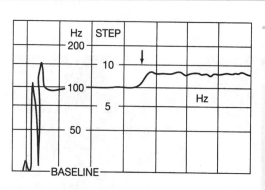

FIGURE **6.16**

Tracing from a Phonatory Function Analyzer

These tracings from the phonatory function analyzer demonstrate how a change in one vocal parameter (pitch, for example) can make a significant change in another parameter (such as rate of airflow). As the pitch level is raised from 100 Hz to a level of 130 Hz, the airflow rate is reduced from 260 mL/sec to a level of 180 mL/sec. Intensity is also increased from 83 to 88 dB SPL.

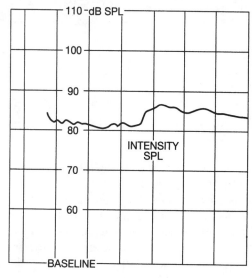

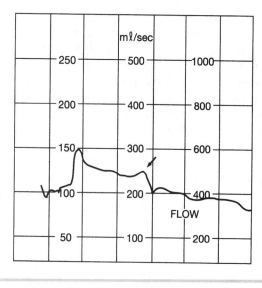

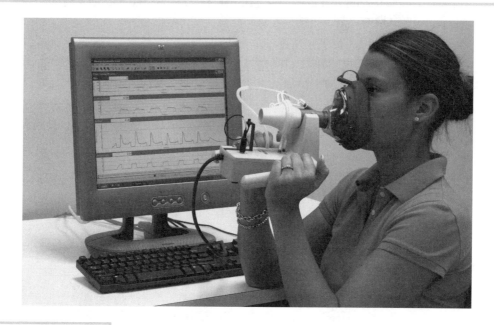

FIGURE **6.17**

A Phonatory Aerodynamic System

Source: Courtesy of KayPENTAX.

pressure level, fundamental frequency, vital capacity, subglottal pressure (derived), glottal resistance, and vocal efficiency, among other parameters.

Three Case Studies Comparing Noninstrumental and Instrumental Assessment Approaches

The studies presented are abbreviated synopses from actual cases. The reports are not complete, but represent the main findings for each case. The observations are scaled on the form in Figure 6.18. Note that baseline observations are charted with circles and that probes are charted with squares.

Case 1. A young adult male with unilateral (right) adductor vocal fold paralysis. See Figure 6.19 for summary findings from both approaches.

Noninstrumental Approach. The case history and ENT information would be very similar for both approaches. In the noninstrumental approach the description of the voice would be most critical. It is important to note that the patient has no difficulty swallowing and can produce an adequate cough.

FIGURE **6.18**

A Clinic Form That Combines Instrumental Acoustic and Airflow Measurements with Perceptual Ratings

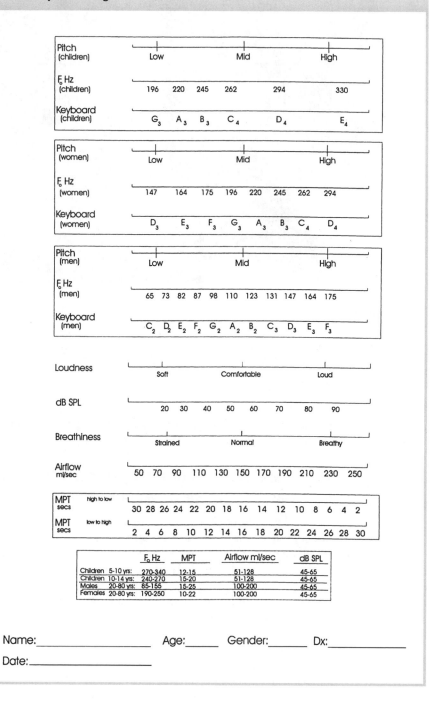

	F_o Hz	MPT	Airflow ml/sec	dB SPL
Children 5-10 yrs:	270-340	12-15	51-128	45-65
Children 10-14 yrs:	240-270	15-20	51-128	45-65
Males 20-80 yrs:	85-155	15-25	100-200	45-65
Females 20-80 yrs:	190-250	10-22	100-200	45-65

Name:_____ Age:_____ Gender:_____ Dx:_____

Date:_____

FIGURE **6.19**

A Clinic Form That Combines Instrumental Acoustic and Airflow Measurements with Perceptual Ratings (Case 1)

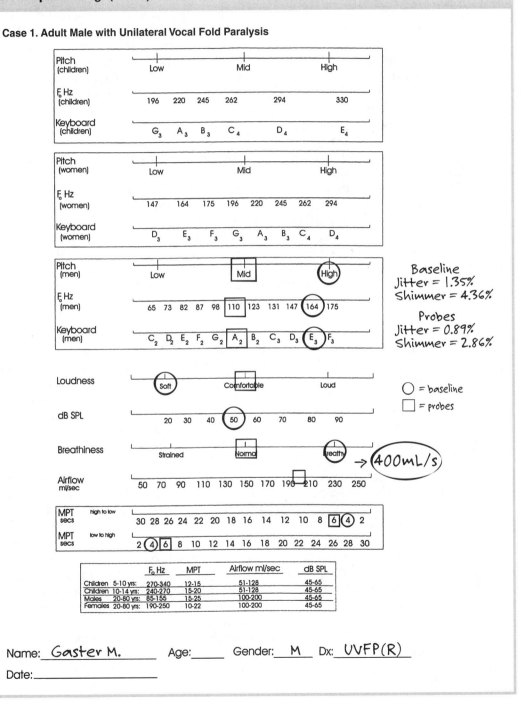

Case 1. Adult Male with Unilateral Vocal Fold Paralysis

Baseline
Jitter = 1.35%
Shimmer = 4.36%

Probes
Jitter = 0.89%
Shimmer = 2.86%

○ = baseline
□ = probes

→ 400mL/s

	F₀ Hz	MPT	Airflow ml/sec	dB SPL
Children 5-10 yrs:	270-340	12-15	51-128	45-65
Children 10-14 yrs:	240-270	15-20	51-128	45-65
Males 20-80 yrs:	85-155	15-25	100-200	45-65
Females 20-80 yrs:	190-250	10-22	100-200	45-65

Name: Gaster M.   Age:_____   Gender: M   Dx: UVFP(R)

Date:_____

The clinician would note that the voice is weak in loudness, extremely breathy, vocally rough in quality (a dry hoarseness), and of short duration of phonation. It may be noted that the patient states that he cannot be heard and that he constantly runs out of breath and must keep taking extra breaths while talking. Duration of phonation may be determined by a stopwatch or by counting the seconds by "one thousand one, one thousand two, one thousand three," and so on. In this case, the duration of phonation is found to be four seconds. The pitch of the voice may also be lower or higher than normal. In this case the voice was high for a male fundamental pitch. Resonance will be observed and the absence of hypernasality noted.

FA.12

Clinical stimulation and the response to clinical probes will be noted on the form as well (Weiss and McFarlane, 1998). For probes, the clinician scales use squares. It may be observed that the extreme breathiness and the low loudness are improved by the head-turning technique and the digital pressure to the larynx technique, both mentioned in Chapter 7. Also a downward pitch shift improves the voice by increasing loudness without extra effort and further reduces breathiness. It is noted that phonation time is extended to 6.5 seconds. An audio recording of the evaluation and the response to clinical facilitation techniques will be made. An oral examination will be completed and the results, likely negative, will be noted. The ENT report of vocal fold paralysis will be used because the clinician will likely not have access to videolaryngostroboscopy.

Instrumental Approach. The instrumental approach with the same young male with unilateral right vocal fold paralysis would be reported in a different manner on the same form. The airflow rate may be reported as 400 mL/sec, rather than as "extremely breathy in quality." The "weakness in loudness" may be reported as 50 dB SPL from the Phonatory Function Analyzer. The fundamental frequency would be reported as 165 Hz rather than as "high for a male fundamental." Vocal roughness will be reported as a jitter value of 1.35% with a shimmer of 4.36%. These values will be noted on the form rather than the perception of "rough, dry hoarseness." Phonation time will be reported as four seconds. Electroglottographic traces will be reported as short closed phases and long open phases of a ratio of 1:4 in time. The irregularity of the waveform from one cycle to the next will be noted. The videostroboscopic results were of a shorter appearing left vocal fold fixed in the paramedian position. The right vocal fold adducts and abducts normally. The left vocal fold is lacking tone and flutters during phonation, giving rise to an asymmetrical vocal fold vibration and an open glottal chink during phonation. With application of the lateral digital pressure technique and head turned to the left the glottal gap is markedly reduced and airflow improves to 200 mL/sec, F_0 lowers to 110 Hz, and jitter and shimmer are reduced to 0.89% and 2.86%, respectively.

The perceptual report is longer than the instrumental report because instrumentation has allowed us to be parsimonious in using words. The instrumental approach has also has allowed us to quantify our findings. This makes comparison of performance at subsequent sessions much easier.

Case 2.   An adult female with muscle tension dysphonia. See Figure 6.20 for summary findings from both instrumental and noninstrumental approaches.

FA.19

FA.23

Noninstrumental Approach.   This woman demonstrated extreme strain and effort during phonation attempts. She had a vocal quality with marked strained–strangled aspects. Her airflow rate appeared low but phonation time was also short, at about five seconds. Voice pitch was low and her rate of speaking was slow. Vocal loudness was generally low but at times was explosive.

Response to clinical stimulation was very positive (Weiss and McFarlane, 1998). With yawn–sigh and tongue protrusion /i/ and upward pitch shifts the voice was much less effortful to produce. The strained–strangled quality was greatly diminished. Phonation time was increased to 12 seconds. The patient reported that this voice was much less effortful to produce and she felt freer during talking than she had in months. Her voice sounded normal in vocal quality and pitch.

Instrumental Approach.   Acoustical analysis revealed a jitter score of 1.60% and a shimmer value of 3.241%. The fundamental frequency was 165 Hz. Duration of phonation was five seconds. The airflow rate was 75 mL/sec. EGG traces were irregular with long closed phases and short or absent open phases. During videostroboscopy the vocal folds were tightly pressed together during phonation with some overlapping of the folds along the glottal margins. Some shortening of the vocal folds was noted as the epiglottis and arytenoids were brought closer together. The false vocal folds were brought into activity overlapping the true vocal folds, making them appear only half their true width. Clinical stimulation using yawn–sigh, tongue protrusion /i/, and upward pitch shifts reduced the excessive glottal valving and extended phonation to 12 seconds. Using the same clinical facilitation techniques during acoustical analysis, the jitter and shimmer were normalized at 0.62% and 2.12%, respectively. Pitch was normalized at 210 Hz and airflow was normalized at 160 mL/sec.

Case 3.   A seven-year-old female presenting with dysphonia associated with vocal abuse and overuse. See Figure 6.21 for summary findings from both instrumental and noninstrumental approaches.

Noninstrumental Approach.   This second grader engages in a number of school and after-school activities, such as choir, piano lessons, girls' clubs, and after-school day care. She has a five-year-old brother. The client's mother, a family physician, reported that the client's voice was moderately hoarse even as a toddler. Perceptually, the voice was low in pitch and hoarse with brief phonation breaks. Phonation time was five seconds. The client engaged in frequent throat-clearing behaviors.

FIGURE **6.20**

A Clinic Form That Combines Instrumental Acoustic and Airflow Measurements with Perceptual Ratings (Case 2)

Case 2. Adult Female with Muscle Tension Dysphonia

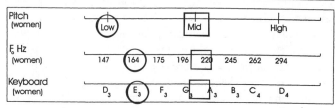

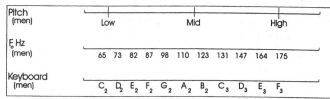

Baseline
Jitter = 1.60%
Shimmer = 3.241%

Probes
Jitter = 0.62%
Shimmer = 2.12%

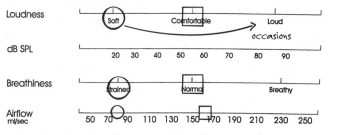

○ = baseline
☐ = probes

	F₀ Hz	MPT	Airflow ml/sec	dB SPL
Children 5-10 yrs:	270-340	12-15	51-128	45-65
Children 10-14 yrs:	240-270	15-20	51-128	45-65
Males 20-80 yrs:	85-155	15-25	100-200	45-65
Females 20-80 yrs:	190-250	10-22	100-200	45-65

Name: Penny M.   Age:_____   Gender: F   Dx: muscle tension dysphonia

Date:_____

FIGURE **6.21**

A Clinic Form That Combines Instrumental Acoustic and Airflow Measurements with Perceptual Ratings (Case 3)

Case 3. Female Child with Vocal Abuse and Overuse

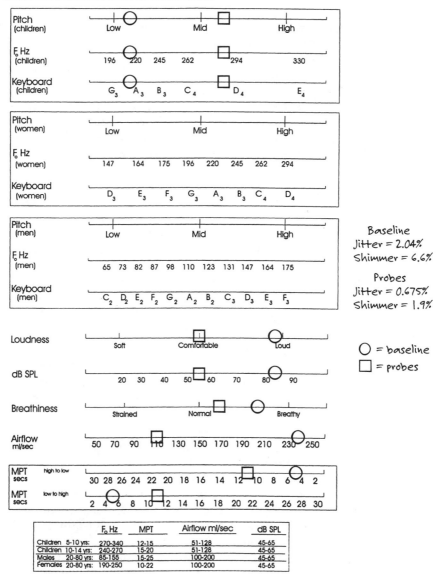

Baseline
Jitter = 2.04%
Shimmer = 6.6%

Probes
Jitter = 0.675%
Shimmer = 1.9%

○ = baseline
□ = probes

	F_o Hz	MPT	Airflow ml/sec	dB SPL
Children 5-10 yrs:	270-340	12-15	51-128	45-65
Children 10-14 yrs:	240-270	15-20	51-128	45-65
Males 20-80 yrs:	85-155	15-25	100-200	45-65
Females 20-80 yrs:	190-250	10-22	100-200	45-65

Name: D.E.   Age: 7 yrs   Gender: F   Dx: Bilateral Vocal Fold Nodules

Date:

FA.10
FA.8
FA.25

Voice intervention was initiated. Increased water intake was recommended and the client was encouraged to employ sniff swallow and silent cough to replace the abusive habits of coughing and throat clear. The client was seen for five sessions of voice therapy. Techniques used were yawn–sigh to relax the pharynx and lower the larynx and pitch shift up to establish "best pitch." Tone focus was also introduced to draw vocal resonance into the facial mask. Auditory feedback using the loop player mode of the Facilitator was a powerful motivator for this client, and she was visibly pleased when she maintained a healthy pitch in a confidential voice tone.

Instrumental Approach.   Acoustic analysis revealed a jitter score of 2.04% and a shimmer score of 6.6%, both of which are above normal limits. F_0 was 217 Hz, lower than normal limits for a seven-year-old female. Airflow was 230 mL/sec, which suggests air escape at the level of the glottis. Videostroboscopy showed small bilateral nodules at the juncture of the anterior third and posterior two-thirds of the vocal folds.

Clinical stimulation using yawn–sigh, pitch shift up and confidential voice were effective in increasing F_0 to 287 Hz with jitter of .675% and shimmer of 1.9%. Perceptually, the voice was still slightly low in frequency for a child, but vocal quality was clear with no phonation breaks. The client was able to reiterate the rationale for all techniques. She reported that she no longer shouts at friends or family and she uses her good "humming" voice when practicing the piano.

SUMMARY

The voice evaluation is the time when the clinician first meets the voice patient, providing the opportunity for observation and testing. The evaluation begins when the patient is observed in the waiting room and continues as part of each therapy session, particularly as the clinician continually searches with the patient for new vocal behaviors. The clinician must continue to evaluate and observe the patient's respiratory, phonatory, and resonance functions. Whenever possible, these functions should be quantified with instrumentation. Auditory–perceptual judgments are also extremely valuable in describing the patient's voice disorder and the manner in which it is produced. The patient's perception of voice handicap is also an important factor to assess. The patient's voice data are used for comparison purposes, to quantify vocal changes from the first visit through subsequent therapy sessions to the final outcome session. Patient performance, both as observed and as measured, is offered to the patient as continuing feedback, helping the patient become aware of voice performance. The evaluation enables the voice clinician to decide on which management steps to take for the patient. If voice therapy is indicated, the evaluation will help the clinician develop a therapy plan and predict the patient's outcome prognosis.

Thought Questions

1. What are the purposes of conducting a voice assessment?
2. How can a voice screening process be implemented in a school setting?
3. Which elements would you include in a voice assessment and why?
4. Is the noninstrumental assessment approach valid?
5. What purpose does the instrumental assessment of voice serve?

7

Voice Therapy

- Describe the reasoning for the suggestion that there is no one voice technique or program that is facilitative for all patients with the same voice problem

- Define the concept of "diagnostic probe" and explain its importance in voice therapy

- Identify the rationales and procedural approaches for the facilitating techniques introduced

There is no set voice therapy regimen. Rather, voice therapy is highly individualized, depending on the cause of the problem, its maintaining factors, the motivation of the patient, and the availability of appropriate management and treatment. Some voice problems may require only the management of professionals outside the profession of the speech–language pathologist (SLP), such as a laryngologist who may successfully treat a small oral cancer by laser surgery. Or the problem of unilateral vocal fold paralysis may be managed by both the laryngologist and the SLP, who will see the patient at different times during the recovery process. Many voice problems are best managed by the SLP alone, who provides the needed voice therapy and required long-term follow-up. For example, the SLP may help the patient with functional aphonia regain voice with voice therapy and then provide the follow-up that may be required by the patient for maintaining normal voice.

What is offered for management and therapy (and by whom) is dictated by the presenting causal and maintaining factors that were identified at the time of the initial diagnostic evaluation. Even during voice therapy, there must be a continuous search for a possible change in the maintenance factors of the voice problem, which could then dictate a different management or therapy offering.

While many of the management strategies differ among voice patients according to whether their problems are organic, neurogenic, or functional, our voice therapy approaches may not be differentiated according to such causal factors. For example, if the patient is exhibiting a problem in breath control, while the cause of the problem may get primary attention, the techniques for using more efficient breath for voice are selected from a pool of approaches for improving breath control. Perhaps the most commonly observed voice problems are related to vocal hyperfunction for which there are many therapy approaches designed to "take the work" out of speaking. A voice therapy approach for a particular person with vocal hyperfunction would be selected from an array of such approaches, with the selection again related to causal and maintaining factors. A young man who exhibits hard glottal attack might profit from learning to reduce his rate of speech, opening his mouth a bit more, learning more of a *legato* (smooth, easy flow) style of voicing, and practicing vocal chanting. Accordingly, his SLP would select those therapy approaches that help facilitate this easy, smooth style of voicing.

The authors were once approached by a computer scientist who suggested that the voice diagnostic–evaluation data could be fed into a software program, which would automatically tell the SLP what therapy methods to use with a recommended sequence of application. Such a cookbook approach to voice therapy is not possible. Rather, the SLP uses the presenting data and observations for decisions regarding management, selecting a particular approach for a trial beginning (known as a diagnostic probe). The patient's response to the probe and its effect on voice determine if that therapy approach will be used or eliminated in therapy or if the approach can be combined with other approaches. Rarely is a particular voice therapy technique applied in isolation. For example, if a louder voice produces a clearer voice with less perturbation, combining work on increasing respiratory volume, extending expiratory durations, improving patient posture, and increasing mouth opening could all be combined with increasing loudness in a treatment session.

There are some differences in overall management and voice therapy among preschool children, school-age children, adolescents, and adults. The age of the person and the physical size of vocal mechanisms, coupled with cognitive understanding of the goals of therapy, will often dictate what can be done. Let us look separately at some of the issues shaping management and voice therapy for children and adolescents–adults.

VOICE MANAGEMENT AND THERAPY FOR CHILDREN

When the preschool child with a voice disorder is brought to the voice clinic, the problem usually has a physical cause. The functional components of the voice problem at this age are minimal. Consequently, most of the early management emphasis is on evaluation. A sudden hoarseness, perhaps accompanied by laryngeal stridor (noise on inhalation), may cause concern that the child may have a serious laryngeal disease, such as papilloma or laryngeal web. Even at very young ages, the otolaryngologist skilled in endoscopy can use a pediatric endoscope and view the larynx. If papilloma or web and other laryngeal diseases were identified, the primary management of the problem would be medical–surgical. If the hoarseness appears to be related to vocal fold thickening or nodules, which have developed after continuous vocal hyperfunction, some parent counseling may usually be in order. Direct voice therapy with the child may be deferred until the preschooler is cognitively able to understand the importance of curbing particular hyperfunctional behaviors, such as yelling and making continuous "funny" noises. Voice therapy might well be delayed until kindergarten or first grade. The primary voice management role in the preschool child is the identification and possible treatment of laryngeal disease rather than as a preliminary evaluative step for voice therapy.

CS.10

The most common voice problem in the school-age child is hoarseness related to vocal hyperfunction. On endoscopy, such children will usually reveal the presence of vocal fold thickening or vocal nodules or polyps. Occasionally, other laryngeal diseases may be identified. This is why management and voice therapy cannot be initiated until the cause of the problem is identified. The organic and neurogenic causal factors discussed in Chapters 3 and 4 will require special medical–surgical management and voice management–therapy consistent with such diagnoses. Again, let us say that the majority of voice problems seen in the school-age population are related to vocal hyperfunction. The overall thrust of voice therapy for vocal hyperfunction in school-age children is identifying their voice abuses and voice misuse (see facilitating approach 8) and reducing the occurrence of such behaviors.

The clinician can probably do nothing more effective than identify those situations in which the child is vocally abusive, such as yelling at a ballgame, screaming on the playground, crying, imitating noises below or above his or her speaking pitch range, and so on. Many children maintain their vocal pathologies simply by engaging in abusive vocal behavior for only brief periods each day. It is often not possible to identify these vocal abuses through interview methods or by observing the child in the therapy room; rather, the child must be observed in various play settings, in the classroom, and at home. This need for extensive observation requires that clinicians solicit the help of the children themselves to determine where they might be yelling or screaming. Teachers can provide some helpful clues about the child's vocal behavior both on the playground and in the classroom. Meeting with parents will often reveal further situations of vocal abuse, and the parents may be asked to listen over a period of time for abusive vocal behavior in the child's play or interactions with various family members. At times, we have had good luck using siblings or peers to help us determine what a child does vocally in certain situations.

Once the abusive situations are isolated, clinicians should obtain baseline measurements of the number of times a vocal abuse is observed in a particular time unit (an hour, a recess period, a day, and so on). Figure 7.1 shows a vocal abuse graph, which plots the number of abuses a child had recorded over a period of two weeks.

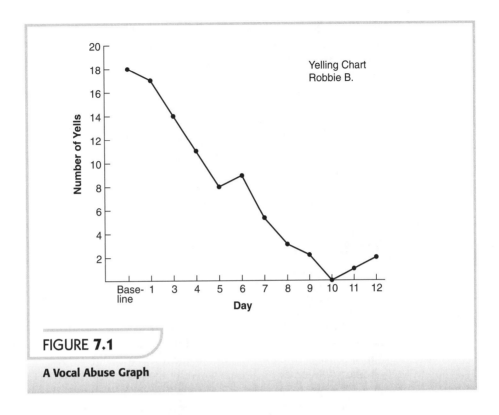

FIGURE **7.1**

A Vocal Abuse Graph

Notice that the first plot on the abscissa is the first day's baseline measurement, which tells on the ordinate how many times the child caught himself yelling on that particular day—for this child, 18 separate yells. The overall contour shows a linear decrement in voice yelling, which is a somewhat typical curve for young children. Having to monitor his offensive behavior seems to motivate the child to reduce it. The child may keep a card in his pocket on which to mark down each occurrence; at the end of the day, he tallies that day's occurrences and plots the total figure on the graph. The review of the plotting graph is a vital part of the therapy, and the child's pride in his graph (which usually shows a decrement in the behavior) helps him continue to curb the vocal abuse. Some children require assistance in making this kind of plot, and sometimes we ask teachers, parents, or friends to also keep tally cards to record the number of events they observed in a particular time period. If children are given proper orientation to the task and clearly know why they must reduce their number of vocal abuses, their tally counts seem to be higher, and perhaps more valid, than the counts of external observers.

Another variation of the tally method requires the child to take his tally card for the date and plot his voice abuse-misuse against that reported by another child or the clinician. For example, in *The Boone Voice Program for Children* (1993) are play materials for a hot-air balloon race in which the clinician "races" the child in plotting changes (in this case abuse–misuse) with hot-air balloons across a sky backdrop. Generating some kind of reward, such as winning the balloon race, helps the child to become more aware of the desirability of curbing voice abuse–misuse.

An important prelude to the tally method—indeed, to any form of speech therapy, particularly voice therapy—is for the clinician to explain to the child what the problem is, what the child seems to be doing wrong vocally, and what can be done about it. Obviously, a child must first know that there is a voice problem (rarely does a child recognize such a problem independently) before he or she can do anything about it. Such explanations are also especially important because most children with voice problems are not self-referred. Their dysphonias have been discovered by someone else. To the child, there may be no problem.

VOICE THERAPY FOR ADOLESCENTS AND ADULTS

The abusive vocal behaviors of adults are likely to be more difficult to isolate than those of children. It is the relatively rare adult voice patient whose vocal abuses are bound only to particular situations. Preachers or auctioneers whose voice problems appear only on the job may be excellent examples of vocal misuse; however, dysphonic adolescents or adults generally have hyperfunctional sets toward phonation. They work to talk in most situations. Sometimes, the exaggerated effort experienced by some voice patients toward vocalization is related to a generalized tension that may become more acute in particular situations, such as when they speak to authority figures or when they try to make favorable impressions on their listeners. A more generalized anxiety might best be treated through counseling or psychological therapy. It has been the authors' observation, however, that even patients with a more generalized anxiety can often take the tension out of their voices by employing voice therapy approaches that seem to open and relax the structures of the airway. Many adult voice patients appear capable of producing an optimum voice, providing someone (the clinician) will only help them "find" it.

Therefore, the primary task of voice clinicians is to explore with patients the various therapy techniques that might produce that "good" voice. We advocate the same approach with adults as we do with children: using facilitating techniques as therapy probes. The approach that works is then used as a therapy practice approach. Once the patients are able to produce a model of their own best voice, this model and the techniques used to achieve it become the primary focus of voice therapy.

Voice clinicians also provide patients with needed psychological support, and together they explore the use of various facilitating techniques to be used in particular situations. Hierarchies of stress can often be identified (Boone and Wiley, 2000; Wolpe, 1987), and behavioral approaches used at these times of stress may minimize symptoms. Patients are taught to isolate those situations in which they experience poor voice and to substitute at those times more optimum forms of behavior, that is, easier voice.

Voice disorders in adolescents and adults often have a negative impact on their lives because they may interfere with life interactions and employment. Some patients become desperate over their vocal problems and seek professional help. The family physician is often the first professional who identifies a voice problem as a disorder that needs the expert help of an otolaryngologist or speech–language pathologist. The physician subsequently refers the patient for a voice evaluation that, more often than not, involves the evaluation–diagnostic procedures described in Chapter 6. Voice therapy is often the recommended step after the diagnostic evaluation.

VOICE THERAPY FACILITATING TECHNIQUES

In this text, we call our therapy approaches *facilitating approaches* or *techniques.* That is, the selected therapy technique facilitates a "target" or a more optimal vocal response by the patient. The techniques may be used with patients having various kinds of voice disorders: organic, neurogenic, or functional. Part of voice therapy is searching with patients to find the facilitating approach that seems to help them produce the desired vocal response. Many patients with the same voice disorder, such as functional dysphonia, may require different therapy approaches for the same problem. It is important to remember that no *one* specific therapy approach is facilitative for all patients with the same voice problem.

The experienced voice clinician will have available many voice therapy techniques to use for particular voice problems with certain patients. In addition to the current list of 25 approaches in this edition of *The Voice and Voice Therapy,* the SLP should be aware of the many other management and therapy approaches described in the literature: Andrews and Summers (2002), Aronson (1990), Boone (1997), Boone and Wiley (2000), Case (2002), Colton and Casper (1996), Greene and Mathieson (1991), Kotby (1995), Morrison and Rammage (1994), and Stemple (2000).

The facilitating approaches in Table 7.1 are listed alphabetically. After each approach, a notation (×) is made to indicate the voice parameters that the particular approach has the potential to influence. For example, approach 1, auditory feedback, can have impact on both loudness and quality, with less influence on voice pitch. Accordingly, for the three columns in Table 7.1 (pitch, loudness, and quality) only the loudness and quality columns are marked with an (×). Other techniques, such as 25, yawn–sigh, influence all three parameters of pitch, loudness, and quality, and each column is marked with an (×). Experienced voice clinicians often combine therapy approaches in their search with the patient in finding the target voice. Each of the 25 facilitating approaches in Table 7.1 is presented from the following four perspectives: (1) kinds of problems for which the approach is useful; (2) procedural aspects of the approach; (3) typical case history showing utilization of the approach; and (4) evaluation of the approach.

TABLE **7.1**	Twenty-Five Facilitating Approaches in Voice Therapy		
	Parameter of Voice Affected		
Facilitating Approach	*Pitch*	*Loudness*	*Quality*
1. Auditory feedback		×	×
2. Change of loudness	×	×	×
3. Chant–talk		×	×
4. Chewing	×	×	×
5. Confidential voice		×	×
6. Counseling (explanation of problem)	×	×	
7. Digital manipulation	×		×
8. Elimination of abuses		×	×
9. Establishing a new pitch	×		×
10. Focus	×	×	×
11. Glottal fry	×	×	×
12. Head positioning	×		×
13. Hierarchy analysis	×	×	×
14. Inhalation phonation	×	×	
15. Laryngeal massage	×		×
16. Masking	×	×	
17. Nasal/glide stimulation			×
18. Open-mouth approach		×	×
19. Pitch inflections	×		
20. Redirected phonation	×	×	×
21. Relaxation	×	×	×
22. Respiration training		×	×
23. Tongue protrusion /i/	×		×
24. Visual feedback	×	×	×
25. Yawn–sigh	×	×	×

1. Auditory Feedback

Kinds of Problems for Which the Approach Is Useful.   Many voice patients profit from using some kind of auditory feedback in and out of voice therapy. Those patients who displayed a window of voice improvement during the evaluation session (such as when masking was used as a diagnostic probe resulting in an immediate improvement in voice) will often benefit from the use of auditory feedback during therapy sessions. Regardless of the causal factor of the disorder (organic, neurogenic, or functional), the patient's voice may improve with such feedback. There are different kinds of auditory feedback that may enhance patient response, such as using real-time amplification and letting patients hear themselves on headphones as they are speaking. Voice improvement is best secured by listening real-time on amplification equipment that has a speech–voice range focus, for

FA.1

example, commercially available instruments such as the Hearit (1995) or the Facilitator (1998) (Figure 7.2). Some motor speech patients might profit from the use of an auditory metronome that can pace either an increased or decreased rate of response modeling for the patient; for example, a metronome set at about 60 words per minute can result in a marked slowing down of the Parkinson's patient's speech rate, which may increase both voice quality–volume and articulation intelligibility. Most voice patients profit from auditory modeling, hearing either their own voice on auditory playback or an external model (perhaps a speaking pitch note or the clinician's voice). Auditory modeling, to be effective, must be immediate. The clinician may stop recording on a cassette, rewind, and play for the patient a recording of the model and the patient response. The auditory playback is easier on loop-playback recorders, such as the tape-loop Phonic Mirror or the solid-state loop auditory feedback mode found on the Facilitator.

Procedural Aspects of the Approach.   Let us separate the application approaches for three forms of auditory feedback: real-time amplification, metronome pacing, and loop playback.

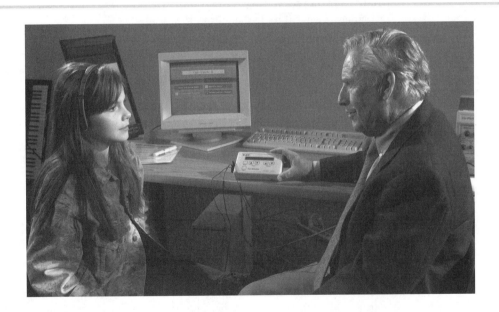

FIGURE **7.2**

Kay Facilitator, Model 3500

The Facilitator is an auditory feedback device with five modes of feedback: real-time amplification, loop feedback, delayed auditory feedback (DAF), masking (speech range), and metronomic pacing.

1. Real-time amplification of speech and voice enables one to hear oneself more clearly than would be possible without such self-amplification and auditory focus. Real-time amplification requires the clinician to use an amplifier, microphone, and headset with the patient. The clinician uses a cassette recorder, a boom box, or an amplifying instrument that provides real-time feedback as the patient speaks.

   a. The patient is asked to listen closely on the headphones to what he or she will be saying. Usually another facilitating approach is used, such as chanting or focus, that the patient will use while speaking. The patient then listens closely to the sound of the voice or speech while he or she is using the approach.

   b. The patient is asked to evaluate the appropriateness of his or her response. If adjustments are made, they are listened to with real-time amplification again.

2. The clicks or beats of a metronome may provide good auditory pacing for those patients who need to decrease or increase their rate of speech.

   a. The rate of clicks per minute is set on the instrument. All wind-up or electronic metronomes have a setting switch. On the Facilitator, the click pacing ranges from 50 to 150 clicks per minute.

   b. The best pacing practice is achieved by the patient matching the clicks by shortening or prolonging the vowel duration of the practice material. Changing vowel duration is a preferred way to change rate rather than altering pause duration between words or phrases.

3. Loop playback allows the patient to hear immediately what was just said. The Phonic Mirror and Language Master were designed for immediate replay feedback. The authors have constructed cassette loops that provide immediate auditory feedback without the need to rewind the tape (Boone, 1982). The more recent Facilitator (1998) has a solid-state loop system that allows the patient who wears a headset an immediate playback (from 1 to 6 sec) of what was just said. These procedures are used for immediate playback on the Facilitator:

   a. The patient wears a headset and lapel microphone. The mode switch on the Facilitator is pushed to LOOPING READY. To record a model and/or patient response, the RECORD button is pressed and released.

   b. The STOP/PLAY button is pressed to stop the recording. Press the STOP/PLAY button again and the recording playback will begin. Tapping this button again will provide another playback as often as one wishes to hear it.

   c. The patient is asked to evaluate the immediate playback. The clinician, who may wear another headset with microphone, provides some feedback specific to the appropriateness of the patient's response. The patient may be asked to repeat the utterance, and steps (3a) and (3b) are repeated.

Typical Case History Showing Utilization of the Approach.   J. W., a 49-year-old social worker, had a two-year history of functional dysphonia. At the time of the initial interview it was found that elevating her pitch slightly at the end of a phrase or sentence seemed to eliminate all hoarseness. Loop playback was very effective in helping her realize that raising pitch slightly in an upward inflection cleared the hoarseness from her voice. Working with her SLP using loop playback, she practiced repeating sentences in two different ways: one, with the usual downward inflection (which caused hoarseness), and two, saying them with upward inflection. Using immediate loop feedback in a few practice sessions appeared to be a primary approach in developing better functional voice outside the clinic, especially in her work as a social worker.

Evaluation of the Approach.   Voice improvement is often enhanced by listening closely to one's voice. The use of auditory feedback is often an important step in therapy for articulation, language, fluency, and voice disorders. Real-time amplification, loop playback, and using external metronomic pacing can be effective auditory aids in voice therapy. A holistic approach to correcting a voice disorder, such as listening to one's voice, is often preferred over fractionating various voice components (breathing, pitch, loudness, etc.) with separate practice for each component.

2. Change of Loudness

FA.2

Kinds of Problems for Which the Approach Is Useful.   Some patients have voices that have inappropriate loudness, too loud or too soft. Many of the vocal pathologies experienced by children are related to such excesses of loudness as screaming and yelling. Weak, soft voices may develop as a consequence of the prolonged hyperfunctional use of the vocal mechanism that results in the eventual breakdown of glottal approximation surfaces, for example, a patient with vocal nodules who loses much airflow around the nodules and is unable to produce an intense enough vocal fold vibration to achieve a sufficiently loud voice. Some speaking environments require a loud voice, and untrained speakers or singers may push for loudness at the level of the larynx rather than adjust their respiration. Inappropriate loudness of voice is most often not the primary causative factor of a voice problem, but rather a secondary, if annoying, symptom. Reducing or increasing the loudness of the voice lends itself well to direct symptom modification through exercise and practice, and often, if other facilitating techniques are being used, does not even require the use of loudness techniques.

Procedural Aspects of the Approach

1. For a decrease in loudness:

   a. See that the patient has a thorough audiometric examination to determine adequacy of hearing before any attempt is made to reduce voice loudness. Once it has been established that the patient has normal hearing, the following steps may be taken.

   b. For young children, ages three through ten, the change of loudness steps in *The Boone Voice Program for Children* (1993) is useful. Ask the child to develop awareness of five different voices:

- Voice 1 is presented as a whisper.
- Voice 2 is presented as the voice to use when not wanting to awaken a sleeping person, a quiet voice.
- Voice 3 is the normal voice to use to talk to family and friends.
- Voice 4 is the voice to use to talk to someone across the room.
- Voice 5 is the yelling voice to call someone outside.

   c. With patients over ten years old, discuss with the patient the observation that he or she has an inappropriately loud voice. The patient may be unaware of the loud voice and should listen to tape-recorded samples of his or her speech. The best demonstration tape for loudness variations would include both the patient's voice and the clinician's, to provide contrasting levels of loudness. Then ask the patient, "Do you think your voice is louder than mine?"

   d. Focus on making the patient aware of the problem. Once the patient becomes aware that his or her voice is too loud, ask, "What does a loud voice in another person tell you about that person?" Loud voices are typically interpreted to mean that the speaker feels "overly confident" or "sure of himself," or that the speaker is putting on a confident front when he or she is really scared, or that he or she is mad at the world, impressed with his or her own voice, trying to intimidate listeners, and so on. Some discussion of these negative interpretations is usually sufficient to motivate the average patient to learn to speak at normal loudness levels.

   e. Practice using a quiet voice (voice 2 in section b). The practice for the quiet voice can be facilitated by using instruments that give feedback specific to intensity, such as the Vocal Loudness Indicator and the Visi-Pitch. The Vocal Loudness Indicator, for example, has a series of lights that are illuminated by increases in voice intensity. Keeping the instrument at a fixed distance, the patient can quickly learn to keep his or her voice at a lower intensity level to prevent the light (all or a few) from coming on.

2. For an increase in loudness:

   a. Determine first that the inappropriate softness of the voice is not related to hearing loss, general physical weakness, or a personality problem; for these cases, a symptomatic approach is not indicated. The steps that follow are for voice patients who are physically and emotionally capable of speaking in a louder voice.

   b. Discuss with the patient the soft voice. A tape-recorded playback of the patient's and clinician's voices in conversation will usually illustrate for the patient the inadequacy of the loudness. After the patient indicates some awareness of his or her soft voice, ask, "What does a soft, weak voice tell us about a person?" Inadequately loud voices are typically interpreted to mean that the speaker is afraid to speak louder, is timid and shy, is unduly considerate of others, is scared of people, has no self-confidence, and so on. Some discussion of these negative interpretations is usually helpful.

c. By exploring pitch level and fundamental frequency, try to achieve a pitch level at which the patient is able with some ease to produce a louder voice. If the patient habitually speaks near the bottom of his or her pitch range, a slight elevation of pitch level will usually be accompanied by a slight increase in loudness. The Visi-Pitch has been useful in helping patients associate changes in pitch with relative changes in intensity. Certain frequencies produce greater intensities. When the patient finds the "best" pitch level, he or she should practice sustaining an /a/ at that level for five seconds, concentrating on good voice quality. He or she should then take a deep breath and repeat the same pitch at a maximum loudness level. After some practice at this "home base" pitch level, ask the patient to sing /a/, up the scale for one octave, at one vocal production per breath; then have him or her go back down the scale, one note per breath, until he or she reaches the starting pitch.

d. Explore with the patient his or her best pitch, that is, the one that produces the best loudness and quality. Auditory feedback devices (such as loop tape recorders) should be employed, so that the patient can hear what he or she is doing. Some counseling may be needed about the practice pitch used because the patient may be resistant to using a new voice pitch level. Note that the practice pitch level may well be only a temporary one, and not necessarily the pitch level the patient will use permanently. It is important that the work be pursued both in and out of therapy. A change in loudness cannot be achieved simply by talking about it. It requires practice.

e. Sometimes respiration training (which we discuss later in the chapter) is necessary for a patient with a loudness problem. Remember, however, that even though loudness is directly related to the rate of airflow through the approximated vocal folds, little evidence indicates that any particular way of breathing is the best for optimum phonation. Any respiration exercise that produces increased subglottal air pressure may be helpful in increasing voice loudness.

f. For those patients who seem unable to increase voice loudness, we might employ the Lombard effect (Newby, 1972). The Lombard effect is observed when patients reflexively voice at louder levels when reading or speaking against increasing competing noise. For example, as the patient reads aloud the clinician introduces about 75 dB of speech-range masking from the Facilitator (see facilitating approach 16 for application procedures).

3. Occasional patients or people wanting to improve their voices demonstrate little or no loudness variation. Fluctuation in loudness can be helped by:

a. Make a tape recording of the patient's voice. Ask the patient how he or she likes the voice on playback. People who become aware of the monotony of their voices, and who are concerned about it, can usually develop loudness variation (and pitch inflection) with practice.

    b. Use a loop-playback system. Record speech or oral reading and then listen back immediately. Ask the patient about the relative appropriateness of loudness or loudness variation.

    c. Most voice and diction books include practice materials for developing loudness variation in the voice.

Typical Case History Showing Utilization of the Approach.   C. T., a 31-year-old teacher, complained for more than a year of symptoms of vocal fatigue, that is, pain in the throat, loss of voice after teaching, and so on. Laryngoscopy revealed a normal larynx, and the voice evaluation found that the man spoke at "a monotonous pitch and low loudness level, with pronounced mandibular restriction, at times barely opening his mouth." Early efforts at therapy included the chewing approach, with special emphasis given to varying pitch level and increasing voice loudness. The patient was highly motivated to improve the efficiency of his phonation; he requested voice therapy three times a week and supplemented the therapy with long practice periods at home. After nine weeks of therapy, pretherapy and posttherapy recordings were compared, and the patient agreed with the clinician that he sounded "like a new man." Speaking in a louder voice for this patient seemed to have an immediate effect on his overall self-image, resulting in an almost immediate increase in his total communicative effectiveness. Not only did the patient achieve a better-sounding speaking voice, but he reported no further symptoms of vocal fatigue.

Evaluation of the Approach.   Inappropriate loudness of voice penalizes the patient. Happily, many of the facilitating techniques described in this chapter have influence on voice loudness, and inadequate loudness is also highly modifiable. In fact, more often than not the use of various other facilitating techniques will have an indirect effect on voice loudness, obviating the need for loudness techniques per se.

3. Chant–Talk

FA.3

Kinds of Problems for Which the Approach Is Useful.   Voice problems related to hyperfunction are often helped by the chant approach. The chant in music is characterized by reciting many syllables on one continuous tone, creating in effect, a "singing monotone." We hear chanting in some churches and synagogues, performed by clergy and select groups. The words run continuously together without stress or a change in prosody for the individual word segments. In singing, the *legato* is very similar to the chant we use in voice therapy. A common dictionary definition of legato is "smooth and connected with no break between tones." The chant in therapy is characterized by an elevation of pitch, prolongation of vowels, lack of syllable stress, and an obvious softening of glottal attack. Once a patient can produce the chant in its extreme form (such as in a Gregorian chant), it can usually be modified to resemble conversational phonation. We have used chanting with other facilitating approaches, such as chewing, open mouth, and yawn–sigh.

Procedural Aspects of the Approach

1. The chant talk approach is explained to the patient as a method that reduces the effort in talking. It is important to point out to the patient that the method will only be used temporarily as practice and will not become a permanent and different way of talking. Demonstrate chant–talk by playing a recording of a religious chant. Then imitate the recording by producing the same voicing style while reading any material aloud.

2. Urge the patient to imitate the same chant voicing pattern. Most patients are able to do this with some degree of initial success. For those who cannot chant in initial trials, present a chant recording again and then follow it with the patient's own chant production. Some lighthearted kidding is useful to tell the patient that the chant is a different way of talking and will only be used briefly as a voice training device. If the patient cannot chant after several attempts, use another facilitating approach. For those patients who can chant, go on to step 3.

3. The patient should now read aloud, alternating the regular voice and the chant voice. Twenty seconds has been found to be a good time for each reading condition. Ask the patient to read aloud first in the normal voice, then in a chant, then back to normal voice, then in a chant, and so on.

4. Record the patient's oral reading. On playback, contrast the different sound of the normal voice with the chanted voice. Discuss the pitch differences, the phonatory prolongations, and the soft glottal onset.

5. Once patients are able to produce chant talk with relative ease, they should try to reduce the chant quality, approximating normal voice production. Slight prolongation and soft glottal onset should be retained as the patient reads aloud in a voice with only slight chant quality remaining.

Typical Case History Showing Utilization of the Approach. C. C. was a 28-year-old woman who sold telephone directory advertising. She began to experience increased dysphonia and "dryness of throat," particularly toward the end of a busy day of calling on customers. On endoscopic examination, she was found to have bilateral vocal nodules with unnecessary supraglottal participation during phonation. She spoke at an inappropriately low pitch, with mandibular restriction and noticeable hard glottal attack. Twice a week she received voice therapy designed to "take the work out of phonation." The chewing approach, coupled with the chant–talk approach, dramatically changed her overall voicing style. She was able early in therapy to incorporate the soft glottal attack of the chant into her everyday speaking voice. Other approaches, such as open mouth and yawn–sigh, were added with various self-practice materials she could use. The patient reported that she practiced throughout the day in her car, driving between appointments. In about twelve weeks, videoendoscopy revealed that the nodules had disappeared and that her supraglottal larynx stayed open during normal voicing. There was no evidence of hard glottal attack at the time of her clinic discharge.

Evaluation of the Approach.   The chant–talk approach is easy for most patients to use. Initially, it is important to let the patient know that chanting is only a temporary behavior, designed to take the work out of phonation. We have found that the method works well with children, who seem to enjoy the "different" way of talking. For those patients who need to reduce hard glottal attack, the chanting approach seems to produce dramatic results for softening voicing onsets.

4. Chewing

FA.4

Kinds of Problems for Which the Approach Is Useful.   We see many people with vocal hyperfunction who appear to speak through clenched teeth with very little mandibular or labial movement. Such patients profit from using the chewing approach. We often kiddingly ask such patients, "Have you ever been a ventriloquist?" We then reply to their usual answer in the negative with "You certainly could be because you barely move your mouth when you speak." Many hyperfunctional voice patients, after being asked the ventriloquist question, develop immediate insight as to their relative lack of mouth opening. Chewing is helpful for the patient who speaks with great tension and hard glottal attack. During simultaneous voicing and chewing, we often hear less strain in the voice, easier glottal attack, and an improvement in voice quality.

Procedural Aspects of the Approach

1. We first do what is necessary to help the patient become aware of the need for greater mouth opening while speaking. Following the ventriloquist question, we may view talking on a real-time video monitor or by looking in a mirror. Immediate video playback after talking is a good method for instructing the patient specific to the relative amount of mouth opening he or she is using.

2. The clinician and patient look in a mirror as the clinician demonstrates exaggerated chewing. Care is given to have both good vertical and horizontal movements of the mouth. We pretend that we are chewing a stack of three crackers at one time with an open mouth. Ask the patient to imitate exaggerated chewing as has been demonstrated. Point out to the patient the amount of mouth opening by saying something like, "You see we let our jaw drop down with our lips open wide. If we were actually chewing crackers, the crumbs would all drop out of our open mouth." Spend as much time as needed to develop good open-mouth chewing.

3. We now add light voice to the chewing. Here we have to be careful to avoid the same kind of monotonous sound, like "yam-yam-yam," that can come from chewing in the same pattern while voicing. To mix the sounds (and the mouth movements) up a bit, we may have the patient say in a chantlike way such nonsense words as "ah-la-met-erah" or "wan-da-pan-da." Stay with such nonsense words until the patient masters the simultaneous chewing–speaking. It should be noted here that most children like to do chewing and take easily to the approach.

Some adults may resist doing it, or be unable to do it; if so, the approach should be abandoned and other approaches used, such as the open-mouth approach.

4. Once simultaneous chewing–speaking is established, ask the patient to count and chew. It will take several practice attempts before the patient can do it. Listen and watch the first attempts on video playback. Tell the patient at this point that the chewing is "a means to the end of producing a more relaxed voice." The patient should be counseled that the exaggerated chewing is only used temporarily and that we will soon cut down the movements to resemble more "the mouth movements of normal speakers."

5. Now use words and phrases for practice chewing. When the patient can do this, we would then practice sentences. Avoid going too fast. Go back to earlier levels if the chewing seems to be "fading."

6. After several weeks of practice in chewing, the patient should be taught how to diminish the exaggerated chewing to resemble more normal mouth movements. Practicing oral reading with chewing is a good final step. Videotaping the practice session will allow the patient to study his or her success on video playback.

7. Ultimately, the patient just "thinks" the chewing method. By this time, the patient has developed an awareness of what oral openness and jaw movement feel like and has experienced the vocal relaxation that accompanies the feeling.

Typical Case History Showing Utilization of the Approach. S. J., a 44-year-old realtor, began to experience extreme vocal fatigue toward the end of her working day. At the voice evaluation, she reported, "Sometimes I lose my voice altogether at the end of the day, or after I talk a lot, it hurts right here" (as she pointed to the general hyoid area). As she volunteered her history, little mouth opening was observed with her voice sounding at an inappropriate high pitch with the ends of sentences characterized by "squeezed phonation." On endoscopy, her vocal folds showed "posterior redness, suggestive of reflux with no middle or anterior pathology noted." A diagnosis of "muscular tension dysphonia" was made with a special notation made relative to "speaking through clenched teeth." Early in voice therapy, the patient worked on developing better respiration skills for voicing and developing more natural oral movements (less mandibular restriction). While there was some initial resistance by the patient to using the chewing approach, after she began to experience increased oral relaxation as she practiced the chewing, she incorporated greater oral movements into her everyday speaking pattern. The patient experienced a very good voice result from both reduction of her reflux by a medical regimen and eliminating her dysphonia and vocal fatigue from voice therapy (with early emphasis given to using the chewing approach).

Evaluation of the Approach. The chewing approach is not a panacea for all voice problems, but its positive effectiveness in reducing muscular tension dysphonia or vocal hyperfunction is observed soon after it is applied. It appears that when oral structures are involved in the automatic function of chewing, according to Brodnitz and Froeschels (1954) who first introduced the technique, these oral structures (facial muscles, mandible, tongue) appear capable of "more synergic, relaxed movement." It appears that relaxing the overall vocal tract while chewing also relaxes the phonatory function of the larynx and pharynx. By employing a commonly used action, such as chewing, the patient is able to achieve relaxation of the vocal tract from a holistic or *gestalt* point of view, without attempting to relax particular muscles. For the voice patient who appears to be talking between clenched teeth, the chewing approach is a good way to develop more open, natural oral movements. This approach may be contraindicated for the patient with TMJ (temporomandibular joint) syndrome.

5. Confidential Voice

FA.5

Kinds of Problems for Which the Approach Is Useful.   Using a soft, confidential voice as an alternative to using a voice produced by much effort and hyperfunction was first described as the "confidential voice" by Colton and Casper (1996). It is similar to the soft voice recommended for children to use as the "quiet voice," the second voice level of loudness that allows voicing at a quiet level "not loud enough to awaken someone sleeping near by" (Boone, 1983). Both children and adults seem to be able to speak in the easy, confidential voice, which makes the approach useful in reducing overall vocal hyperfunction. The confidential voice with its increased breathiness not only reduces voice loudness but affects breath control, slows down speaking rate, and seems to create a more open, relaxed airway. The technique employs light voice (not whispering) and is used in a prescribed time period for reducing hyperfunction in functional dysphonia and in vocal hyperfunction resulting in vocal fold thickening and vocal nodules. The confidential voice is explained to both children and adults as a temporary way of "talking, a means to an end" for developing a better voice.

Procedural Aspects of the Approach.   Much time can be saved in voice therapy by first seeing if the child or adult can imitate the SLP in producing the breathy, confidential voice. If this easy voice can be produced, the clinician explains how it will be used:

1. Repeat the confidential voice model and be sure the client understands how to produce it, a breathy voice with less loudness, as if one wouldn't want to awaken a person sleeping nearby. We do not want a whisper, but use a breathy, light voicing.

2. The breathy, light voice uses up more air. The slightly parted vocal folds and the open airway allow a greater volume of air to pass through than is normally experienced. Therefore, we explain that fewer words are said on one expiration when using the easy voice.

3. Its temporary use is then explained. As often as one can find settings to use the breathy, confidential voice, the client should be encouraged to use it. There will be

situations where such a light voice cannot be used, such as with a salesperson explaining a product to a customer. As soon as possible, however, the client should revert back to using the easy voice. It is important to let the client know about the temporary use of the confidential voice, perhaps by saying, "we will use this confidential voice only for a few weeks, or for as long as it seems to take to break up the effortful, hyperfunctional voice you have been using."

4. Specific instruction should be given for set time periods when the client does oral reading in the confidential voice.

5. It has been the authors' experience that both children and adults are able to produce the confidential voice with relative ease and soon enjoy voicing without "all the work" they previously used in voice production.

For those children and adults who cannot imitate the clinician easily in producing the confidential voice, we use the steps taken for developing a "soft" voice from *The Boone Voice Program for Children* (Boone, 1993) or *The Boone Voice Program for Adults* (Boone and Wiley, 2000).

1. An awareness is developed that divides voice loudness into five levels: (1) whisper, (2) soft voice, (3) normal conversational voice, (4) louder, projected voice, and (5) yelling. Using the voice examples and cartoons from either the child- or adult-level programs, we select the second level, soft voice, as our target voice.

2. The clinician then reads aloud the voice examples at the second level of loudness, producing in effect the confidential voice. The client is asked to imitate the clinician, which may require some individualized coaching. Phrases and sentences are then practiced aloud at the soft voice level.

3. Once the client can produce the breathy, light voice with consistency, we follow the five steps described above in therapy.

Typical Case History Showing Utilization of the Approach.   D. B. was a 40-year-old teacher who taught computer science and computer applications. She experienced an increasing hoarseness that began to interfere with her teaching effectiveness. On endoscopy, she was found to have small bilateral vocal nodules. Following a 14-day period of voice rest, enforced by her laryngologist, she began voice therapy. The confidential voice was one of the first voice therapy techniques introduced, with which she had initial success. She found that she could use the easy breathy voice in all situations, including in her computer classes after using a small voice amplifier with a free-field speaker. Other voice therapy approaches were combined with confidential voice, including work on improving respiration, improving her head–neck posture, increasing greater mouth opening, increased hydration, and elimination of her tendency to clear her throat. After seven weeks, her voice therapy regimen (including the use of the confidential voice) was terminated with her vocal nodules "remarkably reduced" and the patient experiencing a normal voice in and out of the classroom.

Evaluation of the Approach.   The use of the confidential voice replaces the hyperfunctional behaviors that the patient has been using in most voicing attempts. While using the confidential voice, nasoendoscopic viewing confirms that the vocal folds are slightly apart in their total anterior–posterior length, the laryngeal body remains lower, and the supralaryngeal mechanisms are relaxed and open. The voice sounds free of squeezing or tightness. The easy, breathy voice was one of several techniques used to reduce vocal hyperfunction in 39 adults with functional dysphonia; 23 subjects (59%) experienced voice improvement (Boone, 1974). The results of using the confidential voice by five patients with vocal nodules was compared (Verdolini-Marston, Burke, Lassac, Glaze, and Caldwell, 1995) with five nodule patients in a control group not using confidential voice; the confidential voice group improved in both voice quality and in reduction of the vocal nodules. Our clinical experience has found that the use of the confidential voice breaks up the hyperfunctional set the patient has been using for voicing, giving time for the elimination of undesirable vocal events and replacing them with more optimal vocal behaviors.

6. Counseling (Explanation of Problem)

FA.6

Kinds of Problems for Which the Approach Is Useful.   One cannot easily separate the person from his or her voice. Some voice problems may be among the visible symptoms of someone with serious personality problems, or sometimes the voice problem may be the cause of psychological maladaptive reactions. Counseling the voice patient, including direct explanations of the voice problem, may be more effective with the patient than applying various symptomatic voice therapy techniques.

Putting the voice problem in its proper perspective can often free the patient from overwhelming concern. Patients with hyperfunctional voice disorders, in particular, profit from hearing the clinician describe the voice problem in words they can understand. Clinical experience has taught these authors that if they can help individuals know why they have the voice problem, sometimes nothing more is needed to change a phonation style or to curb vocal abuse–misuse. In the case of those dysphonias that are wholly related to functional causes (such as hyperfunction), it is important that clinicians not confront patients with the implication that they "could talk all right if they wanted to." Instead of saying, "You are not using your voice as well as you could," a clinician might say, "Your vocal folds are coming together too tightly." The latter statement absolves the patient of the guilt he or she might experience if the clinician indicated that the patient was doing things "wrong." The patient will be much more receptive to a statement that puts the blame on the vocal folds. For patients with structural changes of the vocal folds, such as nodules or polyps, it may be necessary to explain that the organic pathology may well be the result of prolonged misuse, and that by eliminating the misuse, the patient will eventually experience a reduction of vocal fold pathology.

Procedural Aspects of the Approach.   Counseling the patient is highly individualized. One of the most common counseling approaches in voice therapy is helping the patient to put his or her voice problem in its proper perspective. For some patients, the voice problem is the cause of all of their ills, such as poor job performance, social inadequacy, or general unhappiness. The clinician must have some sensitivity to the depth of the patient's overall attitude and self-image. If the clinician senses psychological or social problems well beyond his or her counseling–psychological training to deal with such problems, referral should be made to professional counselors, psychologists, or psychiatrists. More often than not in voice therapy, a direct explanation of the patient's problem proves to be most effective.

In voice problems related to vocal hyperfunction, it is important to identify for the patient those behaviors that maintain the dysphonia. However, no exact procedure can be laid down; each case has its own rules. For problems related to abuse and misuse of the voice, identify the inappropriate behavior and demonstrate to the patient some ways in which it can be eliminated. In the vocal abuse reduction section of our voice program for children (Boone, 1993), we put much focus on having the child cognitively approach the problem of vocal abuse. By using comic pictures with an accompanying story text, we help the child understand the consequences of continued abuse and emphasize what can be expected (a better voice) if he or she reduces or eliminates such abuses. A voice program for adults (Boone and Wiley, 2000) provides descriptions of vocal hyperfunction and resulting voice problems of functional dysphonia and dysphonia related to vocal nodules or vocal polyps. Excellent illustrations are presented in a workbook–computer program on voice and voice disorders (Blue Tree Publishing, 2002), well-suited for providing information to adult voice patients.

For truly organic problems, such as unilateral adductor paralysis, the same explanations must be made, but in terms of inadequate and adequate glottal closure. Most voice patients want to understand what their problems are and what they can do about them. Make use of medical and diagnostic information, but explain in language the patient can understand. Such imagery as "your vocal cords are coming together too tightly," or "you seem to place your voice back too far in your throat," may lack scientific validity but may help the patient understand the problem. Make explanations brief and to the point, but take care not to put the patient psychologically on the defensive during the first visit. If, after the evaluation, it appears that some psychological or psychiatric consultation is necessary, further diagnostic–therapy sessions may have to be held before the patient can agree to find out more about his or her feelings.

Typical Case History Showing Utilization of the Approach. C. V., a 62-year-old widow, came to the clinic with a voice problem that first resembled spasmodic dysphonia. As she volunteered her history, her voice sounded tight, strangled; it sounded as if she were crying. She differed from the typical patient with spasmodic dysphonia in the diagnostic session and early therapy periods by demonstrating normal voice repetition skills, and she could count or read aloud with normal phonation. Spontaneous narratives, however, about her former work as a department store buyer or details about her personal life were portrayed vocally with great struggle, sometimes accompanied by actual tearing. Early in voice therapy, her SLP was sensitive to the continuous observation that her voice symptoms were part of an overall picture of loneliness and general unhappiness about life. The woman was referred to a counseling psychologist, who, together with the SLP, has helped the patient make a happier life adjustment and consequently experience a better-sounding voice for most situations.

Evaluation of the Approach.   With a little guidance by the clinician in helping the patient understand his or her voice problem, what causes it, and what can be done about it, the typical voice patient can often make progress in overcoming the voice problem. Both children and adults profit from an explanation of their voice problem and from understanding how particular behaviors, like yelling or clearing one's throat excessively, keep their voices in trouble. Sometimes an explanation of the problem is the primary treatment with no other facilitating approaches required. For those patients who need much practice with various approaches, they seem to make better progress when they understand the rationale behind what they are practicing. Voice clinicians must remain sensitive to the psychological needs of voice patients and recognize that some of their patients have personal needs greater than improving their voices per se. Such patients should be referred appropriately to other counseling or psychological professionals.

7. Digital Manipulation

FA.7

Kinds of Problems for Which the Approach Is Useful.   Finger pressure on the thyroid cartilage can be applied by the clinician in different ways for different problems. For males, who for functional reasons are using higher F_0 values than they should, light pressure anteriorly on the thyroid cartilage appears to nudge the thyroid cartilage back slightly, shortening the overall length of the vocal folds. This shortening thickens the folds, resulting in a lower F_0. This anterior pressure approach is particularly effective for postadolescent males whose pitch levels seem to remain at prepubescent levels. Another form of digital manipulation is placing the fingers lightly on the thyroid cartilage and monitoring the vertical positioning of the larynx. During the swallow or in a fear–tension state or when singing notes toward the upper end of one's singing range, the overall larynx appears to rise; lowering of the larynx is achieved during the yawn–sigh (Boone and McFarlane, 1993) or singing at the lower end of one's range or during a very relaxed state. The digital monitoring of laryngeal height is a good technique for anyone who appears to have excessive laryngeal vertical movement or who is concerned about laryngeal posturing at high or low levels. Analysis of voice therapy effectiveness for patients with unilateral vocal fold paralysis (McFarlane et al., 1991, 1998) is another form of digital manipulation found to be effective. McFarlane and others found that finger pressure on the lateral thyroid cartilage wall can often produce better vocal fold approximation, resulting in stronger phonation.

Procedural Aspects of the Approach.   The three digital procedures used in voice therapy are quite distinct from one another, both in the procedural steps used and the kind of voice problems for which they are helpful. We list the steps separately for each of the three procedures:

1. Digital pressure for lowering pitch.

    a. With the exception of some men with falsetto voices, patients will respond to digital pressure by producing a lower voice pitch. Ask the patient to prolong a vowel (/a/ or /i/). As the vowel is prolonged, apply slight finger pressure on the thyroid cartilage. The pitch level will drop immediately.

    b. Ask the patient to maintain the lower pitch after the fingers are removed. If the patient can do this, he or she should continue practicing the lower pitch. If the high pitch quickly reverts back, repeat the digital pressure.

    c. If the method is used to let the patient hear and feel a lower pitch, the patient should practice producing the lower pitch with and without digital pressure on the thyroid cartilage.

2. Monitoring the vertical movements of the larynx.

    a. For a patient with excessive pitch variability and tension related to much vertical movement of the larynx, demonstrate how to place the fingers on the thyroid cartilage and monitor laryngeal vertical movement while phonating.

    b. Ask the patient to produce a pitch level several full musical notes off the bottom of his or her lowest note. Keeping the fingers on the thyroid cartilage, ask the patient to lower pitch one note at a time to the lowest note in his or her pitch range. Usually, the larynx will lower its position in the neck at the low end of the pitch range. Then ask the patient to sing one note at a time up to the top of the singing range, exclusive of falsetto. Toward the top of the scale, the patient should feel (through the fingertips) a slight elevation of the larynx. Review both the lowering and rising of the larynx at the extremes of the pitch range.

    c. Once the patient has experienced vertical movement in the preceding steps, point out that in production of a speaking voice that is relatively free of strain, no vertical movement of the larynx should be felt during digital monitoring. Oral reading and speaking should be developed with little or no vertical laryngeal movements. Practice in oral reading with encouraged pitch variability can then be monitored by slight digital pressure of the thyroid cartilage with the patient's confirming (hopefully) no vertical movement.

3. Unilateral digital pressure for patients with unilateral vocal fold paralysis.

    a. While there appears to be a slight phonation improvement by pressing on the thyroid lamina on the side of the paralysis, this is not always found. We begin, however, by having the patient posture the head straight forward (looking slightly down rather than upward). The patient is asked to phonate and extend a vowel. While the patient phonates, the clinician exerts medium finger pressure on the lateral thyroid wall on the side of the vocal fold paralysis. If a louder, firmer voice is produced with this pressure, continue various phonation tasks, coupled with finger pressure on the thyroid cartilage on the side of the involvement.

b. If louder voice was not achieved in step (a) above, the patient continues to look forward while the clinician applies pressure to the opposite side of the thyroid cartilage (pressing the side opposite the vocal fold paralysis). Attempt various phonation tasks while exerting this lateral finger pressure.

c. If lateral pressure to either thyroid lamina while the patient looks ahead has not produced an improvement in voice, provide lamina pressure with the head turned to one side. If the head is turned to the left, first apply pressure to the left lamina; if unsuccessful, keep the head turned left with pressure then given to the right lamina. If this produces better voice, continue phonation tasks with the head turned to the left and finger pressure on the side that seems to produce the best voice.

d. The last posture is for the head turned to the right with each side pressed in an attempt to find the better, more functional voice.

e. It should be noted again that it has been our experience that one cannot predict which head posture (straight ahead or turned laterally) and/or which side receiving finger pressure will produce a better-sounding voice, whether or not the left or right vocal fold is paralyzed. More often than not, however, digital manipulation following steps a–d will often provide for the patient a better, more functional voice.

Typical Case History Showing Utilization of the Approach. J. F. was a 17-year-old male who had been raised exclusively by his mother until her sudden death about a year before. Since that time he had lived with a maternal uncle who was concerned about the boy's effeminate mannerisms and high-pitched voice. Laryngeal examination revealed a normal adult male larynx. The boy was found to have a habitual pitch level of around 200 Hz, well within the adult female range, but below the level of falsetto. The most effective facilitating technique for producing a normal voice pitch was to apply digital pressure on the external thyroid cartilage. The young man was able to prolong the lower pitch levels with good success, but any attempt at conversation would be characterized by an immediate return to the higher pitch. After three therapy sessions, he was able to read aloud using the lower pitch but was unable to use the lower voice in conversation except with his male clinician. Subsequent psychiatric evaluation and therapy were initiated for "identity confusion and schizoidal tendencies." Voice therapy was discontinued after two weeks, when it was clearly demonstrated that the patient could produce a good baritone voice (125 Hz) whenever he wanted. Unfortunately, follow-up telephone conversations several months after therapy revealed that he was using his high-pitched pretherapy voice exclusively.

Evaluation of the Approach. The effectiveness of any one of the three digital manipulation approaches can be determined immediately. Either the anterior digital pressure to the thyroid cartilage will lower voice pitch or it will not. If the speaking pitch is lowered with digital pressure, it affords an excellent "window" for the patient (such as a young man with puberphonia) to experience producing a lower-pitched voice. Tracking the vertical movements with light finger pressure can often help the patient appreciate the amount of unnecessary laryngeal movement he or she may be experiencing. Finally, in the search for a more functional voice after unilateral vocal fold paralysis, digital pressure on the thyroid lamina with or without head turning may uncover a functional voice. Developing such an uncovered voice in the patient with unilateral vocal fold paralysis may obviate the need for various surgical procedures in the quest of restoring a functional voice (McFarlane et al., 1991, 1998).

8. Elimination of Abuses

FA.8

Kinds of Problems for Which the Approach Is Useful.   There are many ways that one can abuse or misuse the voice. *Vocal abuse* comprises various behaviors and events that have some kind of deleterious effect on the larynx and the voice, such as

1. Yelling and screaming
2. Speaking against a background of loud noise
3. Coughing and excessive throat clearing
4. Smoking
5. Excessive talking or singing
6. Excessive talking or singing while having an allergy or upper respiratory infection
7. Excessive crying or laughing
8. Weight lifting with effortful "grunts"

Vocal misuse means improper use of voice, such as

1. Speaking with hard glottal attack
2. Singing excessively at the lower or upper end of one's range
3. Increasing vocal loudness by squeezing out the voice at the level of the larynx
4. Speaking at excessive intensity levels
5. Cheerleading (Case, 2002)
6. Speaking over time at an inappropriate pitch level
7. Speaking or singing (such as a prolonged show rehearsal) for excessively long periods of time

We could, obviously, add other abuses and misuses to such a list. Identification and reduction of vocal abuse–misuse are primary goals in voice therapy for hyperfunctional disorders such as functional dysphonia with or without such physical changes as vocal nodules, polyps, or contact ulcers. Therapy cannot be successful until contributory vocal abuse–misuse can be drastically reduced. Optimum usage of the voice, such as the vocal hygiene program outlined in Chapter 8, also requires identifying possible abusive voice situations and making deliberate efforts to minimize their occurrence.

Procedural Aspects of the Approach

1. Time must be given early in voice therapy to identifying possible vocal abuse. Once a particular vocal abuse is identified, the patient and clinician should develop a baseline of occurrence. This will often require that the clinician hear and observe the patient in and out of the clinic environment, such as on the playground, at the pulpit, or in a nightclub. The number of times the particular event occurred must be tallied.

2. Children with vocal abuse must become aware of the impact of such abuses on their voices. With children we use the "Vocal Abuse Reduction Program" (Boone, 1993), which recommends: an explanation of how additive lesions occur, using the story *A Voice Lost and Found;* a review of the child's abuses; and a systematic reduction of the child's abuses, using the voice tally card, the voice counting chart, and the hot-air balloon race (p. 7). The focus of the reducing abuse program is to make the child cognitively aware of the relationship of vocal abuse–misuse to increasing symptoms of voice. The story in the program is pictorially illustrated with various vocal behaviors related to changes of "the little bumps on the vocal cords."

3. Discuss identified vocal abuses with the patient, emphasizing the need to reduce their daily frequency. Assign to the patient the task of counting the number of times each day he or she engages in a particular abuse. Perhaps a peer or sibling could be brought in, told about the situation, and asked to join in on the daily count. Depending on the age of the patient, a parent or teacher, spouse, or business associate might be asked to keep track of the number of abuses that occur in their presence. At the end of the day, the abuses should be tallied for that day.

4. Ask the patient to plot his or her daily vocal abuses on a graph. Along the vertical axis, the ordinate, the patient should plot the number of times the particular abuse occurred, and, along the base of the graph, the abscissa, the individual days, beginning with the baseline count of the first day. Instruct the patient to bring these graphs to voice therapy sessions. Keeping a graph usually increases the patient's awareness of what he or she has been doing and results in a gradual decrement of the abusive behavior. The typical vocal abuse has a sloping decremental curve, indicating its gradual disappearance. Greet any decrement in the plots of the people observing the patient, but particularly in those compiled by the patient, with obvious approval.

Typical Case History Showing Utilization of the Approach.   Joyce was a 27-year-old secretary who complained of a voice that was often hoarse and that tired easily every day. Subsequent indirect laryngoscopy confirmed a slight bilateral thickening at the anterior–middle third junction. A detailed history and observation of the patient found that she constantly cleared her throat. The throat clearing had become a habit. She rarely felt that she was able "to bring up any mucus" but just cleared her throat in an attempt to make her voice clearer. A high-speed motion picture depicting throat clearing was shown to the patient. She was counseled to try to reduce its occurrence. The patient subsequently began to tally her throat clearing and coughing as they occurred, plotting them on a graph at the end of the day. Within two weeks, she was able to change her throat-clearing habit. Her vocal quality improved immediately and she never needed formal, long-term voice therapy.

Evaluation of the Approach.   Identifying vocal abuses and attempting to eliminate them by plotting their daily frequency on a graph are effective in helping young children with voice problems. Adolescents are equally guilty of vocal abuses and profit from keeping track of what they are doing. Typical adult abuses, such as throat clearing, are often eliminated after a week or two of graph plotting by motivated patients. The effectiveness of this approach, in fact, is highly related to the skill of the clinician in motivating the patient to eliminate the abusive behavior. The value of the plotting is more in developing awareness of the frequency of the problem than in the actual count per se. Reduction of vocal abuse has become a primary part of most voice therapy programs for children (Andrews and Summers, 2000; Boone, 1993; Stemple, Gerdeman, and Glaze, 1994) and for adults (Boone and Wiley, 2000; Case, 2002; Morrison and Rammage, 1994).

9. Establishing a New Pitch

FA.9

Kinds of Problems for Which the Approach Is Useful.   Although it is well established that there is no absolute optimum pitch at which a particular person should speak, some people with voice problems may profit from speaking at a different pitch level. A change of pitch will often have positive effects on voice, such as improving vocal quality and loudness. Speaking at the very bottom of one's pitch range requires too much force and effort. Similarly, speaking habitually toward the top of one's range can be vocally fatiguing. Because a number of instruments available today can portray fundamental frequency in real time (while one is phonating), awareness and feedback of one's ongoing pitch level play prominent roles in establishing new pitches through therapy (Watts, Murphy, and Barnes-Burroughs, 2003).

Procedural Aspects of the Approach

1. If pitch needs to be raised or lowered, describe where the patient is and where the target pitch is. The methods for determining habitual pitch and pitch range described in Chapter 6 can be applied here. Make a tape recording of the patient producing various pitches, including feedback about the old pitch and the projected target pitch. The playback should always be followed by some discussion comparing the sound and the feeling of the two pitches.

2. Most voice patients can imitate their own pitch models, once they have been produced by the appropriate facilitating technique. Occasionally patients cannot initiate a pitch to match a model, as Filter and Urioste (1981) found in testing college

women with normal voices. A useful model can be produced by having the patient extend an /i/ at the target pitch level for about five seconds and recording the phonation on a loop recorder. The patient will immediately hear the target production. The loop tape playback will provide the patient with a continuous playback of his or her own voice model of the target pitch. There are many advantages to using the patients' own voices as their voice models, in that they already have voicing experience producing the sounds they are now trying to match. Remain with the loop model /i/ for considerable practice before introducing a new stimulus.

3. Several excellent instruments available today can provide real-time display of fundamental frequency, both with a digital read-out and on a display screen on a monitor: PM 100 Pitch Analyzer, Phonatory Function Analyzer, Visi-Pitch, and B & K Real-Time Frequency Analyzer (see reference section at end of book). Usually, these instruments permit the clinician to display patient voice values specific to frequency and intensity. The PM 100 and Visi-Pitch both offer split-screen capabilities, whereby a voice model can be put on an upper screen and the patient's production displayed on a lower screen, permitting comparisons between model and trial productions. Any instrument that can display fundamental frequency information can provide valuable feedback to a patient attempting to establish a new voice pitch.

4. Using any of the four instruments described in step 3 above, the patient can receive exact feedback relative to the frequency he or she is using. Any deviation below or above the target F_0 can be given in immediate feedback. Of great benefit for the patient is developing the immediate awareness when he or she is producing the target F_0.

5. Establishing a new pitch is facilitated by working first on single words, preferably words that begin with vowels. Each word is repeated in a pitch monotone (using the target pitch). Occasionally a patient has more difficulty using the new pitch with certain words. Any such "trouble" words should be avoided as practice material because what is needed at this stage of therapy is practice in rapidly phonating a series of individual words at the new pitch level.

6. Once the patient does well at the single-word level, introduce phrases and short sentences. It is usually more productive at this stage to avoid practice in actual conversation because the patient is better able to use the new phonation in such neutral situations as reading single words, phrases, and sentences. When success is achieved at the sentence level, assign the patient reading passages from various voice and diction books. Success in using the new pitch level can be verified by using the instruments described earlier in step 3.

7. After reading well in a monotone, the patient may try using the new pitch in some real-life conversational situations. In the beginning he or she may have more success talking to strangers, such as store clerks; patients often find it difficult to use the new pitch level with friends and family because their previous "sets" may prevent them from utilizing their new vocal behavior. Whatever conversational situation works best for the individual should be the one initially used.

8. It is helpful in therapy to record the patient's voice as he or she searches to establish a new and different pitch level. When the patient is able to produce a good voice at the proper pitch level, his or her own "best" voice can then become the therapy model.

Typical Case History Showing Utilization of the Approach.   John, a 10-year-old boy, was referred by his public school speech clinician for a laryngeal examination because of a six-month history of hoarseness. The findings included a normal larynx and a "low-pitched dysphonic voice." John could readily demonstrate a higher phonation, which was characterized by an immediate clearing of quality. In the discussion that followed the tape-recorded playback of his "good" and "bad" voice, John stated that he thought he had been trying to speak like his older brother. The clinician pointed out to him that his better voice was more like that of other boys his age, and that the low-pitched voice he had been using was difficult for others to listen to. In subsequent voice therapy with his school clinician, John focused on elevating his voice pitch to a more natural level. His success was rapid, and therapy was terminated after six weeks.

Evaluation of the Approach.   The pitch of the voice changes constantly, according to the speaker's situation. In some patients, however, the pitch level appears to be too high or too low for the overall capability of the laryngeal mechanism. In other people, an aberrant pitch level is just one manifestation of the total personality. Patients with additive masses to the folds (nodules, papilloma, polyps, and so on) may have lower pitch levels than normal because the thicker vocal folds vibrate more slowly, emitting a lower fundamental frequency. As the lesion is reduced or eliminated, the frequency of the voice becomes higher, perhaps approaching normal limits. For patients with additive laryngeal lesions due to vocal hyperfunction, it is often best to work slowly toward increasing pitch level to approximate levels of the patient's age and sex peers. Some patients use aberrant pitch levels because of personality factors. Counseling such patients and helping them want to change pitch levels might well have to precede actual symptomatic therapy to alter pitch. Typically, however, voice patients who may need to change pitch levels can do so rather quickly, after experiencing marked improvement in overall voice quality because of pitch change.

10. Focus

FA.10

Kinds of Problems for Which the Approach Is Useful.   Good focus of the voice is characterized by the voice coming "from the middle of the mouth, just above the surface of the tongue" (Boone, 1997, p. 71). Problems in "horizontal" voice focus occur when the tongue is too far forward or too far backward within the mouth. The "thin" or baby-sounding voice is produced by carrying the tongue high and forward. The back-focused voice, sounding like the country bumpkin voice, is produced by carrying the tongue elevated in the back of the mouth.

The most common focus problem we see in patients with voice disorders is the voice sounding as if it were deep in the throat. Many patients focus on their throats as the anatomical site of their problem. Such patients profit from resonant therapy or the front-focus approach because it shifts their mental imagery from the throat to the upper vocal tract (Boone, 1997; Verdolini, 2000).

Perkins (1983) has written that "voice that feels focused high in the head" is a more efficient voice, and it can survive extensive vocalization. The clinician helps the patient focus on the area of his or her face under the cheeks and across the bridge of the nose. Most patients with chronic dysphonia experience both difficulty finding their voices and continued expectancy of vocal failure. They clear their throats continually, they make phonation rehearsals, and they worry about the poor vocal quality they are likely to have the next time they attempt to speak. For these patients successful voice clinicians often employ two techniques, respiration training and placing the voice in the facial mask, for two reasons: (1) to improve respiratory control and resonance; (2) to transfer the patient's mental focus away from the larynx and place it with the activator (respiration) and the resonator (supraglottal vocal tract).

Procedural Aspects of the Approach

1. An explanation of focus is facilitated by having the patient review Figure 7.3 with the clinician. Determination is first made as to what kind of remedial focus is needed: Is the voice too far forward, too back, or sounding deep in the throat? Although cited in the Figure 7.3 line drawing, a nasal focus is not presented as a focus problem.

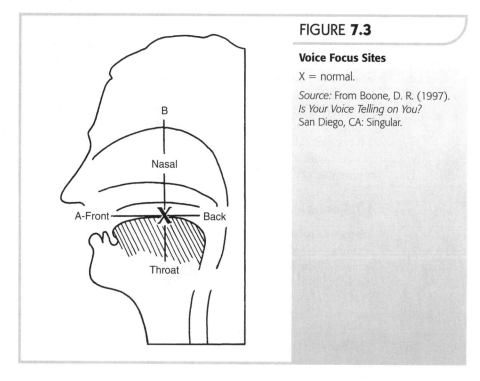

FIGURE **7.3**

Voice Focus Sites

X = normal.

Source: From Boone, D. R. (1997). *Is Your Voice Telling on You?* San Diego, CA: Singular.

2. For anterior focus, the clinician points to the left side (labeled "Front") of the horizontal line A in Figure 7.3, saying to the client, "It appears that your voice sounds too far forward in your mouth. This seems to be caused by carrying your tongue high and forward in your mouth. This makes the voice sound babyish or thin." If possible, the clinician should imitate a thin, front sounding voice, commenting afterward, "I made the thin voice with my tongue carried forward."

    a. Front-of-the-mouth focus can often be corrected by producing back-of-the-mouth sounds in rapid succession. We ask the patient to repeat "kuh-kuh-kuh-kuh" in a rapid series, stressing the back consonant /k/ and other low back vowel sounds like "kah," "guh," and "gah."

    b. For other exercises designed for correcting anterior focus, the clinician might use the exercises from Boone's *Is Your Voice Telling on You?* (1997, pp. 79–80).

    c. Compare the old thin voice with the back voice, using some kind of loop or recorded feedback.

3. For posterior-focused voice, the clinician points to the right end of the A line in Figure 7.3 marked "Back." We say to the patient, "Your voice sounds back in your mouth, which seems to come from your tongue placed too far back. We can bring your tongue forward by practicing some front-of-the-mouth sounds."

    a. We seem to get posterior-to-anterior shift of focus quicker when only whisper is used on the first practice words. The patient is instructed to repeat front-of-the-mouth words like *peep, pipe.* Each word is said rapidly four or five times, like "peep-peep-peep-peep-peep."

    b. TH (voiceless) words like *this* or *that* are whispered in rapid succession, four or five times.

    c. /s/ words like *see* and *sat* are whispered in a rapid series.

    d. The whispered series for each word is then repeated with light voice. Posterior focus exercises may be found in Boone (1997, pp. 80–81).

4. Poor vertical focus, with the voice sounding as though it is focused down deep in the throat, produces poor vocal quality. Of the three focus problems (front–back–throat), the throat focus voice is the most common problem seen in the voice clinic. Getting the voice "out of the throat" is a problem of mental imagery. Although the clinician and the patient can hear the low-throat voice focus, it is not possible to find an exact anatomic site where the low voice is produced. Rather, we use the imagery of "placing the voice in the facial mask" or in the middle of the face, as shown in the drawings of Figure 7.4. Or we tell the patient, referring back to Figure 7.3, "Your voice should sound like it's coming from the ×, where the two lines cross, or from the surface of your tongue."

    a. Time should be given in developing the imagery of taking the voice "out" of the throat and "placing" it in the front of the face, or the facial mask (Verdolini, 2000). Many clinicians and voice scientists profess skepticism over the construct of focus; however, functionally a change of focus can

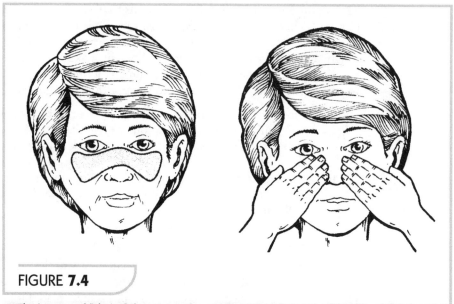

FIGURE **7.4**

The imagery of "placing" the voice in the middle of the face is helped by using these two pictures.

Source: From Boone, D. R. (1993). *The Boone Voice Program for Children* (2nd ed.). Austin, TX: Pro-Ed.

produce an immediate and dramatic change in the sound of the voice. While physiologically we cannot demonstrate focus, its immediate sound effects produce measurable changes in voice (less perturbation, formant shifts, quality differences).

b. Give as much time as possible to step a above. A good way to begin higher focus is with increased nasalization. Have the patient say "one-a-one-a-one" with exaggerated nasality. Place the fingers along the bridge and sides of the nose to feel the sound vibrations in the nose. Use other monosyllabic nasal words like *mom, me, many,* and exaggerate their nasality.

c. If the patient confirms feeling the vibrations of the nasal consonants and the nasalized vowels, practice reading short nasal sentences with exaggerated nasal resonance, such as "many men want some money." Practice reading /m-n-ng/ phrases and sentences. Contrast the feeling of the higher-focused nasal voice with the lower throat voice. The two voices should sound and feel different.

d. If the nasal consonants have facilitated a higher focus from the throat focus, introduce some high front vowels and words like *baby, beach, take,* emphasizing the resonance in the facial mask.

e. This is a good time to listen critically to the higher-focused resonance. Use the loop playback of the Facilitator, or listen to the voice and look at the tracings on the Visi-Pitch. Contrast the old lower focus with the higher mouth focus, contrasting the sound and the "feel" of the two voices. Oral reading and conversation in the voice clinic should emphasize the feeling of higher focus and the "set" the patient assumes to achieve it.

Typical Case History Showing Utilization of the Approach. Lilly was a 49-year-old financial planner who decided that her voice was "too small for the kind of work I do." A subsequent voice evaluation found her to have a habitual voice pitch around 260 Hz (near middle C) with a thin, front-of-the-mouth resonance. An endoscopic examination found her to have a normal larynx. When she listened to her voice on cassette playback, she commented, "That's the kind of baby voice I always seem to have." Our subsequent voice therapy emphasized developing a more posterior focus to her voice. In a few therapy sessions, she developed a voice that sounded like it came from "further back," with a noticeable improvement in overall voice resonance. She was also able to lower her voice pitch two full notes to 195 Hz (near an A3). After eight therapy sessions, she consistently showed a more mature voice with normal resonance. On a two-year follow-up interview, she continued to demonstrate a normal voice.

Evaluation of the Approach. For the patient with a thin, front voice or a back, "bumpkin" voice, or a low in the throat voice, changing one's voice focus appears to be an easily attained goal. Contrasting the sound of the voice from front, back, or low with a voice that sounds like it is coming from the middle of the mouth or higher in the facial mask is a vital step in using focus in therapy. If the patient can change the sound focus of his or her voice after clinician instruction and modeling, the impact on improving voice is almost immediate. Successful use of focus can be coupled with other therapy approaches, such as auditory feedback, establishing a new pitch, nasal–glide stimulation, and the open-mouth approach. Occasional voice patients will be unable to hear the difference between a deep-focused voice and a higher-placed facial mask voice; for such patients, the focus approach cannot be used.

11. Glottal Fry

FA.11

Kinds of Problems for Which the Approach Is Useful. True glottal fry is produced in a relaxed manner with very little airflow and very little subglottic air pressure (Zemlin, 1998). Glottal fry, considered a normal voice register, is valuable for patients with vocal nodules as well as for patients with other hyperfunctional problems such as polyps, cord thickening, functional dysphonia, and even spasmodic dysphonia and ventricular phonation. Although glottal fry can be an extremely powerful facilitating technique to improve voice in the dysphonic patient and is a useful diagnostic vocal probe, it has a second use, as well: It can be an index of vocal fold relaxation. In order to produce a glottal fry of 65 to 75 Hz, which is desirable, the vocal folds must be relaxed. A patient may not always be able to achieve this fry in the first session, but the accomplishment of a "good fry" of about 70 or 75 Hz is an index that the larynx has been relaxed. The glottal fry can be produced on either inhalation or exhalation. After producing glottal fry phonation for 5 to 10 seconds and then being asked to say a phrase such as "easy does it," a patient with nodules often experiences normal or near-normal vocal quality for the first time in months.

Procedural Aspects of the Approach

1. A common pencil eraser or very dry hard raisin can represent a vocal nodule. When placed between the pages of a hardback book, the eraser keeps the pages apart with a gap on either side of the eraser; likewise, nodules produce a gap between the vocal cords. If the eraser is placed between two marshmallows instead of between the pages of a book, the marshmallows "wrap around" the mass of the eraser. In glottal fry, the compliant vocal cords can "wrap around" the nodules and improve approximation. A clinician can see this with stroboscopic videoendoscopy and demonstrate it to the patient.

2. Ask the patient to let out half of his or her breath and then say /i/ softly, holding it until it fades away slowly. Encourage the patient to stretch the /i/ as long as possible.

3. Once the patient has a well-sustained /i/ in the glottal fry mode, have him or her open the mouth medium wide and protrude the tongue. Then have the patient make the tone "larger" by "opening the throat." The desired tone is a deep, resonant, slow series of individual pops, which we describe as sounding "like dragging a stick along a picket fence."

4. Have the patient attempt to produce the same tone on inhalation as on exhalation. Some people are better able to produce the glottal fry on inhalation. Also have the patient alternately reverse the tone—first on exhalation, then on inhalation. Next, have the patient say words such as *on* and *off* and *in* and *out* in the glottal fry mode. Suggest that the patient slightly prolong these words and say them on both inhalation ("on," "in") and exhalation ("off," "out"), alternately back and forth between ingressive and egressive airflow. Record the glottal fry so the patient has a model or target.

5. When the patient is able to produce these words well and can produce the sustained /i/ or /a/ in glottal fry, ask him or her to say "easy does it," "squeeze the peach," or "see the eagle" in a normal voice. These are almost always produced with greatly improved or normal vocal quality. The patient will generally be able to say only a few words with the improved quality and will then need to go back to the glottal fry mode. Record these phrases and contrast them with the patient's typical voice. Also ask the patient to judge the two.

6. When the correct glottal fry is learned, instruct the patient to practice for a few minutes several (ten or more) times each day. To assist the patient in practice, suggest that he or she tie practice to the environment—for example, by producing the

fry each time he or she sees a bus or a red car, or during the last two minutes of each hour. The patient must be producing the fry appropriately before you allow practice.

Typical Case History Showing Utilization of the Approach.   Mark, a 10-year-old boy, and Brian, an 11-year-old boy, were referred for voice evaluation by an oto-laryngologist who had diagnosed bilateral vocal nodules. Both boys had low-pitched, hoarse voices with frequent phonation breaks during connected speech. They had had these voices for nearly one year. After teaching glottal fry as just described, we had "contests" to see who could fry the longest and at the slowest rate. We had the boys say words in the fry mode back and forth to each other. We saw each boy twice a week, once together and once individually, for 45-minute sessions. In three months, their voices were normal, and the nodules were completely gone. We should note that with one boy, we reduced vocal abuses during his soccer activity as well.

Evaluation of the Approach.   The approach appears to work because very little subglottic pressure and very little airflow are required to produce the glottal fry. Therefore, there is little stress on the folds. The compliant folds seem to reduce the amount of friction as they meet during phonation. This allows the nodules to be reduced or reabsorbed even though the patient continues to talk. The new talking is produced with far less vocal fold tension.

12. Head Positioning

FA.12

Kinds of Problems for Which the Approach Is Useful.   Basic to good vocal performance (acting, lecturing, singing) is good posture and head positioning. Also, changing head position may facilitate a better voice in patients with various kinds of voice problems. Patients with unilateral vocal fold paralysis will sometimes demonstrate a stronger voice by lateralizing head position, with or without digital pressure on the lateral lamina of the thyroid cartilage (see facilitating approach 7, digital manipulation). Finding optimum head positioning has been found to be helpful in chewing and swallowing with patients with various neurological disorders (McFarlane, Watterson, Lewis, and Boone, 1998). The symptoms of dysarthria involving both speech and voice may be minimized in a particular patient by a specific head position. We find that a patient with symptoms of vocal hyperfunction can often experience a better, more relaxed voice by placing the head in a different position. Several distinct head positions can be tried in therapy in an attempt to find one that facilitates better voice:

1. Normal straight ahead
2. Neck extended forward with head tilted down, face looking up
3. Neck flexed downward with head tilted down, face looking down
4. Neck flexed unilaterally with head tilted to either the left or right, with tilted face looking forward
5. Head upright and rotated toward left or right, face looking in that direction

Any one head position may change pharyngeal–oral resonating structures in such a way that a change in vocal quality (either better or worse) may occur.

Procedural Aspects of the Approach

1. Introduce the approach by demonstrating various head positions, either by photograph, video, or live demonstration. A simple explanation of the technique should accompany the demonstration: "Sometimes changing the positions of our heads can improve the sound of our voices. The head can be tilted either down or back, or to the left or right. Sometimes we can improve the sound of our voices simply by turning our heads to one side or the other. No one head position seems to help everyone. Let us try a few and listen to any changes in voice we hear."

2. The best voicing task to use to search for head position influence is the prolongation of vowels, such as /i/, /ɪ/, /ɛ/, /æ/, /o/, or /u/. Once a helpful position is discovered, any kind of voice practice material can be used.

3. Many gradations in positioning are possible between the normal head position and one of the extreme head positions described previously. For example, when flexing the neck and bringing the head down in a gradual movement, perhaps at the beginning of the movement, a voice change can be noted. As soon as change can be noted, if it is to occur, the head should be kept at that position without going to the full range of the movement.

4. Neurologically impaired patients may experience some oral–pharyngeal asymmetry from their disease, that is, one side of the neck or oral cavity may function better than the other side. A particular lateral movement of the head may make a sudden and noticeable improvement in voice in such patients. If so, then ask the patient to practice voice material with the head in the lateral position. Head positioning, particularly to one side, is often effectively combined with lateral digital pressure (facilitating approach 7) on the thyroid lamina, searching with the patient to find the position that seems to increase subglottal pressure, resulting in a louder, more functional phonation (McFarlane et al., 1998).

5. Patients with vocal hyperfunction, that is, patients who use too much effort to talk, often profit most from neck flexion with the chin tucked down toward the chest. Such downward carriage of the head seems to promote greater vocal tract relaxation. If an easy, target voice is achieved with neck flexion, this head-down position should be held during voice practice attempts.

Typical Case History Showing Utilization of the Approach. Mary was a 55-year-old housewife who had had vocal difficulties for the past five years. A subsequent voice evaluation found that she had a moderately severe functional dysphonia accompanied by neck tension with severe mandibular restriction, hard glottal attack, and an inappropriately high voice pitch. Voice therapy was scheduled twice weekly with therapy focus on increasing her mouth opening, developing an easy glottal attack with "a legato phonatory style." The chewing and open-mouth approaches were unsuccessful until changing head position was added to the therapy. Mary was instructed to "tuck in her chin," flexing the anterior neck muscles with her face looking downward. Keeping her chin down, she was able to reduce neck tensions; she experienced immediate improvement in vocal quality. In subsequent therapy sessions, she developed an awareness that much of her past vocal strain was related to her tendency to hyperextend her neck; by using the opposite head position with anterior neck flexion, she was able to produce voice with relatively little strain. This change of head position, coupled with other therapy techniques designed to promote greater oral openness and ease of vocal production, helped Mary reestablish a normal voice.

Evaluation of the Approach.   Changing to another head position by flexing or extending the neck can have an immediate positive effect on voice quality. Such an approach is seldom used in isolation but rather usually in combination with other voice therapy approaches, such as using the open-mouth approach or digital manipulation. Whereas patients such as Mary with severe functional tensions often profit from anterior neck flexion, voice problems caused by some neurogenic diseases are often minimized by using some of the other head positions described earlier, in this section. Lateralization of the head by looking to one side or the other can often produce a stronger voice in patients with unilateral vocal fold paralysis. Changing head positions to facilitate better voice requires much trial and error. If a particular head position works, it should be used; if not, other head positions should be tried.

13. Hierarchy Analysis

FA.13

Kinds of Problems for Which the Approach Is Useful.   In hierarchy analysis, the patient lists various situations in his or her life that ordinarily produce some anxiety and arranges those situations in a sequential order from the least to the most anxiety provoking. Individual patients may instead prepare a hierarchy of situations, ranging from those in which they find their voices best to those in which they find them worst. This technique is borrowed from Wolpe's (1987) method of reciprocal inhibition, which teaches the patient relaxed responses to anxiety-evoking situations. After identifying a hierarchy of anxiety-evoking situations, the patient begins by employing the relaxed responses in the least anxious of them and, in therapy, works his or her way up the hierarchy, thereby eventually deconditioning his or her previously established anxious responses. The identification of hierarchical situations (less anxiety–more anxiety; worst voice–best voice) is a useful therapeutic device for most patients with hyperfunctional voice problems, which by definition imply excessive overreacting. Patients with functional dysphonia, or with dysphonias accompanied by nodules, polyps, and vocal fold thickening, frequently report that their degrees of dysphonia vary with the situation. Such patients may profit from hierarchy analysis. Case (2002) reports effective use of hierarchy analysis for particular aspects of voice, such as pitch or loudness.

Procedural Aspects of the Approach

1. Begin by developing in the patient a general awareness of the hierarchical behavior to be studied. If, for example, the patient is to be asked to identify those situations in which he or she feels most uncomfortable, discuss with the patient the symptoms of being uncomfortable. Or if the patient is going to develop a hierarchy of situations in which he or she experiences variation of voice, discuss and give examples of a good voice or a bad voice. Explain that the patient must develop a relative ordering of situations, sequencing them from "good" to "bad." Some patients are initially resistant to this sort of ordering, perhaps because they never realized that there are relative gradations to their feelings of anxiety or relative changes in their quality of voice. They may not be aware that the degree of their anxiety or hoarseness is not constant.

2. Although the majority of voice patients are soon able to arrange situations into a hierarchy, a few require practice sequencing some neutral stimuli. On one occasion, a woman was taught the idea of sequential order by arranging five shades of red tiles from left to right, in the order of the lightest pink to the darkest red. Having done this, she was then able to sequence her voice situations, proceeding gradually from those in which her voice was normal to those in which it was extremely dysphonic.

3. As a home assignment, have the patient develop several hierarchies with regard to his or her voice. One hierarchy might center on how the patient's voice holds up with the family, another on how it is related to the work situation, and a third on what happens to it in varying situations with friends. After these hierarchies have been developed by the patient at home, review them in therapy.

4. In therapy, use the "good" end of the hierarchical sequence first. That is, begin by asking the patient to recapture, if possible, the good situation. The goal of therapy is to duplicate the feeling of well-being or the good voice that the patient experienced in the situation rated as best. Efforts should be made in therapy to recall the good factors surrounding the more optimum phonation. If the patient is successful in re-creating the optimum situation, his or her phonation will sound relaxed and appropriate. The re-created optimum situation thus serves as an excellent facilitator for producing good voice. After some success in re-creating the first situation on the hierarchy, capturing completely his or her optimum response (whether this is relaxation or phonation or both), the patient will then be able to move on to the second situation. Again the goal is to maintain optimum response. The rate of movement up the hierarchy will depend entirely on how successfully the patient can re-create the situations and maintain optimum response. By using the relaxed response in increasingly more tense situations, the patient is conditioning himself or herself to a more favorable, optimum behavior.

5. Although some patients can re-create situations outside the clinic with relative ease, some cannot. As soon as possible, have the patient practice the optimum response outside the clinic under good conditions, so that he or she will eventually

be able to use it in the real world in more adverse situations. The patient must not lose sight of the goal of maintaining the good response in varying situations outside the clinic.

6. Not all patients can go all the way up the hierarchy, maintaining good voice at each level. Such patients should be counseled that most people experience anxiety or poorer voice in some situations, such as at the highest level of the hierarchy. Some practice might be given at one step lower in the hierarchy where good performance is still maintained.

Typical Case History Showing Utilization of the Approach.   Jamie was a 28-year-old transsexual who was in counseling for gender transference from male to female. As part of her overall gender-change program it was recommended that she "receive speech–voice therapy to develop a more feminine speaking style." In voice therapy, Jamie reported that her out-of-clinic voicing was continually changing, "very dependent on what kind of situation I find myself in." Jamie was employed full-time as a secretary–receptionist in an area agency for aging. Her speech–language pathologist worked with her to develop this nine-step hierarchy in which she found she had the best female voice all the way down to the level where it seemed hardest to convey her femininity:

Best Voice

1. I always have my best new voice with my mother.
2. The director of our agency. She is always a great listener to everyone.
3. I answer the phone at work with a very good voice.
4. The doctor at the clinic doesn't listen as well as he should. He wants me to try harder to be a woman.
5. Some salespeople are hard to talk to and especially car mechanics.
6. I think some people at the church are bigots.
7. I still date my old girlfriend who doesn't understand me anymore.
8. Meeting new men tends to make me nervous and my speech breaks down.
9. Talking with my dad is hardest. He won't accept me and still calls me Jim.

Worst Voice

Evaluation of the Approach.   Most voice patients report great variability in voice quality, depending on how much they have been using the voice, the time of day, and the psychodynamics of the speaking situations. Hierarchy analysis is often helpful for dealing with vocal inconsistencies experienced while talking with different people in various situations. By analyzing the hierarchical situations in which voice deteriorates or improves, the patient develops an awareness of those situational cues that are causing voice changes. Perhaps for the first time, the patient realizes that voice quality is not a constant and that vocal quality fluctuations are somewhat dependent on how relaxed one feels or how comfortable one is with his or her listeners. Therapy then focuses on using the best voice found low on the hierarchy. The patient attempts to use that optimum voice in those situations in which he or she has previously experienced difficulty. Hierarchy analysis is consistently useful in voice therapy.

14. Inhalation Phonation

FA.14

Kinds of Problems for Which the Approach Is Useful.   Patients who have functional aphonia and functional dysphonia often profit from inhalation phonation. It introduces the high-pitched inhalation voice, which, according to Lehmann (1965), is always produced by true vocal fold vibration. This can be a helpful technique for the patient who perseverates using ventricular phonation and often demonstrates difficulty "getting out of it." Likewise, it can be helpful for the patient with functional dysphonia who has developed some maladaptive voice that seems to resist change. On videoendoscopy, when the voice patient is asked to produce an inhalation voice, we see the true folds in a stretched position (lengthened in their respiratory length) suddenly adducted and set in vibration. It is the relative thinness of the folds on inspiration that seems to produce the high-pitched voice. The ease with which most patients can produce the technique (inhaling with voice and exhaling with a near-matched voice) makes the approach readily useful in establishing or reestablishing true vocal fold vibration.

Procedural Aspects of the Approach

1. This particular approach, which is similar to masking, is perhaps better demonstrated than explained. Demonstrate inhalation phonation by phonating a high-pitched sound while elevating the shoulders. It is important to time the initiations of the inhalation with shoulder elevation. Elevate the shoulder so you can mark for the patient the contrast between inhalation (shoulders raised) and exhalation (shoulders lowered).

2. After demonstrating several separate inhalations with simultaneous shoulder elevation and phonation, say, "Now, I'll match the high-pitched inhalation voice with an expiration voice." Inhale, raising the shoulders and simultaneously humming in a high pitch, then dropping the shoulders on exhalation and producing the same voice. Repeat the inhalation–exhalation matched phonations several times.

3. Ask the patient to make an inhalation phonation. He or she should repeat the inhalation phonation several times. Now again repeat the inhalation–exhalation matched phonation, taking care to make the associated shoulder movements. Then tell the patient, "Now drop your shoulders on expiration, making the same high-pitched voice as you do it." With a little practice, most patients are able to do it.

4. After the patient has produced the matching hum, say, "Now, let us extend the expiration like this." Demonstrate a continuation of the high pitch, sweeping down from your falsetto register to your regular chest register on one long, continuous

expiration. Repeat this several times. Then say to the patient, "Once I've brought my vocal cords together at the high pitch, I then sweep down, keeping them together, to the pitch level of my regular speaking voice."

5. If the patient is unable to produce this shift from high to low, repeat the first four steps. If the patient can make the shift down to the regular speaking register, say, "Now you're getting your vocal cords together for a good-sounding voice." Take care at this point not to rush the patient into using the "new" voice functionally. Rather, have the patient practice some similar hum phonations. After some practice just phonating the hum, give the patient a word list containing simple monosyllabic words for "true" voice practice.

6. Once the patient is able to produce inspiration–expiration without difficulty, he or she should be instructed to no longer use the pronounced shoulder movements. Elevating and dropping the shoulders are only necessary to mark the difference between inspiration and expiration.

7. Stay at the single-word practice level until normal voicing is established. We often spend several therapy periods practicing the new phonation as a motor practice drill without attempting to make the voice conversationally functional. You might say, "Now we're getting the vocal folds together the way we want them." This places the previous aphonia or ventricular phonation "blame" on the mechanism rather than on the patient. Counseling with the patient at this time is important. The motor practice gives the patient time to adjust to the more optimum way of phonating.

Typical Case History Showing Utilization of the Approach.   Derek, a five-year-old boy, was found to have small bilateral vocal nodules. His speech clinician placed him on complete voice rest, which unfortunately was enforced for five continuous months. At the end of five months, the nodules had disappeared, and Derek was instructed by both the physician and the speech pathologist to resume normal phonation. Despite all his efforts, Derek could only whisper. He became completely aphonic but whispered easily to all people with much animation and relative comfort. This functional aphonia remained for two months, after which he was instructed, "Go back and talk the normal way." Derek gestured that he wanted to use his voice but could not "find it." Therapy efforts for restoring phonation were begun about seven months after Derek's phonations had ceased. Inhalation phonation was initiated, and at the first therapy session Derek was able to produce a high-pitched inhalation sound and to follow his clinician well by matching the inhalation with an expiration sound. He was able to use an expiration phonation, appropriate in both quality and pitch, by the end of the first therapy session. He was scheduled for two other appointments within a 24-hour period, during which he practiced producing his regained normal voice. He was counseled that his "voice is working now and you'll never have to lose it again." The boy has had normal phonation since his voice was restored using the inhalation phonation technique. Counseling to curb yelling and other vocal abuses appeared to be successful, as Derek has experienced no return of the bilateral vocal nodules.

Evaluation of the Approach.   Some patients who experience either aphonia, dysphonia, or ventricular phonation for any length of time lose their ability to initiate normal true fold phonation. The longer the aphonia or dysphonia persists, the harder it might be to use normal voice. Inhalation phonation is a simple way to produce true cord approximation and voicing. The high-pitched voice on inhalation probably results from the folds being longer in their inhalation posture, and even though they may adduct on command, they remain in their longer configuration. This elongated posture thins them, resulting in the higher-pitched phonation. The important part of the approach, however, is matching the inhalation voicing with exhalation voicing. Once the patient can produce the exhalation voice without the inhalation prompt, the inhalation practice is no longer needed.

15. Laryngeal Massage

FA.15

Kinds of Problems for Which the Approach Is Useful.   This particular approach follows the procedures, modified slightly, for manual circumlaryngeal therapy, as presented by Aronson (1990), which offer gentle manipulation and massage of the larynx. The approach is recommended for use with patients with functional voice disorders in which structural or neurogenic causal factors cannot be identified. While the most commonly used professional term for such voice disorders is *functional dysphonia,* a few authors have recommended that these functional disorders be classified as *psychogenic dysphonia* (Aronson, 1990) or *muscle tension dysphonia* (Morrison and Rammage, 1994). As introduced earlier in this text, we use the term *functional dysphonia* generically to include hoarseness without identified structural or organic cause, ventricular dysphonia, puberphonia, falsetto, and voicing with discomfort (pain, scratchy throat, etc.). Stress, psychological conflict, and overall systemic tension often appear to worsen the symptoms of functional dysphonia. Manual circumlaryngeal therapy offers gentle laryngeal manipulation and massage, resulting in lower laryngeal carriage and greater intrinsic–extrinsic laryngeal muscle relaxation.

There are two studies in the literature (Roy, Bless, Heisey, and Ford, 1997; Roy and Leeper, 1993) that both report successful use of manual circumlaryngeal therapy as a primary therapy for patients ($N = 17$ and 25, respectively, in the two studies) with functional dysphonia. Of startling clinical significance is that positive reduction of voice symptoms was achieved for each patient in only one therapy session using this laryngeal manipulation–massage therapy. Although the present authors can report good results with this technique, we have also achieved lower laryngeal posturing with greater muscle relaxation using the yawn–sigh technique (Boone and McFarlane, 1993). Therefore, in our clinical practice, we employ the yawn–sigh first for the patient with a high larynx and laryngeal tension. If the patient is not successful employing the yawn–sigh, our next approach is the use of manual circumlaryngeal therapy as described by Aronson (1990).

Procedural Aspects of the Approach

1. The first step is a screen for a high larynx and likely excessive laryngeal–neck muscle tension. If not present, other facilitating approaches are used. If present, we continue.

2. The yawn–sigh is first attempted (see facilitating approach 25). If a lower larynx and greater muscle relaxation are achieved by using the yawn–sigh, we do not apply laryngeal manipulation and massage.

3. We follow Aronson's procedures for reducing "musculoskeletal tension associated with vocal hyperfunction":

    a. Encircle the hyoid bone with the thumb and middle finger. Work back posteriorly until the major horns are felt.

    b. Apply light pressure with the fingers in a circular motion over the tips of the hyoid bone.

    c. Repeat this procedure with the fingers from the thyroid notch, working posteriorly.

    d. Find the posterior borders of the thyroid cartilage (medial to the sternocleidomastoid muscles) and repeat the procedure.

    e. With the fingers over the superior borders of the thyroid cartilage, begin to work the larynx gently downward and laterally at times.

    f. Ask the patient to prolong vowels during these procedures, noting changes in quality or pitch. Clearer voice quality and lower pitch indicate relief of tension. Because of possible fatigue, rest periods should be provided.

    g. Improvement in voice is immediately reinforced. Practice should be given in producing voice in vowels, words, phrases, and sentences.

    h. Discuss with the patient how voice tension has been reduced. Repeat the procedures. Can the patient maneuver his or her own larynx to a lower position?

4. We find out whether the patient can experience the same lowering of the larynx with muscle relaxation by producing the yawn–sigh. We discuss how both techniques can be used when excessive laryngeal tension is experienced.

Typical Case History Showing Utilization of the Approach.   Carl was a 23-year-old graduate student in speech and hearing sciences who complained to his clinical supervisor that in certain situations he experienced "such tightness in my throat, I can hardly get my voice out." A subsequent voice evaluation found him to have unnecessarily high carriage of his larynx accompanied by some evidence of functional dysphonia. He was asked to read Aronson's description of therapy for "musculoskeletal tension (vocal hyperfunction)" (1990, p. 339). Subsequently, the supervisor conducted a full one-hour manual circumlaryngeal therapy session with Carl that had an immediate result of lowering his laryngeal posture and relaxing his voice, resulting in "a voice that was always there with greater intensity and less perturbation." Carl was followed over an 18-month period (while in graduate school) and was able to maintain a normal voice following the one session of laryngeal ma-nipulation and massage.

Evaluation of the Approach.   One only has to see a demonstration of this manipulation–massage technique to be impressed with its sudden effectiveness in reducing muscular tension and producing a more relaxed, lower-pitched, resonant voice. We have been impressed with the results of laryngeal massage. Aronson has described his approach as "maneuvering the patient's laryngeal and hyoid anatomy," which fits the term *massage,* described as "the act of rubbing, knead-ing, or stroking the superficial parts of the body with the hand" (Blakiston, 1985, p. 913). The studies by Roy and Leeper (1993) and Roy and colleagues (1997) sug-gest short-term benefits from using laryngeal massage or manual circumlaryngeal therapy with functional dysphonic patients.

16. Masking

FA.16

Kinds of Problems for Which the Approach Is Useful.   Patients with functional aphonia are often able to produce normal phonation under conditions of auditory masking. Using masking with patients who have functional dysphonia will often reveal a "window" of improved phonation. It appears that many such patients pro-duce faulty voices because of poor real-time auditory monitoring. The use of mask-ing in both diagnostic testing and therapy will often reveal changed phonation states that can then be recorded and used as voice models in subsequent therapy. The masking facilitating approach uses a voicing–reflex test, which audiologists administer as the Lombard test (Newby, 1972). The normal hearing patient will increase voice loudness reflexively when hearing a masking noise. In fact, the Lombard test was first introduced as a method of finding voice in patients with functional aphonia. When asked to phonate in a loud-noise background, patients with functional aphonia sometimes used light voice. In the voice–reflex situation, the patient wears earphones and is asked to read a passage aloud. As the patient is reading, a masking noise is fed into the earphones. The louder the masking, the louder is the patient's voice. At loud masking levels the patient cannot monitor well either the loudness or the clearness of his or her voice. Some patients with func-tional dysphonias actually experience clearer voices when they cannot monitor their productions because of loud masking. Some care should be given to the amount of masking intensity that is used, particularly when using white or pink noise masking (ASHA, 1991). The use of speech-range masking, such as that provided by the Facilitator (1998), permits effective masking at relatively low intensity levels.

Procedural Aspects of the Approach

1. The masking approach is best used without any prior explanation. The in-creased voicing experienced under masking conditions is produced on a reflexive, nonvolitional basis.

2. Masking should be presented with the patient wearing headphones and not presented free-field. The patient is seated by a masking source, such as the white noise of an audiometer or the speech-range masking of the Facilitator. The patient is asked to read aloud and to keep reading no matter what kind of interruption he or she may hear. We typically have the patient read (or very young children are asked to count) about ten seconds, introduce masking for five seconds, go back to reading without masking, then reintroduce masking. We record the patient's oral reading, and on playback we can hear the changes in voice that are introduced when masking occurs.

3. A recording should be made as the patient reads aloud. An aphonic patient's whisper may change to voice under conditions of masking. It is important to have recorded the emergence of voice, which the patient can use in step 5. The dysphonic patient (functional, ventricular, or puberphonic) should also be recorded while using the masking approach. Marked differences in voice quality between the absence and presence of masking conditions will probably be evident.

4. Five- or ten-second exposures to masking are introduced to the patient bilaterally. The intensity levels should be in excess of 70 dB SPL, which is sufficiently loud to mask out the patient's own voicing attempts. Whenever an aphonic patient hears the loud masking, he or she may attempt some feeble vocalization. Under masking a dysphonic patient will produce a louder voice and often a voice with more normal vocal quality as well.

5. Do not use the masking method beyond the trial stage with those few voice patients who do not demonstrate the voice–reflex effect. If it works well, and produces voice improvement, the method may be used as part of every therapy period. You might then experiment by having the patient listen to recordings of himself or herself, to see whether the patient can match volitionally his or her voice under masking conditions. Recordings can then be made contrasting the voice without masking (attempting to re-create the same voice as heard under masking) and the voice with masking. Try to have the voices sound alike.

6. A patient may profit from reading aloud under masking conditions, and then having the masking abruptly ended to see if he or she can maintain the better voice. Many other variations using the masking noise can be initiated by inventive clinicians.

Typical Case History Showing Utilization of the Approach. Lillian was a nine-year-old girl who had a history of vocal nodules that had been previously treated successfully with voice therapy. Several months after therapy had been terminated as successful (no nodules, normal voice), Lillian developed a severe influenza that left her with no voice. She was completely aphonic and could communicate only by whispering and using good facial expressions and gestures. The aphonia continued for one month (over the December holiday break) before she returned to the voice clinic. The masking approach was used with Lillian after attempts at modeling and request for voice failed. Lillian was asked to read aloud under conditions of 70-dB masking. Her reading attempts were recorded on a 20-second loop tape. As soon as masking was introduced, light phonation was heard and recorded on the loop cassette. The masking and oral reading were stopped, and Lillian was asked to hear her good voice on the tape. The child clapped her hands in joy that she now had a returned voice. Further masking followed by ear training was used as her voice became stronger. After two follow-up therapy sessions, Lillian was discharged with a normal voice. The pushing approach—producing the word *patch* with sudden extension of arms—was then demonstrated for Lillian to use "if you ever lose your voice again." Hopefully, her "believing" in pushing as a protection against future voice loss will function as a placebo effect and prevent any recurrence of aphonia. Lillian has had no voice problem in the five years since the one month of aphonia.

Evaluation of the Approach.   The masking approach is most helpful with aphonic patients. It is also helpful for patients with some form of functional dysphonia or young men with puberphonia. If the masking noise is loud enough, in excess of 70 dB SPL, patients cannot hear their voices to monitor phonation. If required to continue speaking by reading aloud under conditions of masking, patients will often produce relatively normal voices. Clinicians should use some care in confronting the patients on audio playback with their "good" voices. Improved voices under conditions of masking should be used as the patients' models for their own imitation phonations. Clinicians should use the masking approach with some degree of eclecticism—that is, if the approach works, use it; if it does not, quickly abandon it.

17. Nasal/Glide Stimulation

FA.17

Kinds of Problems for Which the Approach Is Useful.   Clinicians frequently note that in voice therapy certain stimulus sounds seem to facilitate an easier-produced, often better-sounding voice. This is particularly true working with children and adults having problems of vocal hyperfunction. Watterson, McFarlane, and Diamond (1993) have found in studying 15 adult voice patients with vocal hyperfunction and 15 matched control subjects that nasal and glide consonants facilitated better voicing patterns and were judged by the hyperfunctional subjects as "easier" to produce. The concept of differences in vocal effort has been also investigated by Bickley and Stevens (1987) and Baken and Orlikoff (1988), generally finding that supraglottal resonance–articulatory postures have a direct relationship to laryngeal physiology and function. Using words that contain many nasal and glide consonants, usually coupled with other therapy techniques, often helps the patient produce desired "target" vocalizations. Using nasal/glide consonants as therapy stimuli is particularly useful for patients with functional dysphonia, spasmodic dysphonia, and dysphonias related to fold thickening, nodules, and polyps.

Procedural Aspects of the Approach

1. Most therapy techniques require the patient to say something. For example, in the open-mouth approach or in practicing focus, the patient is given a few stimulus words to say. Words that contain nasal or glide consonants will often produce the best-sounding voice or the voice that appears made with the least amount of effort (as compared with words containing other consonants).

2. The clinician can find a number of monosyllabic and polysyllabic words containing nasal consonants for the patient to practice saying as the response when using various facilitating approaches. Here are a few examples: *man, moon, many, morning, many men, moon man, manual lawnmower, Miami millionaire, morning singing.*

3. A variation of the technique is to use nasal monosyllabic words and introduce an /a/ between each word. Ask the patient to say three words in a row with the neutral /a/ between each word. For example, "man a man a man" or "wing a wing a wing."

4. We use the same procedure for words containing glide consonants. It has been found, however, that nasal consonants combine very well with the /l/ and /r/ phonemes, and many of our glide words contain nasal consonants: *loll, lil, rare, rah, lilly, arrow, marrow, married, married women, one lonely memory, Laura ran around, remember many lawmen.*

5. Using monosyllabic /l/ and /r/ words with an /a/ between them seems to produce good voice, such as "lee a lee a lee" or "rah a rah a rah."

Typical Case History Showing Utilization of the Approach. Louise was a 66-year-old housewife who was forced to divorce her husband of some 42 years. She experienced a number of somatic symptoms following the divorce, including a severe functional dysphonia. Endoscopic–stroboscopic examination revealed a high carriage of the larynx with moderate vocal fold compression. The yawn–sigh approach was found to be effective in lowering her larynx and encouraging a more optimal vocal fold approximation. Under the sigh condition, she was asked to say various words. It was found that words with many nasal and glide consonants facilitated the easiest-produced and best-sounding voice. Intensive self-practice and twice-weekly voice therapy for nine weeks, supplemented by concurrent psychological counseling, resulted in a good functional return of normal voice.

Evaluation of the Approach. Clinicians are always looking for voicing tasks that facilitate good voice production. Recent research has validated that certain sounds, particularly nasal and glide consonants, facilitate voice production. Among patients with vocal hyperfunction, nasal/glide consonant words are perceived by patients as producing voice with less effort (Watterson et al., 1993). Word stimuli containing many nasal/glide consonants appear to facilitate in voice therapy a voice that sounds better and is produced (according to patient self-evaluation) with less effort.

18. Open-Mouth Approach

FA.18
CS.7

Kinds of Problems for Which the Approach Is Useful.   Encouraging the patient to develop more oral openness often reduces generalized vocal hyperfunction. Opening the mouth more while speaking and learning to listen with a slightly open mouth allow the patient to use his or her vocal mechanisms more optimally. The open-mouth approach promotes more natural size–mass adjustments and more optimum approximation of the vocal folds, and this helps correct problems of loudness, pitch, and quality. Opening the mouth more is also recommended to increase oral resonance and to improve overall voice quality. The voice also sounds louder. Developing greater openness should be part of any voice therapy program wherein the patient is attempting to use the vocal mechanisms with less effort and strain. This approach is often combined in treatment with other therapy approaches.

Procedural Aspects of the Approach

1. Have the patient view himself or herself in a mirror (or on a video playback, if possible) to observe the presence and absence of open-mouth behavior. Identify any lip tightness, mandibular restriction, or excessive neck muscle movement for the patient.

2. Children seem to understand quickly the benefits of opening the mouth more to produce better-sounding voices. In our voice program for children (Boone, 1993), we use a brief story that illustrates two boys, one who talks with his mouth closed and one who speaks with his mouth open. We then introduce a hand puppet and ask the child if he or she has ever been a ventriloquist. The ventriloquist is described as someone who does not open the mouth, in contrast to the puppet, who makes exaggerated, wide-mouth openings.

3. The ventriloquist-puppet analogy (Figure 7.5) also works well with adults. Let the patient observe the marked contrast between talking with a closed mouth and talking with an open one. Ask the patient to watch himself or herself speak the two different ways in a mirror. Instruct the patient that what he or she is attempting will at first feel foreign and inappropriate. The initial stages of letting the jaw relax are frequently anything but relaxed.

4. To establish further this oral openness, ask the patient to drop the head toward the chest and let the lips part and the jaw drop open. Once the patient can do this, have him or her practice some relaxed /a/ sounds. When the head is tilted down and the jaw is slightly open, a more relaxed phonation can often be achieved (Boone and Wiley, 2000).

5. In order for patients to develop a feeling of openness when listening, and as a preset to speaking, they must first develop a conscious awareness of how often they find themselves with tight, closed mouths. One way to develop this awareness is to have patients mark down, on cards they carry with them, each time they become aware that their mouths are closed unnecessarily. The marking task itself is often enough to increase a patient's awareness, and over a period of a week the number

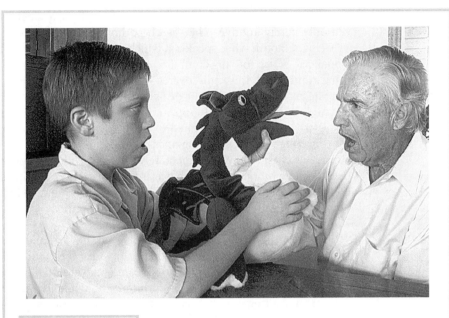

FIGURE **7.5**

Open-Mouth Approach

Clients understand quickly the benefits of opening the mouth to produce better sounding voices. Here, the approach is facilitated in a fun and whimsical manner using a puppet.

of mouth closings will decrease notably. Another way of developing an awareness of greater orality is to have patients place in their living environments (on a dressing table, desk, or car dashboard) a little sign that says OPEN or perhaps has a double arrow or any other code that might serve as a reminder.

6. Greater oral openness requires a lot of self-practice to overcome the habit of talking through a restricted mandible. Steps 3 and 4 facilitate greater mouth opening and are good practice tasks. After some practice in using greater mouth opening, the patient should confirm what it looks like by viewing video playback in practice sessions. Practice materials for improving greater mouth opening may be found in practice kits for children (Blonigen, 1994; Boone, 1993) and in voice books such as Andrews (1995), Boone (1997), Brown (1996), Case (2002), Colton and Casper (1996), and Stemple, Gerdeman, and Glaze (1994).

Typical Case History Showing Utilization of the Approach.   J. J., a 17-year-old high school girl, was examined by a laryngologist about one year after an automobile accident in which she had suffered some injuries to the head and neck. Laryngoscopic examination found all visible laryngeal structures normal in appearance and function, despite the fact that since the accident the girl's voice had been only barely audible. The speech pathologist was impressed "with her relatively closed mouth while speaking, which seemed to result in extremely poor voice resonance." Voice therapy combined both the chewing and the open-mouth facilitating approaches. It was discovered in therapy that for three months after the automobile accident the girl had worn an orthopedic collar that seemed to inhibit her head and jaw movements. It appeared that much of her closed-mouth, mandibularly restricted speech was related to the constraints imposed upon her by the orthopedic collar. When using the open-mouth approach with her head tilted down toward her chest, she was immediately able to produce a louder, more resonant voice. The open-mouth approach was initiated before beginning chewing exercises, and both achieved excellent results. Therapy was terminated after six weeks, with much voice improvement in both loudness and quality.

Evaluation of the Approach.   The voice, both normal and dysphonic, improves in quality with greater mouth opening. On opening the mouth a bit more, the voice usually improves immediately. Besides opening the mouth more while speaking, the approach also encourages slight mouth opening while listening. A gentle opening of less than one finger wide between the central incisors keeps the teeth apart and generally fosters a relaxed oral posture. The open-mouth approach has been particularly effective with performers who often open their mouths well during performance (acting, singing) but may forget the importance of opening their mouths during conversation.

19. Pitch Inflections

FA.19

Kinds of Problems for Which the Approach Is Useful.   The prosodic and stress patterns of the normal speaking voice are characterized by changes in pitch, loudness, and duration. In some individuals, the lack of pitch variation is noticeable because the resulting voice is monotonous and boring to listeners. Speaking on the same pitch level with little variation, which for the average speaker is impossible to maintain, requires the inhibition of natural inflection. It is usually observed in overcontrolled people who display very little overt affect. Fairbanks (1960), who describes pitch variation as a vital part of normal phonation, defines inflection and shift: "An *inflection* is a modulation of pitch during phonation. A *shift* is a change of pitch from the end of one phonation to the beginning of the next" (p. 132). Voice therapy for patients with monotonic pitch seeks not only to establish more optimum pitch levels but also to increase the amount of pitch variability. Any voice patient with a dull, monotonous pitch level will profit from attempting to increase pitch inflections. Many patients with functional dysphonia related to vocal hyperfunction appear to speak with little pitch fluctuation, often part of a pattern of oral and mandibular tightness with the lips and mandible in a fixed, nonmoving pattern. The SLP typically combines work on increasing loudness (intensity) with efforts to increase pitch variability; working on pitch alone is difficult without influencing loudness variations.

Procedural Aspects of the Approach

1. The patient must first become aware of his or her vocal monotony in playback of a recorded utterance or on loop playback on an instrument like the Facilitator. Play samples of lack of pitch variability and follow with samples of good pitch variability, as provided by the clinician. Follow the listening with evaluative comments.

2. Begin working on downward and upward inflectional shifts of the same word, exaggerating in the beginning the extent of pitch change. Helpful sources for increasing pitch variation may be found in Boone (1997), Boone and Wiley (2000), Brown (1996), McKinney (1994), Morrison and Rammage (1994), and Stemple and Holcomb (1988), among many others.

3. Using the same practice materials, have the patient practice introducing inflectional shifts within specific words, keeping loudness levels about the same.

4. Pitch inflections can be graphically displayed on many instruments such as the Visi-Pitch or PM 100 Pitch Analyzer. Set target inflections for the patient, to see if the patient can make his or her pitch level reach the same excursions or movement as the target model on the scope.

5. Record and play back for the patient various oral reading and conversational samples, critically analyzing the productions for degree of pitch variability.

Typical Case History Showing Utilization of the Approach.   Dr. T., a 51-year-old economics professor, received severe course evaluations from his students, who complained of his "monotonous" voice. On a subsequent voice evaluation, during both conversation and oral reading, he used "the same fundamental frequency with only minimal excursion of frequency." His voice was indeed monotonous, not only in pitch but in loudness, as well. He also used the same duration characteristics for most vowels. Dr. T. was highly motivated to improve his speaking voice and manner of speaking. Subsequent therapy focus was on increasing pitch inflections and improving loudness variations. He was provided with audiocassette tapes, which he practiced daily, matching the target model productions with his own voicing attempts. After six weeks of voice therapy and intensive self-practice, Dr. T. demonstrated improvement in both his conversational and lecture voices. Unfortunately, his lack of overall animation and boring affect still resulted in poor course evaluations. However, his conversational voice with increasing pitch inflections appeared to make a much more favorable impression on those around him.

Evaluation of the Approach.   Voice quality in functional dysphonias is often improved when overall effort in speaking is reduced. Speaking for an extended period of time in a monotone is tiring (to both the speaker and the listener). People who wish to improve the quality of their speaking voices can often profit from increasing pitch variability as they speak. Using auditory feedback, listening to one's voice on playback, appears to be a good way of improving pitch variability in one's voice.

20. Redirected Phonation

FA.20

Kinds of Problems for Which the Approach Is Useful.   Some children and adults with voice problems experience difficulty "finding" their voices. This is particularly more common among patients with functional aphonia or functional dysphonia in their attempts to find interactive phonation. In redirected phonation, the SLP searches with the patient to find some kind of vegetative phonation (coughing, gargling [Boone, 1983], laughing, throat clearing) or some kind of intentional voicing ("playing" the comb or kazoo, humming, singing, trilling [Colton and Casper, 1996], or saying "um-hmm" [Cooper, 1990]). If the patient has the capability of voicing one or more of these noncommunicative (other than "um-hmm") sounds, the sound(s) might be redirected into production of the speaking voice. Upon hearing the unintended phonation for speaking, the clinician counsels the patient, "Now your vocal folds sound like they are coming together well when you make that sound on the kazoo (or other voiced production)." This is usually followed by recording the phonation, such as the gargle or the "um-hmm," and then using it as the patient's beginning intentional voicing model.

Procedural Aspects of the Approach.   The search for random phonations that can be redirected to the speaking voice for patients with functional aphonia or functional dysphonia is obviously highly individualized. While some patients will "uncover" phonation on nontalking tasks, many patients will never be able to reveal any phonation, no matter what the task may be. Since there appears to be no preference for introduction of particular behaviors that may reveal phonation, we are listing alphabetically nine phonatory behaviors that have been reported as useful for redirecting phonation to the speaking voice:

1. *Coughing.* Asking the functional aphonic patient to cough has long been used (Van Riper and Irwin, 1958) to uncover a vegetative phonation that might be redirected to the "lost" speaking voice. The patient produces a cough on command and is then instructed to prolong the cough with an extended vowel. See Chapter 5 for further description of ways to use the cough in searching for the voice in functional aphonia.

2. *Gargling.* The voice used in gargling can often be extended after the gargling ceases. During the gargle, the patient places the gargle solution in the mouth, tilts the head back, and agitates the solution in the back of the throat by making a prolonged expiratory phonation. The patient is asked to hold the gargle expiration for five seconds. Back vowels and /k/ and /g/ are then introduced "on top" of the gargle. Keeping the same tilted upward head position, the patient is then asked to produce a "dry" prolonged gargle sound, using these back phonemes. The gargle voice is then redirected to communicative phonation practice materials.

3. *Humming.* An occasional dysphonic patient may develop a voice with less perturbation by humming a song. The clinician explains to the patient that "we are going to listen to a certain song you may know, and as we hear it, we'll hum

together the tune we hear." If the patient can hum along, the humming should be recorded and used as a possible target voice. In searching for the patient's best voice, we have on occasion found the voice during humming (and immediately afterward) as the best voice to build on in therapy.

4. *Laughing.* Humor and laughing can play an important part in voice therapy, particularly with the patient who displays excessive muscular tension while voicing. The typical patient does not realize that his or her laughter is a form of voicing. The laugh is recorded, presented on playback, and discussed from the points of view of pitch, loudness, and quality. Spontaneous laughter is usually relaxed and can provide for the patient a sharp contrast to a hyperfunctional voice, both in sound and overall body tension.

5. *Playing the comb or kazoo.* An occasional patient with functional aphonia can produce voice while playing on a comb or blowing a tune through a kazoo. The aphonic patient may be unaware that his or her musical attempts when playing the comb or kazoo are producing vocal fold vibration, or voicing. The skilled SLP does not confront the patient with the discrepancy of a musical sound (voice) with no speaking voice. Instead, the patient is instructed to articulate a word (using nasal/glide words) "on top of" the tune being played. If this can be done, attempts are made to produce the same sounds without the tune of the comb or the kazoo.

6. *Singing.* Singing can sometimes be redirected as speaking voice phonation. Occasional patients with functional dysphonia present clearer voices with less perturbation while singing. If this can be demonstrated, an early therapy task is to combine singing and speaking by singing practice sentences. Similar to procedures used during chant–talk, the goal is to eventually phase out the singing as a prelude to using the speaking voice. Efforts should be made, however, to still use the improved breath control, ease of production, and better vocal quality that was used while singing.

7. *Throat clearing.* Many voice patients clear their throats continually in their search for clearer phonation. In fact, typical vocal hygiene programs eliminate habitual throat clearing as part of the program. For the functional aphonic patient, however, we may use throat clearing in our search for a speaking voice. If the aphonic patients can clear their throats, we ask them to do it with intention. Toward the end of the throat clearing, the patient is asked to continue the effort by prolonging a low back vowel. This vocalization is then used as a "starter sound" for production of monosyllabic words beginning with low back vowels. We have redirected a vegetative phonation into a speaking voice.

8. *Trilling.* For the typical person, producing a trill is a difficult task. If a voice patient can produce the trill, it can be a most helpful technique for developing a better voice. The trill is produced by the tongue tip on the alveolar ridge with the anterior tongue oscillating in the outgoing airstream. Colton and Casper (1996) have written, "The trill appears to 'jump start' the vibratory behavior of the vocal folds" (p. 289). The trill seems to produce for most voice patients the best voice

they are capable of making and is therefore useful in voice therapy for functional dysphonia and in improving the sound of the injured voice.

9. *Um-hmm.* We call "um-hmm" the voice of agreement. When person A is listening to person B in conversation, person A may agree with speaker B by saying "um-hmm" in an automatic "natural way." Much of Cooper's (1990) direct voice rehabilitation and training focuses on redirecting the patient's utterance of "um-hmm" into an easy and improved speaking voice. The voice produced by the "um-hmm" voice is reported by Cooper to be spoken at an appropriate pitch level with good facial mask resonance. We redirect this automatic phonation with dysphonic patients, using the "um-hmm" as a starter phonation, followed by other nasalized words on the same breath, such as "um-hmm one; um-hmm man; um-hmm many." Let the patient have an immediate auditory feedback of his "um-hum" productions by using a loop playback system, such as the loop mode of the Facilitator. Introduce phrases and sentences, monitoring the patient's productions to have the same pitch and quality heard on the single words.

Typical Case History Showing Utilization of Approach. Sister Catherine was a 42-year-old nun who lost her voice while on a month-long renewal tour, where she had to give daily lectures at a number of parochial schools. Subsequent laryngoscopy found her to have a normal larynx and the speech–language pathologist found her to have "functional aphonia." Attempts at coughing and inhalation phonation were unsuccessful in early therapy attempts to help her "find" her voice. The gargle approach was introduced with immediate results. She was able to produce an expiratory phonation while gargling, with her head tilted back and her mouth wide open. The clinician rewarded her early gargle phonations with attempts like "now your cords are coming together." The Sister was reassured that her vocal folds could come together well and produce voice on expiration. After several repetitions with the gargle, voice was sustained without the need of gargling water. At the first therapy session when gargle was successfully introduced, counseling and explanations about voice were all provided; toward the end of the session, Sister Catherine was able to produce good voice consistently, coupling her phonation attempts with chanting and the open-mouth approach. Within four therapy sessions, she reported having her normal voice back again.

Evaluation of the Approach. In redirected phonation, the SLP searches with the patient to find some kind of voicing, such as coughing or playing a kazoo, and then taking that phonation and redirecting it into the speaking voice. For the patient with functional aphonia, the search for any kind of vocal fold vibration is often the first step in voice therapy. Any phonation uncovered is then applied to the speaking voice. The dysphonic patient has often adapted a number of poor voicing behaviors that might be better replaced by "um-hmm" or one of the other eight nonverbal phonations described here. Each behavior is made automatically by the patient, and once it has been redirected to the speaking voice, it is no longer needed. The search for nonverbal phonations is often part of the voice evaluation and is frequently used in the early phases of voice therapy.

21. Relaxation

FA.21

Kinds of Problems for Which the Approach Is Useful.   It is not possible for most students, working adults, and retirees to have a world that is free of tension. As Eliot (1994) has written in describing the need for relaxation and a reduction in life's stresses, "When you can't change the world, you can learn to change your response to it" (p. 87). Because encountering stress is part of the human condition, what becomes important is how we react to stresses. Our patients with hyperfunctional voices often develop vocal symptoms as part of their stress reaction. Among the particular voice symptoms Boone (1997) related to stress are diplophonia, dry throat and mouth, harshness, elevated pitch, functional dysphonia, and shortness of breath. Accordingly, a frequent goal in voice therapy is to take the "work" out of phonation by using such voice therapy techniques as the openmouth and yawn–sigh approaches along with symptomatic relaxation.

Symptomatic relaxation methods might well relax components of the vocal tract but may not lead to overall relaxation from stress reduction (Feldman, 1992). It is usually useless to imply to voice patients that if they "would just relax," their voice symptoms would lessen and their voices improve. If our patients could relax, they would. The clinician must recognize that a certain amount of psychic tension and muscle tonus is normal and healthy; however, some individuals overreact to their environmental stresses and live with "a fast idle," expending far more energy and effort than a situation requires. When such psychic effort is causative or coupled with voice symptoms, some encouragement for increasing the patient's relaxation abilities is in order. By relaxation, therefore, we mean a realistic responsiveness to the environment with a minimum of needless energy expanded.

Procedural Aspects of the Approach

1. For children, we develop an understanding of principles of relaxation, following some of the recommendations and materials offered by Wilson (1987) or Andrews and Summers (2002). For adults, it is helpful to have voice patients read the chapters on stress management and methods for reducing stage fright in Boone (1997) or read about posture and release in Brown (1996).

2. Introduce to the patient the concept of differential relaxation as outlined by Feldman (1992). The classical method of differential relaxation might be explained to the patient and applied. Under differential relaxation, the patient concentrates on a particular site of the body, deliberately relaxing and tensing certain muscles, discriminating between muscle contraction and relaxation. The typical procedure is to have the patient begin distally, away from the body, with the fingers or the toes. Once the patient feels the tightness of contraction and the heaviness of relaxation at the beginning site, he or she moves "up" the limb (on to the feet or hands, and thence to the legs or arms), repeating at each site the tightness–heaviness discrimination. Once the torso is reached, the voice patient should include the chest, neck, "voice box," throat, and on through the mouth and parts of the face. With some patients, we start the distal analysis with the head, beginning with the scalp and then going to the forehead, eyes, facial muscles, lips, jaw, tongue, palate, throat, larynx,

neck, and so on. Some practice in this progressive relaxation technique can produce remarkably relaxed states in very tense patients.

3. Various biofeedback devices can help the patient develop a feeling of relaxation. Such feedback as galvanic skin response, pulse rate, blood pressure, and muscle responsiveness through electromyographic tracings all seem to correlate well with patients' feelings of anxiety and tension. By performing a particular relaxed behavior, such as yawning, a patient can confirm his or her particular arousal state by the biofeedback data. Using such biofeedback devices, the patient can soon learn what it "feels" like to be relaxed or free of tension.

4. Wolpe (1987) combines relaxation with hierarchy analysis. The patient responds to particular tension-producing cues with a relaxed response, such as feeling a heaviness or warmth at a particular body site, and maintains a relaxed response in the tension situation. The patient may instead develop a situational hierarchy specific to tension and voice by attempting to use a relaxed voice at increasingly tense levels of the hierarchy, as outlined in the adult voice program by Boone and Wiley (2000).

5. Head rotation might be introduced as a technique for relaxing components of the vocal tract. The approach is used in this way: The patient sits in a backless chair, dropping the head forward to the chest; the patient then "flops" his or her head across to the right shoulder, then lifts it, then again flops it (the neck is here extended) along the back and across to the left shoulder; he or she then returns to the anterior head-down-on-chest position and repeats the cycle, rolling the head in a circular fashion. A few patients will not find head rotation relaxing, but most will feel the heaviness of the movement and experience definite relaxation in the neck. Once a patient in this latter group reports neck relaxation, he or she should be asked to phonate an "ah" as the head is rolled. The relaxed phonation might be recorded and then analyzed in terms of how it sounds in comparison to the patient's other phonations.

6. Open-throat relaxation can also be used. Have the patient lower the head slightly toward the chest and make an easy, open, prolonged yawn, concentrating on what the yawn feels like in the throat. The yawn should yield conscious sensations of an open throat during the prolonged inhalation. If the patient reports that he or she can feel this open-throat sensation, ask him or her to prolong an "ah," capturing and maintaining the same feeling experienced during the yawn. Any relaxed phonations produced under these conditions should be recorded and used as target voice models for the patient. Encourage the patient to comment on and think about the relaxed throat sensations experienced during the yawn.

7. Wilson (1987) includes an excellent presentation on various relaxation procedures for use with children, developed by Wilson and other authors, which seem to have equal applicability to adults. Most of the procedures described can immediately increase relaxation and reduce tension associated with speaking.

8. Ask the patient to think of a setting he or she has experienced, or perhaps imagined, as the ultimate in relaxation. Different patients use different kinds of imagery here. For example, one patient thought of lying in a hammock, but another person reacted to lying in a hammock with a set of anxious responses. Settings typically considered relaxing are lying on a rug at night in front of a blazing fire, floating on a lake, fishing while lying in a rowboat, lying down in bed, and so on. The setting the patient thinks of should be studied and analyzed; eventually, the patient should try to capture the relaxed feelings he or she imagines might result from, or may actually have been experienced in, such a setting. With some practice—and some tolerance for initial failure in recapturing the relaxed mood—the average patient can find a setting or two that he or she can re-create in his or her imagination to use in future tense situations.

Typical Case History Showing Utilization of the Approach. M. Y., a 34-year-old missile engineer, developed transient periods of severe dysphonia when talking to certain people. At other times, particularly in his professional work, he experienced normal voice. Mirror laryngoscopy revealed a normal larynx. During the voice interview, the speech pathologist was impressed by the man's general nervousness and apparently poor self-concept. In exploring the area of interpersonal relationships, the patient confided that in the past year he had seen two psychiatrists periodically but had experienced no relief from his tension. Further exploration of the settings in which his voice was most dysphonic revealed that his biggest problem was talking to store clerks, garage mechanics, and persons who did physical labor; some of his more relaxed experiences included giving speeches and giving work instructions to his colleagues. Subsequent voice therapy included progressive relaxation. Once relaxed behavior was achieved, the patient developed a hierarchy of situations, beginning with those in which he felt most relaxed (giving instructions to colleagues) and proceeding to those in which he experienced the most tension (talking with car mechanics). After some practice, the patient was able to recognize various cues that signaled increasing tension. Once such a cue occurred, he employed a relaxation response, which more often than not enabled him to maintain normal phonation in situations that had previously induced dysphonia. As this consciously induced response continued to be successful, the patient reported greater confidence in approaching the previously tense situations, knowing he would experience little or no voice difficulty. Voice therapy was terminated after eleven weeks, when the patient reported only occasional difficulty phonating in isolated situations and increased self-confidence in all situations.

Evaluation of the Approach. The popularity of many relaxation and stress-reduction programs today is probably due in part to their offering people with excessive tensions some relief from their agonies. Symptomatic voice therapy focuses on faulty voices and sometimes the tensions associated with (if not the cause of) the vocal problems. A growing number of voice clinicians feel that direct symptom modification, such as teaching relaxed responses to replace previously tense responses, breaks up the circular kind of response that often keeps maladaptive vocal behaviors "alive." In effect, we talk the same way today that we talked yesterday until we learn a better way to respond. Using the voice in a more relaxed manner with less competitive tension is a "better way to respond."

22. Respiration Training

FA.22

Kinds of Problems for Which the Approach Is Useful.   Singing teachers and vocal coaches often put more emphasis on respiration training for singers and actors than speech–language pathologists do for patients for voice disorders. While training in breath support is vital for the extremes of vocal performance produced by singers and actors, the typical patient with a functional voice disorder may need only some instruction for developing expiratory control (such as avoiding "squeezing" out final words of an utterance because of lack of adequate breath). Hoit (1995), in an excellent article summarizing studies of diaphragmatic–abdominal muscle physiology, makes a strong point for recognizing the difference in muscle function specific to whether the student–patient's body is supine or vertical. It would appear that increasing abdominal muscle participation while the patient is either sitting or standing would have some relevance to the voice patient with vocal hyperfunction. Management of respiratory limitations related to neurogenic voice disorders and pulmonary disease is discussed in Chapter 4 and 8 of this text. The following procedures are useful with functional voice disorders when there is a demonstrated need to improve respiratory function for voice.

Procedural Aspects of the Approach

1. Provide the patient with a simple demonstration on how expiratory air can set up vibration (i.e., place your lips gently together and blow through them, setting up a visual–audible demonstration). If the clinician has difficulty doing this, moistening the lips will often facilitate the vibration and its audible sound. Continue with the explanation by discussing with the patient how our outgoing air passes between the vocal folds, setting them into vibration, which we hear as voice.

2. After the patient is aware that the outgoing airstream sets the vocal folds in vibration to produce voice, a brief explanation of respiratory physiology is presented in words the patient can understand. For example, Case (2002) begins by saying in effect that as our chest gets bigger, the air comes into the lungs. As the chest becomes smaller, the air comes out, passing through the larynx. The steps for "getting bigger" and "smaller" are then described, often combined with demonstration, with the patient practicing taking in a breath and letting the breath out slowly.

3. Demonstrate a slightly exaggerated breath, as used in sighing. The sigh begins with a slightly larger-than-usual inhalation (like a yawn) followed by a prolonged open-mouth exhalation, usually with light, breathy voice. Describe the type of

breath used to produce the sigh as the "breath of well-being," the kind of easy breath one might take when comfortable or happy—the sigh of contentment. One of the authors (DB) tells his patients "the kind of noise you make when you first see the Grand Canyon!"

4. Demonstrate the quick inhalation and prolonged exhalation needed for a normal speaking task. Take a normal breath and count slowly from one to five on one exhalation. See if the patient can do this; if he or she can, extend the count by one number at a time, at the rate of approximately one number per half-second. This activity can be continued until the patient is able to use the "best" phonation achieved during the number counts. Any sacrifice of voice quality should be avoided, and the number count should never extend beyond the point at which good quality can be maintained (Boone, 1997).

5. Various duration tasks, such as prolonging vowels, provide excellent practice in expiratory control. Prolonging an /s/, /z/, /a/, /ɑ/, /æ/, or /i/ for as long as possible provides an expiratory measure that can be used for comparison. Take a baseline measurement in the beginning, such as number of seconds a particular phonation can be maintained, and see whether this can be extended with practice. Avoid asking the patient to "take in a big breath"; rather, ask him or her to take in a normal breath of well-being, initiating a lightly phonated sigh on exhalation. See if the patient can extend this for 5 seconds. If so, progressively increase the extension to 8, 12, 15, and finally 20 seconds. The voice patient who can hold on to an extended phonation of a vowel for 20 seconds has certainly exhibited good breath control for purposes of voice. Such a patient would not have to work on breath control per se, but he or she might want to combine work on exhalation control with such approaches as hierarchy analysis (to see if he or she can maintain such good breath control under varying moments of stress).

6. Select from various voice and articulation books reading materials designed to help develop breath control. Give special attention to the patient's beginning phonation as soon after inhalation as possible, so as not to waste a lot of the outgoing airstream before phonating. Encourage the patient to practice quick inhalations between phrases and sentences, taking care not to take "a big breath."

7. With young children who need breathing work, begin with nonverbal exhalations. One way to work on breathing exhalation with little children is to use a pinwheel, which lends itself naturally to the game "How long can you keep the pinwheel spinning?" With practice, a child will be able to extend the length of his or her exhalations (the length of time the pinwheel spins). Another method of enhancing exhalation control is to place a piece of tissue paper against a wall, begin blowing on it to keep it in place when the fingers are removed, and keep blowing on it to see how long it can be kept in place. Both the pinwheel and tissue-paper exercises lend themselves to timing measurements. These measurements should be made and plotted graphically for the child; when a certain target length of time is reached, the activity can be stopped.

8. When working with a singer, actor, or lecturer who needs some formal respiration training, you might take the following steps:

    a. Avoid having the patient lie supine on his or her back for the purpose of observing abdominal protusion on inhalation and abdominal retraction on expiration. As Hoit (1995) summarized, chest wall–abdominal muscle movements while supine are not the same as when sitting or standing in a vertical position. The only time we recommend watching supine abdominal movements is when the patient appears very tense; the tense patient may profit from watching the passive movements of the abdomen as the diaphragm's displacement moving toward the feet works to protrude the abdominal wall.

    b. Formal work on respiration requires good patient posture. Have the patient stand against a wall, with the buttocks and shoulders making some wall contact. Have the patient "stand tall," with the chin slightly tucked in as if the top of the head were suspended by a rope attached to the ceiling.

    c. Have patients place one hand on the central abdomen and one hand laterally low on the rib cage (ninth through twelfth ribs). Instruct them to feel the abdomen and rib cage getting larger on inhalation. On exhalation, feel the abdomen tightening and the rib cage getting smaller. This exercise should be repeated as often as required to give the patient the awareness that on inhalation the chest gets bigger and on exhalation it gets smaller.

    d. The patient is encouraged to feel the abdomen tightening on expiration. Some practice should be given to following inhalation (accomplished primarily through chest wall expansion) by gradual tightening (contraction) of the abdominal muscles. As soon as the patient demonstrates some ability to contract the abdominal muscles on expiration, add phonation activities. The voice patient who has been speaking from the level of the throat, without adequate breath support, will "feel" the difference that a bigger breath makes when phonation is desired. The voice patient who needed respiration training in the first place must have respiration and phonation combined into practice activities as soon as possible.

    e. Ask the patient to prolong vowel sounds coupled with continuant-type consonants with and without abdominal muscle support. Provide immediate auditory feedback, such as by using a loop recorder, so that the patient can contrast the voice differences produced with and without abdominal support.

    f. Develop with the patient the concept of increasing one's air volume by increasing chest expansion. Explain that with greater air volume available for expiration-phonation, it will be possible to say or sing more words per breath without squeezing or strain at the end of a phrase or sentence. It has been demonstrated (Plassman and Lansing, 1990) that subjects with perceptual cues (such as feeling chest wall expansion) can soon develop strategies to reproduce desired and greater lung volumes.

9. For serious problems in respiration, which are often related to such illnesses as emphysema or bronchial asthma, the clinician should enlist the help of

other specialists to help the patient improve efficiency. Physical therapists, respiratory therapists, and pulmonary medical specialists may have the expertise required to assist the patient. The voice clinician can often offer the patient ways of phrasing and using expiratory control to better match what the patient is trying to say and thus can supplement the respiration therapy of these other specialists. For example, we have coordinated a breathing-for-speech program for quadriplegic patients, in which the speech pathologist and the physical therapist work closely with the patient to improve both general respiration and expiratory control for speech phrasing and better voice.

Typical Case History Showing Utilization of the Approach. Libby was a 45-year-old special-education teacher who complained of vocal fatigue as a regular part of her teaching day. She felt that when she was not working, her voice was not a problem. Observation of Libby during her voice evaluation revealed that conversationally she often began to speak without an adequate inspiration. After five or six consecutive spoken words, her voice would become dysphonic and strained. Her voice problems seemed to occur when her air volumes were low and she was experiencing inadequate transglottal airflow. Subsequent voice therapy, designed to reduce the amount of work she was putting into vocalization, gave some priority to increasing her inspiratory volumes, reducing the number of words she attempted to speak on one breath, and teaching her to take "catch-up" breaths when she needed them. Loop recordings were used in therapy to monitor her breath support; she would read a ten-word sentence aloud and then immediately listen to a loop playback of the utterance, judging it for respiratory adequacy and lack of strain. After five weeks of twice-weekly voice therapy working on better respiratory control, Libby developed an easy phonatory style and a voice that served her well in her various life situations, including her teaching.

Evaluation of the Approach. A number of voice patients may profit from some kind of respiration training. At the time of the initial voice evaluation, such patients may have done poorly on air-volume and pressure tests or exhibited poor expiratory control. Vocal attempts by such patients are often strained and involve too much effort; symptoms of vocal hyperfunction are common. A slight increase of inspiratory volume may produce an immediate effect of reducing vocal strain and improving overall vocal quality.

23. Tongue Protrusion /i/

FA.23
CS.1
CS.2

Kinds of Problems for Which the Approach Is Useful. Many hyperfunctional voice problems are improved by the tongue-protrusion approach. This approach is especially helpful for patients with ventricular phonation (dysphonia plicae ventricularis) or "tightness" in the voice, such as when the laryngeal aditus (laryngeal collar) is held in a somewhat closed position. When the tongue is held in a posterior position or the pharyngeal constrictor muscles are contracted to constrict the pharynx, the voice will sound strained or "tight." A patient with such symptoms is asked to produce /i/ with the tongue extended outside of the mouth (but not far enough to cause discomfort). This works to offset the squeezing of the pharynx. The tongue must not protrude so far outside of the mouth that it causes muscle strain in the area under the chin. The /i/ is produced in a high pitch either at the upper end of the patient's normal pitch range or at the lower end of the falsetto register. This approach can be used simultaneously with the glottal fry or the yawn–sigh.

Procedural Aspects of the Approach

1. Demonstrate to the patient what is expected by opening the mouth and protruding the tongue while producing a high-pitched, sustained /i/. Stress that the jaw is to "drop open" comfortably and that the tongue is to be extended comfortably. Many patients are reluctant, at first, to stick out the tongue in the presence of a stranger, so demonstrate and reassure them that this is just what you want. You may touch the patient's chin with the index finger to encourage a little wider jaw opening and say, "Roll the tongue out a little farther."

2. The patient should go up and down in pitch while sustaining the /i/ vowel, with the mouth open and the tongue out. Listen for improved vocal quality. When this is achieved, ask the patient to sustain the tone (McFarlane, Nelson, and Watterson, 1998).

3. Have the patient chant /mimimimi/ at this level with the tongue still out of the mouth. Then instruct the patient to slowly "slip" the tongue back into the mouth while continuing to produce the /mimimimi/.

4. At this point, the pitch is usually still high. Demonstrating a sustained /i/ lowered by three steps from the pitch that the patient was producing often achieves a good quality on the first step or the first two steps, but a return to the poor voice may occur on the third step. Repeat the procedure, but only go down two steps. Sustain the second step. Repeat until the tone is established. You may need to return to the original open mouth and tongue protrusion if the target tone is lost.

5. When the new tone is established, gradually add words to the sustained /i/, for example, *be, pea, me, see the peach,* and *easy does it.*

Typical Case History Showing Utilization of the Approach.
Tammy, a 15-year-old girl, was referred with ventricular phonation of more than 18 months' duration. Her voice, which was consistently hoarse, rough, and low in pitch, was effortful to produce and made her sound like an older male speaker. Tammy had undergone a prolonged bout of flu prior to the onset of the ventricular voice, and she frequently coughed and cleared her throat violently. Strong glottal valving could be heard at times during connected speech. After seven sessions of individual voice therapy using the tongue-protrusion approach just described, Tammy's voice was normal in all situations at home, in school, and at work for the first time in more than 18 months.

Evaluation of the Approach.   This approach appears to work because the tongue, when protruded, pulls its root out of the pharynx and opens the laryngeal aditus. Also, the high pitch is made with a light, breathy approximation of only the true vocal cords. The production of voice with the tongue outside of the mouth is sufficiently novel so as not to trigger the typical pattern of phonation that may have become habituated.

24. Visual Feedback

FA.24
CS.2
CS.9

Kinds of Problems for Which the Approach Is Useful.   With the advent of computer-assisted instrumentation, there is great reliance on the monitor screen as a feedback device. For example, the patient can have a target F_0 line fixed on the screen, and the therapy task is to attempt to match the line with his or her same F_0 production. Converging of the lines is visual reinforcement of a "correct" production. When we presented using various forms of auditory feedback as a facilitating approach, we recognized that the auditory system may well depend on auditory feedback as a primary mode for modifying speech–language–voice behaviors. However, most voice patients also profit from receiving visual feedback relative to respiratory physiology, acoustic parameters of voice, and various digital feedback values (air volumes, pressure flow, F_0, or percentage of nasal resonance, and so forth). For example, patients working on nasalance problems will often profit from using the Kay Elemetrics Nasometer, which provides real-time visual feedback relative to the acoustic balance between oral and nasal resonance; the data generated by the Nasometer can provide visual feedback specific to the success of increasing or decreasing one's nasal resonance. Visual feedback can provide the patient with data specific to his or her voice measurements, as compared with the data found on the same vocal behaviors in the normal population. Visual feedback is valuable in voice therapy with any kind of patient who is working to improve or optimize vocalization.

Any of the evaluation instruments we use in our diagnostic voice evaluations that have visual dials, screens, or readouts can be used for visual feedback. We compare visually the patient's performance under different conditions, such as visual magnetometer tracings on a screen that depict relative abdominal–chest wall movements under voice intensity conditions (i.e., such as the soft voice versus the loud voice). Making photocopies of visual data provides good feedback for the patient or for the parents of a child with a voice problem who may see the child's voice progress as depicted in visual readouts (pitch changes, perturbation changes, etc.). Providing visual feedback for the patient can play a prominent role in voice therapy.

Procedural Aspects of the Approach

1. Visual feedback instruments should be introduced to the patient. In respiration, any of the measuring devices for air volume and pressure flow described in Chapter 6 may be useful, particularly in comparing early performance with performance after therapy. Real-time measurements of respiration, such as how long

one can prolong /s/, can be useful. Magnetometer tracings can be studied as the patient is performing, providing real-time feedback relative to abdominal–chest wall movements. Flexible videoendoscopy can provide the patient with visual confirmation of adequacy of velopharyngeal closure, pharyngeal and supraglottal participation during voicing, and/or detailed visualization of vocal fold movements. Stopping and restarting video playback provides visual feedback of actual oropharyngeal physiology.

2. The term *feedback* implies ongoing monitoring of some kind, giving back performance information to the patient as he or she is performing. Biofeedback (monitoring galvanic skin response, blood pressure, stress, etc.) is generally fed back to the patient visually, providing changing numeric values or changes in the number or color of lights or line tracings. Some forms of biofeedback include tactual or proprioceptive monitoring, both of which have little relevance to voice feedback, as both the pharynx and larynx are not particularly endowed with tactual or proprioceptive receptors. Acoustic and laryngeal physiology monitoring, when converted to visual images, can provide useful feedback, particularly when used jointly with another facilitating approach. For example, look at Visi-Pitch tracings and perturbation numeric values when visually tracking voice production under deliberate changes in loudness (facilitating approach 2). Ask patients to match the visual feedback they may be seeing with the loop auditory feedback of what they have just said.

3. Real-time visual feedback of patient posture, head position, mouth opening, and other body positioning can be viewed in a mirror. Prior to the advent of computer-assisted therapy, much voice therapy was done with the clinician and the patient side by side in front of a mirror. Real-time posturing feedback can also be done with a videocamera with a direct feed into a playback monitor, perhaps with a zoom closeup or a side view that couldn't be accomplished by directly looking into a mirror. The best postural visual feedback is video playback. Particular posture positions, such as verticality of head or degree of mouth opening, are recorded and either played back immediately or deferred as feedback later in the therapy session.

4. Many computer-assisted clinical software programs have vital visual feedback available for patients of all ages. For example, the *Dr. Speech* (Tiger Electronics, 1997) software programs have real-time portrayals (digital, line tracings, cartoons) for such voice parameters as pitch or loudness. Among many other computer-assisted programs is the visual feedback available in the Computerized Speech Lab (CSL) software programs (Kay, 1997) that permit looking at 22 parameters of a single vocalization, and then comparing the data with built-in threshold results.

5. The speech–language pathologist will find an endless number of software programs that can provide visual feedback on some aspect of voice performance. However, try to use only those programs that provide some ongoing auditory feedback coupled with the visual feedback.

Typical Case History Showing Utilization of the Approach.   Bill was a 21-year-old college student with vocal nodules and a severe dysphonia. At the time of his voice evaluation, it was found that he spoke at the very bottom of his pitch range. When he elevated pitch two or three notes, his voice became remarkably clearer. Using the Visi-Pitch we were able to set pitch boundaries within which we wanted him to practice. If he dropped his voice too low, he could see his tracing go below our target lines. Jitter and shimmer values dropped considerably near B2 on a piano keyboard, which we used as a target pitch. Bill profited from his clinical practice on the Visi-Pitch, which provided him with immediate visual feedback relative to both his pitch usage and the perturbation values that shifted with the pitch of his voice. Auditory feedback, particularly loop playback, was also effective for Bill in practicing an easy glottal attack with a slightly higher voice pitch. At the end of eight weeks of twice-weekly voice therapy, endoscopic examination found Bill to have "a normal larynx, free of vocal nodules."

Evaluation of the Approach.   As instrumentation is developed that can portray various aspects (respiration–phonation–resonance) of voice, it can play an important role in providing visual feedback to patients. Once a target behavior has been isolated for a patient, such instrumentation can provide ongoing feedback on the appropriateness of patient production. Feedback presents various visual portrayals (values of frequency, jitter, shimmer, and so forth) of what the patient is hearing. Various facilitating efforts in therapy often produce changes in the sound of voices that are confirmed by different feedback devices. Not to be forgotten for visual feedback are the mirror and video playback. Once an optimal voicing pattern has been established, the use of feedback devices is no longer necessary.

25. Yawn–Sigh

FA.25
CS.1
CS.2
CS.11

Kinds of Problems for Which the Approach Is Useful.   The yawn–sigh is one of the most effective therapy techniques for minimizing the tension effects of vocal hyperfunction. Characteristically, in vocal hyperfunction, we see the larynx rise, the tongue lifted high and forward, the vocal folds tightly compressed, and the pharynx constricted (Boone and McFarlane, 1993). The yawn–sigh provides a dramatic contrast: The larynx drops to a low position, the tongue is more forward, there is a slight opening between the vocal folds, and the pharynx is usually dilated, as seen in Figure 7.6. The yawn–sigh is frequently combined with other therapy approaches for such problems as functional dysphonia, spasmodic dysphonia, and dysphonias related to thickening, vocal fold nodules, and polyps. Any patient who might profit from a lower, more relaxed carriage of the larynx is a candidate to receive either laryngeal massage (following Aronson's [1990] steps for "maneuvering the patient's laryngeal and hyoid anatomy," p. 34) as outlined in facilitating approach 15 or to use the yawn–sigh approach. It has been these authors' experience (Boone and McFarlane, 1993) that if the patient can readily do the yawn–sigh, we do not have a need to use the Aronson maneuvering approach.

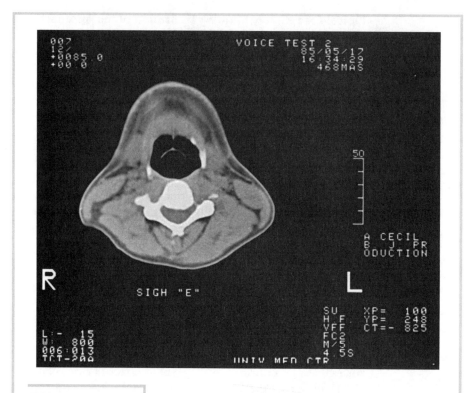

FIGURE **7.6**

A CT Scan

A CT scan depicting the dilated pharynx of a normal subject producing a prolonged /i/ vowel on an expiratory sigh. This CT scan was taken near the apex of the arytenoids, showing the horizontal cross section of the neck and mandible. Vertebral bone is shown in white; the open airway (with a slice of epiglottis across it) is represented in black (absence of tissue).

Procedural Aspects of the Approach

1. With children, explain this approach using the pictures and narrative from Boone (1993). Showing a child the appropriate pictures, we read:

> This girl usually has a tight mouth. She uses too much effort when she speaks. Her voice does not sound good. (Demonstrate) This girl is opening her mouth wide and yawning. She is very relaxed. When she sighs at the end of the yawn, it will be her best voice (p. 141).

2. With teenagers and adults, explain generally the physiology of a yawn; that is, a yawn represents a prolonged inspiration with maximum widening of the supraglottal airways (characterized by a wide, stretching opening of the mouth). You may show the photograph in Figure 7.6 and contrast it with other CT scans of the pharynx taken while subjects were doing other vocal tasks, as displayed by Pershall and Boone (1986). Then demonstrate a yawn and talk about what the yawn feels like.

3. After the patient yawns, following your example, ask the patient to yawn again and then to exhale gently with a light phonation. In doing this, many patients are able to feel an easy phonation, often for the first time.

4. Once the yawn–phonation is easily achieved, instruct the patient to say words beginning with /h/ or with open-mouthed vowels, one word per yawn in the beginning, eventually four or five words on one exhalation.

5. With teenage and adult clients, yawn–sigh exercises are available, with explanations that the patient can read in Boone (1997, pp. 121–126).

6. Demonstrate for the patient the sigh phase of the exercise, that is, the prolonged, easy open-mouthed exhalation after the yawn. Then, omitting the yawn entirely, demonstrate a quick, normal open-mouthed inhalation followed by the prolonged open-mouthed sigh.

7. As soon as the patient can produce a relaxed sigh, have him or her say the word *hah* after beginning the sigh. Follow this with a series of words beginning with the glottal /h/. Additional words for practice after the sigh should begin with middle and low vowels. Take care to blend in, toward the middle of the sigh, an easy, relaxed, relatively soft phonation. This blending of the phonation into the sigh is often difficult for the patient initially, but it is the most vital part of the approach for the elimination of hard glottal contacts.

8. Once the yawn–sigh approach is well developed, have the patient think of the relaxed oral feeling it provides. Eventually, he or she will be able to maintain a relaxed phonation simply by imagining the approach.

Typical Case History Showing Utilization of the Approach.   Jerry, a 47-year-old manufacturer's representative, had a two-year history of vocal fatigue. He often lost his voice toward the end of the workday. After a two-week period of increasing dysphonia and slight pain on the left side of the neck, a consulting laryngologist found that Jerry had "slight redness and edema on both vocal processes." The subsequent voice evaluation also found that he spoke with pronounced hard glottal attack in an attempt to "force out his voice over his dysphonia." Using the yawn–sigh approach, Jerry was able to demonstrate a clear phonation with relatively good resonance. His yawn–sigh phonations were recorded on loop and fed back to him as the voice model he should imitate. Because Jerry reported some stress in certain work situations, the hierarchy analysis approach was used to isolate those situations in which he felt relaxed and those in which he experienced tension. Thereafter, whenever he was aware of tense situational cues, he employed the yawn–sigh method to maintain relaxed phonation. Combining yawn–sigh with hierarchy analysis proved to be an excellent symptomatic approach for this patient because his voice cleared markedly, and no recurrence of the periodic aphonia was evident. Twice-weekly therapy was terminated after 12 weeks, and the patient demonstrated a normal voice and a normal laryngeal mechanism.

Evaluation of the Approach.   The yawn–sigh is a powerful voice therapy technique for patients with vocal hyperfunction. During the yawn–sigh, the pharynx is dilated and relaxed. When the patient is asked to sigh an /i/ or an /a/, the voice comes out with little effort and sounds relaxed. For some patients with continued vocal hyperfunction, the voice produced on the sigh will feel relaxed, in dramatic contrast to the patient's normally tense voice.

SUMMARY

We have included 25 facilitating approaches that can be used in symptomatic voice therapy. While most of them can be used individually, there is clinical advantage to combining certain approaches together with particular patients. For example, a typical voice therapy session might include counseling, use of the confidential voice, head positioning, visual feedback, and the yawn–sigh, combined or used sequentially. Voice therapy for most voice problems requires continuous assessment of what the patient is able to do vocally. The selection of which therapy approach to use is highly individualized for the particular patient, and no one approach is helpful for the same voice problem with every patient.

Thought Questions

1. Which of the 25 facilitating approaches could be used for treating children with vocal hyperfunction? Why would these be useful?
2. Which of the 25 facilitating approaches could be used for treating adults with unilateral vocal fold paralysis? Why?
3. Why is it recommended that the speech–language pathologist *not* establish a preprogrammed therapy sequence for a particular kind of voice disorder, such as functional aphonia? Functional dsyphonia? A neurogenic dysphonia–dysarthria?

8

Management and Therapy for Special Problems

LEARNING OBJECTIVES

- Identify the characteristics of each of the specific voice populations introduced

- Describe behavioral management approaches to each particular voice population

- Explain the role of the SLP in counseling and intervention for individuals with laryngectomy

We have reviewed various voice disorders with many different causes in Chapters 3 through 5: diseases and injuries, neurogenic factors, and misuse of the voice. For example, in Chapter 5, as we discussed voice problems related to vocal hyperfunction, we presented the cause and typical treatment of vocal nodules and vocal fold polyps. Furthermore, specific therapy approaches for nodules and polyps were described in Chapter 7. Neurogenic voice disorders, such as vocal fold paralysis and spasmodic dysphonia, were presented in Chapter 4. In this chapter, however, we consider special voice conditions and their treatment that do not necessarily fall under the headings of previous chapters. We will describe the voice problems and then focus on management strategies and possible voice therapy approaches. Voice resonance, particularly nasalance problems and their management, will be presented in Chapter 9.

In Table 8.1, we have organized the special problems discussed in Chapter 8 into three categories, with problems listed alphabetically under each heading. The text presentation then describes what is important to know about each problem from the perspective of the speech–language pathologist (SLP), followed by some description of possible management and remediation strategies.

TABLE **8.1**	**Management–Voice Therapy for Special Voice Problems**	
Particular Populations	**Respiratory-Based Problems**	**Laryngeal Cancer**
The aging voice	Airway obstructions	Medical intervention
Deaf and hard of hearing	Asthma	Laryngectomy
Pediatric	Emphysema	Counseling and
Professional voice users	Faulty breath control	communication options
Transgender	PVFM	
	Tracheostomy	

MANAGEMENT–VOICE THERAPY FOR PARTICULAR POPULATIONS

The Aging Voice

About one in every eight Americans is 65 years or older, and this number is expected to increase as the "baby boom" generation begins to turn 65 (U.S. Bureau of the Census, 2000). In fact, the size of the older population is projected to double over the next 25 years, growing to an estimated 71.5 million people (U.S. Administration on Aging, 2004). This group represents the fastest growing segment of the U.S. population, with the over-85 group showing the largest percentage increase of any population segment (Barry and Eathorne, 1994). It has been estimated that elderly clients with communication impairments constitute 19% of the caseloads of speech–language pathologists (Slater, 1992). By the year 2050 it is expected that people over age 65 will constitute 39% of the speech–language–impaired population. Therefore, speech–language pathologists must continually seek new methods of prevention, differential diagnosis, and intervention with older adults (Shadden and Toner, 1997).

There are very few epidemiologic studies of the prevalence, risk factors, and psychosocial impact of dysphonia in the elderly. Because studies of the epidemiology of dysphonia in this population have been restricted solely to investigations of those seeking treatment, the true prevalence of voice disorders in the general elderly population remains largely unknown. Roy and colleagues (Roy, Stemple, Merrill, and Thomas, 2007) interviewed 117 people over age 65 using a questionnaire that addressed three areas related to voice disorders: prevalence, potential risk factors, and psychosocial consequences/effects. They reported (p. 628) that the lifetime prevalence of a voice disorder in this population was 47%, with 29% of participants reporting a current voice disorder. The majority of respondents (60%) reported chronic voice problems persisting for at least four weeks. Seniors who had experienced esophageal reflux, severe neck/back injury, and chronic pain were at increased risk. Voice-related effort and discomfort, increased anxiety and frustration, and the need to repeat oneself, were specific areas that adversely affected quality of life. In a similar epidemiologic study of persons under the age of 65, Roy and colleagues (Roy, Merrill, Gray, and Smith, 2005) reported (p. 1998) that the lifetime prevalence of a voice disorder was 30%, with 6% of participants reporting a current voice disorder.

The term *presbyphonia* is often used to describe the clinical condition of elderly patients presenting to the otolaryngologist with gradual weakening of the voice (Kendall, 2007, p. 137). Patients complain of an inability to project the voice over background noise and hoarse voice quality which deteriorates throughout the day. Visual examination of the larynx may reveal mild bowing of the vocal fold margins, a spindle-shaped glottis, prominent arytenoid cartilage vocal processes, and vocal fold edema (Bloch & Behrman, 2001; Pontes, Brasolotto, and Behlau, 2005). Laryngostroboscopy may reveal asymmetry of vocal fold vibration and electroglottography may reveal predominance of the open phase (Winkler and Sendlmeier, 2006). Presbyphonia is correlated with poorer health-related quality of life and a tendency to avoid social situations (Costa and Matias, 2005; Golub, Chen, Otto, Hapner, and Johns, 2006; Verdonck-de Leeuw and Mahieu, 2004).

Presbyphonia is not the most common cause of hoarse voice quality in the elderly population, and may account for hoarseness in less than 10% of patients (Woo, Casper, Colton, and Brewer, 1992). Benign vocal fold lesions such as polyps are the most common cause of hoarseness in elderly patients, followed by malignant lesions, vocal fold paralysis, and functional dysphonia (Kandogan, Olgun, and Gultekin, 2003). Neurologic disorders such as Parkinson's disease and essential tremor are also common, as are inflammatory conditions such as chronic laryngitis from laryngopharyngeal reflux disease (Hagen, Lyons, and Nuss, 1996). A thorough evaluation to rule out organic disease is warranted in any elderly patient presenting with hoarseness. Considering this information, one might well conclude that management and therapy should be more focused on various disease processes than on aging per se.

Because the acoustic features of voice are affected by respiratory, phonatory, and resonance events, each must be appreciated when developing an understanding of the senescent voice (Baken, 2005; Ringel and Chodzko-Zajko, 1987). The first comprehensive studies reporting age-related changes in speech breathing were conducted in the late 1980s by Hoit and colleagues (Hoit and Hixon, 1987; Hoit, Hixon, Altman, and Morgan, 1989). Across these two seminal studies the investigators examined speech breathing in 30 males and 30 females in three age groups (25, 50, 75 years). Speech breathing changes were assessed both from extemporaneous speech and reading. The major findings of Hoit and Hixon (1987) were that elderly males demonstrated larger rib cage volume initiations, larger lung volume excursions, and larger lung volume expenditures per syllable than younger men, particularly during extemporaneous speaking. The major findings of Hoit and colleagues (1989) were that, compared to younger women, elderly females demonstrated larger rib cage excursions during oral reading, increased frequency of inhalation during reading, increased air expenditure during unphonated intervals during reading, and larger lung volume initiations during extemporaneous speaking. The speech breathing changes reported by Hoit and her colleagues correspond with reports that changes in general pulmonary functioning with aging become measurable at around age 40 years (Rochet, 1991).

Much of what is known about the acoustic characteristics of the voices of older speakers is culled from the work of Linville and her colleagues (see Linville, 2001) and Mueller and his colleagues (see Caruso and Mueller, 1997) (see Table 8.2). Many of their findings correlate well with what is known about the effects of aging on the larynx and supraglottal vocal tract (see Colton, Casper, and Leonard, 2006, and Kahane and Beckford, 1991, for extensive reviews of this topic).

In both men and women, speaking fundamental frequency (SFF) changes as an individual moves from young adulthood into old age. However, the pattern of change is quite different for the two genders: SFF in men lowers from young adulthood into middle age and then rises again into old age; in women, SFF remains fairly constant into middle age, then drops slightly and remains unchanged through old age. Maximum phonational frequency range (MPFR) also appears to be altered by the process of aging. Postmenopausal (presumably, middle-aged) women are able to produce

TABLE **8.2**   Synopsis of Voice Changes with Advanced Age

Finding	Literature Source
Speaking fundamental frequency (SFF) raises in men and lowers in women.	Awan (2006); Brown, Morris, Hollien, and Howell (1991); Linville (1996); Xue and Deliyski (2001).
Maximum phonational frequency range (MPFR) is reduced in men and women.	Hollien, Dew, and Phillips (1971); Linville (1987); Ptacek and Sander (1966); Ramig and Ringel (1983).
SFF is less stable in men and women.	Linville, Skarin, and Fornatto (1989); Xue and Deliyski (2001).
Amplitude is less stable in men and women.	Linville (1996); Linville, Skarin, and Fornatto (1989); Xue and Deliyski (2001).
Standard deviations of SFF and amplitude increase in men and women.	Linville and Fisher (1985); Orlikoff (1990); Xue and Deliyski (2001).
Maximum intensity of vowel productions is reduced in men and women.	Morris and Brown (1994).
Perturbation increases (jitter, shimmer, spectral noise) in men and women.	Awan (2006); Decoster and Debruyne (1987); Ferrand (2002); Linville (2002); Linville, Skarin, and Fornatto (1989); Xue and Deliyski (2001)
Formant frequencies are lowered in men.	Benjamin (1997); Linville (2002); Linville and Fisher (1985); Linville and Rens (2001); Liss, Weismer, and Rosenbek (1990); Rastatter and Jacques (1990); Scukanec, Petrosino, and Squibb (1991).

lower basal tones than their younger or older counterparts; however, this does not significantly expand total MPFR capabilities. At the other end of the MPFR, a reduction in the ceiling tone is a well-known finding in female speakers, even for those who have had professional voice training. In men, there does not appear to be an effect of aging on MPFR. Fundamental frequency and amplitude are reported to be less stable in older speakers and the standard deviations of these measures also tend to increase with age. Increased perturbation (that is, jitter, shimmer, spectral noise) in the voices of aging speakers also has been reported. Lastly, speech intensity has been reported to change with aging. Vocal intensity during conversational speech has been reported to increase with aging in men, but not women, and in both genders, reductions of maximum intensity of vowel productions has been reported.

Resonance characteristics of voice vary as a function of aging as well. Centralization of vowels is reported to be a common tendency of older speakers, and as a result, formant frequencies of vowels have been shown to differ in older versus younger speakers (Liss, Weismer, and Rosenbek, 1990). Lengthening of the vocal tract in older speakers is also thought to contribute to changes in formant frequencies (Kahane, 1981), chiefly a lowering of these frequencies across vowels (Linville and Rens, 2001). In addition to investigations into the effects of aging on formant frequencies, the effect of aging on nasal resonance also has been investigated, though not as extensively. Hutchinson, Robinson, and Nerbonne (1978) reported that nasalance in 50-to-80-year-old speakers is higher than the norms of younger speakers reported by Fletcher (1972). Lastly, Scarsellone, Rochet, and Wolfaardt (1999) reported slightly lower nasalance in elderly speakers when their maxillary dentures were removed versus in place, leading these investigators to conclude that existing normative data for nasalance could be applied to elderly speakers regardless of the status of their maxillary dentition.

Some general characteristics of the voices of aged people lead to their identification as older speakers. A number of studies going back to the 1960s have demonstrated a relationship between older speakers' chronological age, sex, and vocal characteristics and listener perceptions of their vocal age (Linville and Fisher, 1985; Ryan and Burk, 1974; Shipp and Hollien, 1969). More recent studies have revealed an association between perceived vocal age and inferred physical attributes of the speaker, as well as between perceived vocal age and the stereotypes of older persons. From this research literature a number of conclusions can be drawn. First, young adult listeners are capable of discriminating between younger and older adult voices with a high degree of accuracy (Huntley, Hollien, and Shipp, 1980; Ptacek and Sander, 1966), though listeners tend to slightly overestimate the age of younger speakers and underestimate the age of older speakers (Ryan and Capadano, 1978). Second, young adults are also quite good at distinguishing relatively minor differences in ages of older speakers, for example, distinguishing among 60-, 70-, and 80-year-olds (Hummert, Mazloff, and Henry, 1999). Third, young adults have a better than chance ability to estimate within five years a speaker's chronological age (Hollien, 1987). Fourth, listeners are able to reasonably estimate an older speaker's weight and height from their voice and can do so almost as well as they can from viewing facial photos (Krauss, Freyberg, and Morsella, 2002). Lastly, listeners perceive older speakers more negatively than younger speakers, particularly on competence dimensions (Hummert et al., 1999).

Tremor, hoarseness, breathiness, voice breaks, decreased loudness, slower speaking rate, and a change in habitual pitch are specific acoustic characteristics that have been identified in perceptual studies of the elderly voice of both males and females (see Ramig and Ringel, 1983, and Gorham-Rowan and Laures-Gore, 2006, for reviews). The changes in habitual pitch, however, appear to be sex-dependent. In middle-aged males an increase in habitual pitch seems to signal advancing age, while in middle-aged (postmenopausal) women a decrease in habitual pitch signals advancing age. These acoustic cues are likely the product of age-related physiological changes to the vocal tract. Some of the physiological changes that have been identified include the lengthening of the vocal tract or oral cavity, a reduction in pulmonary function, laryngeal cartilage ossification, an increased stiffening of the vocal folds, and a reduction in vocal fold closure (see Zraick, Gregg, and Whitehouse, 2006, for review).

It would appear from an overall voice management point of view that efforts to improve the overall physical fitness of the aged patient will often have a positive influence on voice (Orlikoff, 1990; Ramig and Ringel, 1983). Stemple and colleagues have reported that vocal function exercises may improve a patient's laryngeal physiology, potentially improving voice (Thomas and Stemple, 2007). Counseling the patient about the need for good vocal hygiene may be helpful. Direct work on improving respiratory efficiency can help the older person develop better expiratory control, perhaps saying more words per breath. Direct work on increasing the speed of one's speech can have a "rejuvenating" effect on the sound of the older patient's voice. Among other facilitating approaches we have found useful in improving the voice of a motivated older person are auditory feedback, focus, glottal fry, masking, respiration training, and visual feedback. Berg and colleagues have reported that voice-related quality of life improves in patients with age-related dysphonia who participate in voice therapy (Berg, Hapner, Klein, and Johns, 2008).

Deaf and Hard of Hearing

A severe hearing loss will affect voice in both children and adults. Voice is usually not affected in a sensorineural hearing loss until the loss exceeds 50 dB in frequencies under 2000 Hz (Hull, 2001). Severe congenital hearing loss takes the largest toll on development of language with severe impact on voice production. Early recognition of hearing loss among newborns enhances early intervention, which may permit some development of auditory-based language–speech skills, such as spoken language, voice, speaking rate, prosody, and speech articulation. The later in life a severe-to-profound hearing loss occurs, the less impact there will be on a child's voice.

Voice characteristics of deaf or profoundly hard-of-hearing children or adults include an elevated fundamental frequency (F_0), downward formant shifts, varied pitch and loudness changes, and resonance variations (Boone, 1966a; Seifert,

Oswald, Bruns, Vischer, Kompis, and Haeusler, 2002; Subtelny, Whitehead, and Klueck, 1989). In addition to these voice alterations, the child with congenital deafness or the child or adult who acquires profound hearing loss will usually develop a slower rate of speech by prolonging vowels and show variations in the prosody or melody of speech. The earlier the onset of deafness or profound loss, the more severe the aforementioned voice and speech symptoms.

Cochlear implants, one of the preferred treatments for minimizing speech and voice abnormalities in the profoundly hard of hearing, have yielded important information on hearing loss effects on speech–voice production. One such early study (Svirsky, Lane, Perkell, and Wozniak, 1992), used an on–off study of auditory deprivation on voice in adults with cochlear implants; they found that when the implant was turned off for 24 hours, subjects demonstrated elevated fundamental frequencies, increased intraoral pressures, and lowering of the second formant. With the restoration of electrical input via the implant, these acoustic values returned closer to normal values. Among the marked changes in speech and voice that older children experienced after cochlear implants, Seifert and colleagues (2002) found positive changes in voice pitch, elevated second formant, resonance, and rate of speech.

Older children and adults who acquire hearing loss over time may eventually show changes in loudness of voice and in articulation. Voice quality seems to hold well for those who have had normal voice for many years before the onset of hearing loss. Whenever possible, voice training for the severely hearing-impaired child or adult should not begin until efforts are made to provide needed amplification. The optimum fitting of a hearing aid has positive effects on both speech and voice, often preserving voice quality, vowel duration, and normal prosody. Cochlear implants are an option for improving the hearing competence of both children (Eisenberg and Johnson, 2008) and adults (Evans and Deliyski, 2007) with a profound sensorineural hearing loss. Recent introduction of auditory brain stem implants (Eisenberg, Johnson, Martinez, DesJardin, Stika, and Dzubak, 2008) holds promise for future generations with profound hearing loss. Once auditory amplification can be introduced, the SLP and audiologist can initiate some auditory training procedures that have been found to have positive impact on improving voice (Goffman, Etmer, and Erdle, 2002).

Although elevated voice pitch and excessive pitch variability are common findings in those with severe hearing loss, the anatomy and physiology of the larynx and vocal folds are the same as those of the normal hearing population. Hard-of-hearing children profit from developing an awareness of other voices, as well as an awareness of their own pitch levels, by using amplification feedback and instrumental tracings of pitch. Instrumental and software programs that provide good visual feedback of pitch and pitch variability may play primary roles in voice training. Such computer programs can also provide real-time feedback relative to excesses in voice loudness (too loud or not loud enough). The SLP provides display boundaries on the screen for pitch, pitch variability, and loudness, within which one must keep his or her voice values.

A useful voice-training device by the SLP is to provide "cue arrows" pointing in the desired direction of pitch change. For example, for a typical deaf child attempting to lower the voice, cards should be printed with a down arrow. These cards should be placed wherever possible in the child's environment—in the wallet, on the bureau or desk, and so on. Also, the classroom teacher and voice clinician can give the child finger cues by pointing toward the floor. Another method for developing an altered pitch level is to place the fingers lightly on the larynx and feel the downward excursion of the larynx during lower pitch productions and the upward excursion during higher ones. The ideal or optimum pitch is produced by minimal vertical movement of the larynx. Any noticeable upward excursion of the larynx, except during swallowing, will immediately signal that the voice may be at an inappropriately high pitch level. Once an appropriate pitch level has been established, the child may read aloud for a specified time period, placing the fingers lightly on the thyroid cartilage to monitor any unnecessary vertical laryngeal movement.

The typical voice of a deaf child who has had no training in developing a good voice is characterized by alterations in nasal resonance, often accompanied by excessive pharyngeal resonance, which produce a cul-de-sac voice. The major contributing factor to these resonance alterations is the excessive posterior posturing of the tongue in the hypopharynx, which markedly lowers the second formant (Monsen, 1976; Wirz, 1986). The tongue is drawn back into the hypopharynx and creates the peculiar resonance heard in deaf speakers; this back resonance sounds similar to the resonance sometimes heard in speakers with athetoid cerebral palsy, or oral verbal apraxia. The cul-de-sac voice has a back focus to it. In addition, the hearing-impaired child or adult may demonstrate marked variations in nasal resonance—too much nasal focus (hypernasality) or insufficient nasal resonance (hyponasality); such nasal resonance variations may be due in part to the posterior carriage of the tongue, as well as to the inability to monitor acoustically the nasalization characteristics of the normal speaker.

Altering the tongue position to a more forward carriage and tongue protrusion (see Chapter 7) can contribute greatly to establishing more normal oral resonance in the voice. In addition to the procedures outlined in Chapter 7 for altering tongue position, more detailed procedures and therapy materials for both children and adults are available in *The Boone Voice Program for Children* (1993) and *The Boone Voice Program for Adults* (2000). Once the tongue has been placed in a more "neutral setting" (Laver, 1980), the patient needs to practice making vocal contrasts between back-pharyngeal resonance and normal oral resonance. The patient needs to develop an awareness of what it feels like to use the lips, the tongue against the alveolar processes, the tongue on the hard palate, and other front-of-the-mouth postures. Such front focus seems to develop only after intensive practice doing tasks that encourage anterior tongue carriage.

For severely hard-of-hearing children and young adults who have had cochlear implants or who wear hearing aids, computer programs and workbooks are designed not only for auditory processing and for developing listening skills, but the same materials are available for working on speech and voice (Erlmer, 2003; Mokhemar, 2002). Several innovative software programs are also available for children and adults (VoxMetria, 2008; FonoView, 2008).

The deaf speaker must also work to eliminate hypernasality if it is present. The patient first needs to become aware of excessive nasal resonance by reviewing feedback from various instruments that measure airflow and acoustic output simultaneously from both the oral and nasal cavities. How much of the perceived voice is oral and how much is nasal can be determined by the Nasometer, which is a computer-based system that can make an acoustic analysis of the relative amount of nasalance in a voice signal. The patient produces voice that is directed into two microphones separated by a nasal–oral separator. The computer screen provides real-time feedback about the relative acoustic output between the two channels.

Pediatric Voice Problems

As noted in Chapter 1, it is estimated that more than 7.5 million American children have some trouble "using their voices" (National Institute for Deafness and Other Communication Disorders, 2007). Dysphonia can be detrimental to children both psychosocially and academically. In the psychosocial realm, studies have revealed that dysphonic children are perceived by listeners as "weak, slow, or sick" more often than normal-speaking children (Ruscello, Lass, and Podbesek, 1988). Academically, some adverse effects of voice impairment on a child's educational performance can include limited participation in speaking activities, fear of participating in oral reading activities, and limited participation in classroom discussion with peer groups. To address reduced academic performance as a function of dysphonia, Hoffman Ruddy and Sapienza (2004) describe eligibility decisions for students with dysphonia in school-based settings that fall within the framework of the Individuals with Disabilities Education Act (IDEA). These authors outline six school-based service delivery options for the voice disordered child that are effective under IDEA guidelines.

Children differ from adults in the way they produce their voice because pediatric laryngeal anatomy is distinct from adult laryngeal anatomy. As described in Chapter 2, among those differences are the size of the larynx, the proportion of membranous versus cartilaginous structure, and the position of the larynx, which in the child lies between the first and third cervical vertebrae, descending to between the sixth and seventh cervical vertebrae in the adult (Sapienza, Ruddy, and Baker, 2004).

Most etiologies underlying dysphonia or hoarseness in children are benign and generally easy to treat (McMurray, 2003); however, children presenting with hoarse voices must have a thorough voice evaluation because some voice disorders are life threatening (see Chapter 3 and Respiratory Disorders in this chapter). Dysphonia such as that experienced from laryngeal papilloma can present a significant and sometimes fatal airway obstruction. Likewise, cysts, while not life threatening, can cause dysphonia by increasing the mass of the body of the vocal fold. Therefore, it is critical that children with voice disorders be referred to a team of professionals experienced in providing comprehensive evaluation and management.

Once an organic cause is ruled out and the child has been diagnosed with a voice disorder of a functional nature, it is the realm of the speech–language pathologist, the family, educators, and other significant individuals in the child's life to identify the environments in which the abuse–misuse occurs and to develop strategies to reduce these instances of misuse (see Chapter 7). Successful voice clinicians must build into their schedules actual visit to playgrounds, music rooms, churches, and other venues where the child spends his or her day. In reducing one child's vocal abuse, a major factor was visiting the school lunchroom and changing his manner of repeating the phrase, "Do you want white or chocolate milk?" 300 times each day as he passed out the milk during the noisy lunch period. Special attention must be given to the identification of playground screaming and yelling in children. One only has to listen to the noise level of the typical primary school playground to realize that yelling at play appears to be a normal childhood behavior. A child with a voice problem, however, often has a history of yelling a little louder and a bit more often than normal-voiced peers.

In clinic, we review the anatomy and physiology of the laryngeal mechanism using videotapes and DVDs, although still photographs are also powerful visual tools to aid the patient's understanding of the disorder. We use age-appropriate descriptive terminology to discuss the mechanics of normal voice and vocal abuse. Some examples we use are discussing the soreness and redness of palms after clapping hands forcefully and asking the child to describe what his or her vocal folds would feel like if they "clapped" all day. We attempt to videorecord the child interacting with his family in free play or discussion. We review the video and discuss pitch, loudness, and vocal quality. This audio and video feedback indirectly draws everyone's attention to the distinctive qualities of voice, and the child and the family can begin to talk about voice using the same language.

A specific approach that we have found successful with the child population is attempting to pair child voice clients in therapy (Von Berg and McFarlane, 2002a). This arrangement has been found to be conducive to early and lasting success. At the beginning of the therapy session, unstimulated acoustic measures are collected from each child using the Visi-Pitch or similar instrumentation. If the clinic does not have this type of instrument, an analog or digital voice recorder is sufficient. The children listen to their voices and discuss any changes from the previous session. The children discuss vocal parameters using the same vernacular developed during the audio and videorecording of the family session discussed earlier. Each child is challenged to describe techniques that might move the voice closer to a "just right" voice. Facilitating approaches are then introduced, and each is followed by a child production using a novel phrase-generating task. The children analyze each other's productions, which is a powerful way to increase each child's understanding of the dysphonia and how to improve vocal quality. We often videorecord and immediately replay these sessions to take advantage of the children's motivation to critique and repair dysphonias.

Professional Voice Users

The professional user of voice exerts unusual demands on respiration–phonation–resonance. We use the term *professional voice* for the voice of the actor, singer, teacher, salesperson, minister, telemarketer, politician, broadcaster—people whose primary occupation competence (and probable success) is shaped by their voices. The speech–language pathologist often approaches a group of professional performers with a vocal hygiene program, providing some information about normal voice, with emphasis given to avoiding vocal excesses that might impair the voice. Holmberg, Hillman, Hammarberg, Södersten, and Doyle (2001), however, have found that a vocal hygiene program alone is not always associated with good voice. It would appear that a vocal hygiene program needs to be coupled with some voice instruction provided by a vocal coach, singing teacher, or SLP to help the professional voice user maintain a functional professional voice (Broaddus-Lawrence, Treole, McCabe, Allen, and Toppin, 2000).

One of the obstacles we experience in working with the professional voice user is the relative "performance innocence" of the teacher or clinician. The professional uses his or her voice often beyond the normal limits we generally associate with heavy voice use. The teacher or voice clinician who has never performed beyond these supposed limitations may seem unconvincing to the performer in advising how to correct a voice problem. Similar to the voice clinician who wants to communicate with the voice scientist or the scientist who likes to dabble clinically, once we stray beyond our swath of training and competence, our "performance naivete" shows to the performance expert.

Another obstacle to working successfully with the professional voice user is the lack of a meaningful shared language between the performer and the clinician. For example, the actor or singer may have been taught a way of breathing for performance that is at variance with new voice science findings specific to respiratory physiology (as presented in facilitating approach 22 in Chapter 7). Imagery abounds with performers. Yet the clinician cannot take away this imagery without replacing it with descriptions that will enhance performance, as well as encourage using vocal mechanisms in a healthy manner. Rather than attack it directly, the skillful clinician can often use performers' imagery about what they are doing and simply modify it by demonstrating how less muscle effort can produce similar vocal output. Excesses in muscle tension while performing have been categorized by Koufman, Radomski, Joharji, Russell, and Pillsbury (1996), finding that much unnecessary muscle tension occurs supraglotally, particularly among "bluegrass/country and western and rock/gospel singers." When excessive muscle tensions appear in the clinician's judgment to cause laryngeal problems, voice therapy directed toward decreasing these excessive glottal and supraglottal muscle tensions can be effective. Excessive muscle tension can be reduced by using such clinical approaches as auditory feedback, change of loudness, chant–talk, chewing, counseling, focus, changing glottal attack, laryngeal massage, open-mouth approach, relaxation, and yawn–sigh.

One of the best methods of improving voice for the teacher, salesperson, or preacher is using loop auditory feedback (Facilitator, KayPENTAX). For example, the clinician can provide a voice model that the client "matches" with a response. On the Facilitator, once the recording is stopped, the playback button is pushed and the client listens immediately on earphones to what was just said, and the clinician and client evaluate the response. Subsequent recordings can be made until client response meets some evaluative criteria. Having the client match an auditory model (the client's own or that of the clinician) enables holistic use of the vocal mechanisms, which avoids breaking down motor response into separate components. Such fragmenting of response should be avoided when possible (Boone, 1997).

Speaking with immediate auditory feedback on the Facilitator controls for background sound levels, a good practice situation but perhaps unlike the real world of speaking. In many professional voice situations, the performer must speak above unreasonable background sound levels. Among many research studies looking at noise level impact on vocal performance, Ferrand (2006) and Stathopoulos and Sapienza (1993) have found that excessive noise may compromise respiratory function, pitch changes, voice quality, and overall phonatory stability. Using the voice at high intensities to "overcome" high background noise levels, particularly for long periods of time of time, can take a real toll on the professional voice.

When actors, public speakers, politicians, ministers, and broadcasters consult with the SLP for problems with voice, the SLP should have them first complete questionnaires (Portone, Hapner, McGregor, Otto, and Johns, 2007) regarding their use of voice (Voice Handicap Index, VHI) and how the voice problem may affect their quality of life (Voice-Related Quality of Life Measure, V-RQOL). Questionnaire and voice evaluation data should be reviewed to determine what type of voice therapy is indicated. The services of either an SLP or a vocal coach (VASTA, 2008) may then be provided. A blend of both specialties is often an ideal combination for the professional user of voice who is experiencing some vocal difficulties (Zeine and Walter, 2002). Consideration is often given to providing vocal hygiene counseling and information along with voice therapy. Following simple vocal hygiene guidelines often produces immediate benefit for the professional user of voice. Combining vocal hygiene and voice exercises for teachers with self-reported voice symptoms has also been found to produce significant voice improvement (Gillivan-Murphy, Drinnan, O'Dwyer, Ridha, and Carding, 2006).

Singers often experience functional and/or organic problems of voice, and they are often referred to the SLP for consultation and possible voice therapy. A special voice handicap index for singers has been developed (Cohen, Jacobsen, and Garrett, 2007) which provides information relative to the constancy and impact of the problem on singing performance. For the SLP with a limited background in music performance and singing, consideration should be given to consultation with a singing teacher (NATS, 2008). The SLP often finds with professional singers that their vocal problems seem to originate from their activities when not singing, such as excessive throat clearing, smoking, lack of hydration, or talking too much before and after performance (Boone, 1997).

Of all professional performance groups, teachers appear to be the professional group experiencing the most vocal problems. Looking at voice disorders in a population of 550 primary school teachers, Munier and Kinsella (2008) found that "27% suffered from a voice problem, 53% reported an 'intermittent' voice problem, while only 20% had no voice problem." Roy and colleagues (2004, 2005) have found an overwhelming prevalence of voice disorders in teachers compared with other adults in the same age population. Among research studies looking at effectiveness of voice disorder prevention programs for teachers, Duffy and Hazlett (2004) and Bovo, Galceran, Petruccelli, and Hatzapoulos (2007) reported on voice prevention programs with significant voice improvement for experimental subjects (versus control groups) in the programs.

The individual teacher, when consulting with the SLP, sometimes benefits from a classroom visit by the SLP to see and hear the teacher in action. The SLP may find the teacher in the classroom using much vocal hyperfunction while teaching, in sharp contrast to normal voicing efforts in the voice clinic. In a study reviewing outcome effects of three treatments (using a voice amplifier, resonant therapy, or respiratory muscle training) for teachers with voice disorders, Roy and colleagues (2003) found that posttreatment results on the Voice Handicap Index (VHI) yielded positive support for teachers with voice problems using some kind of portable voice amplifier in the classroom. Teachers with clinical voice problems require a full medical and SLP diagnostic evaluation, followed by appropriate medical management and individualized voice therapy designed by the SLP for that particular teacher.

Transgender (Transsexual)

In the past 50 years the SLP has seen a growing number of clients who are seeking a gender identity change. Most are going through a male-to-female (MtF) transition with a desire to feminize their voices and overall communication style. Also, the fewer female-to-male (FtM) clients wish to acquire a more masculine voice and speaking style. The Harry Benjamin International Gender Dysphoria Association (HBIGDA, 2005), working to improve the living conditions of persons with gender identity change, recognizes the benefits of changing one's speech, voice, and general communication style. While for a strict definition of changing one's gender to that of the opposite sex, the term *transsexual* (TS) is more accurate, HBIGDA recognizes that the descriptive term *transgender* (TG) is now more commonly used.

The SLP working in less dense population areas, as opposed to those SLPs working in large cities, will clinically see few TG persons. An actual prevalence or incidence figure in the United States for the TG population in 2008 has not been clearly established (AGA, 2008). Although there is a growing literature base for speech–voice change in the TG patient (Adler, Hirsch, and Mordaunt, 2006), much of what is done clinically is related to positive outcome data where the patient performs more like the "target gender," and the TG patient is pleased by his or her therapy outcome performance (comparing pre- and post-VHI scores). Group evidence-based practice data are difficult to generate because of the relative scarcity of TG patients in one clinical setting, costs, the fragility of the social–psychological situation emerging around the patient, and the influence of other associated treatments (such as hormone), among other reasons (Oates, 2006).

In a private practice situation, the senior author of this text (DB) has created and used a gender speech–voice presentation scale, in which the client's communication style is scaled on ten behaviors, as seen in Figure 8.1.

At the initial voice diagnostic session, a video recording is made of conversation and an oral reading passage. The TG client and the SLP watch and listen to the playback. We spend the balance of the time going over each of the ten variables, rating the different parameters of performance by circling a score in black

FIGURE **8.1**

Gender Speech–Voice Presentation
A rating scale used in an SLP private practice for documenting communication style for transgender clients (MtF) and (FtM).

Name: _____   **Date:** _____

	M			Target			F			Comments
Altered Lexicon	1	2	3	4	5	6	7	8	9	
Breathiness	1	2	3	4	5	6	7	8	9	
Facial Expression	1	2	3	4	5	6	7	8	9	
Gesture	1	2	3	4	5	6	7	8	9	
Intonation	1	2	3	4	5	6	7	8	9	
Pitch	1	2	3	4	5	6	7	8	9	
Pitch Flexibility	1	2	3	4	5	6	7	8	9	
Rate	1	2	3	4	5	6	7	8	9	
Volume and Loudness	1	2	3	4	5	6	7	8	9	
Vowel Prolongation	1	2	3	4	5	6	7	8	9	

Summary/Plan:

ink. The target value for each variable is in the middle of the scale, the 5 value. The MtF client is scored on the left side of the scale, from 1 to 5; the FtM scale is on the right, 9 down to 5. For example, a very masculine client desiring to move toward femininity would score many 1 or 2 values in the beginning. With some therapy and much practice, TG clients will move toward the 5 value. During selected future therapy sessions, the scale is readministered and values are circled in different ink colors. Successful therapy outcome can be not only seen and heard, but illustrated by visible changes on the rating scale.

Using the ten behaviors on the presentation scale, let us consider some literature support for typical feminine and masculine speech, voice, and communication styles. The typical listener to TG speech and voice identifies pitch as the biggest variable to change. The FtM client can lower voice pitch from taking male androgen hormones, which also causes other masculinizing effects like increased muscle definition, greater appetite, and increased body and facial hair. The estrogen hormones that are taken by the MtF have no effect on vocal folds with no contributing changes to pitch or voice quality. Voice presents the "greatest challenge for up to 90% of transitioning MtF clients" (Bowers, Adler, Hirsch, and Mordaunt, 2006, p. 96). In voice therapy for the MtF client, we concentrate on elevating voice pitch (often up to F3 or G3) and increasing pitch variability and intonation, such as raising pitch at the end of a phrase or sentence (Gelfer and Schofield, 2000).

Both speaking rate and voice volume have "gender-marking" function in communication (Boonin, 2006). The adult female speaks at a slower rate than her male counterpart. In our therapy with the MtF client, we work to prolong vowels and take intra-phrase pauses to slow overall speaking rate slightly under the normal rate of 145–175 words per minute (Fitzsimmons, Sheahan, and Staunton, 2001). A slightly faster rate is encouraged for the FtM client. Voice volume is slightly higher for adult males than for females. In our therapy with TG clients we encourage voice intensity levels that are consistent with the target gender (Oates and Dacakis, 1983).

The overall gender presentation is affected by the language and gesture the client uses in conversation, at work, and at play. Biologic females may use greater adjective–adverb descriptors than biologic males. Males tend to use more controlling direct sentences with less conditional words like "I believe," "maybe," or "perhaps." The SLP interested in language differences (Hooper, 2006) between the sexes can identify some of the polarities that can be avoided or incorporated by persons in gender transition. Language pragmatics are accompanied by typical nonverbal behaviors that are somewhat different between the sexes, such as body posture, facial expression, eye contact, or hand gestures (Hirsch and Van Dorsel, 2006).

The TG person in transition is usually experiencing difficult psychological and social problems. These problems often outweigh the patient's need for voice change. Accordingly, the SLP must look at the transgender patient from a counseling perspective with the need to provide strong psychological support. When the patient is ready to change communication style to match his or her desired gender change, the SLP has much to offer with voice therapy.

MANAGEMENT–VOICE THERAPY FOR RESPIRATORY-BASED VOICE PROBLEMS

Respiratory problems often influence how a child or adult is able to use voice. Severe problems in respiration often require lifesaving medical–surgical intervention. In milder breathing problems, the SLP can often play both a diagnostic and therapeutic role, working closely with the pulmonary medicine physician and the respiratory therapist. Let us consider a few respiratory problems and their overall management, including possible voice therapy.

Airway Obstructions

The voice clinician may encounter a number of children and adults with voice problems related to airway obstructions. Although obstructive airway problems require medical–surgical intervention and management, the speech–language pathologist may play an important part in both identification and management of the disorder. The two basic contributing causes of airway obstruction (O'Hollaren, 1995) are structural and lesion mass airflow interference and abnormal laryngeal movement interference.

Airflow Interference. There are both infectious and noninfectious causes of laryngeal-mass obstruction to airflow. Severe involvement of the epiglottis and supraglottal structures is almost always the result of a bacterial infection, treatable with appropriate antibiotic therapy. Depending on the size of the supraglottal swelling, inspiratory and expiratory breathing can be seriously compromised. Subglottal obstruction from disease is most often seen in croup, a viral disease, usually characterized by inhalation stridor. Once croup is differentiated from such problems as paradoxical vocal fold dysfunction (which is often confused with asthmatic stridor), effective treatment includes "hydration, humidification, racemic epinephrine, and corticosteroids" (O'Hollaren and Everts, 1991). Airway obstruction can be caused by such space-occupying lesions as papilloma, granuloma, carcinoma, or large cysts—all described in Chapter 3. Once such lesions are identified as compromising the airway, effective medical management may include radiation therapy to reduce the lesion size or surgical reduction or removal of the lesion. The obstructive lesion is watched closely and, when it becomes too large, such as is often observed in juvenile papilloma, a surgical approach restores required airway competence. The voice clinician often plays an important role with the postsurgical mass-lesion patient, establishing the best voice possible with voice therapy (despite a scarred and abnormal glottal margin).

Vocal Fold Paralysis. The most common laryngeal movement obstruction to in and out air movement within the airway is laryngeal paralysis, unilateral or bilateral. In Chapter 4, we looked at the multiple possible causes of vocal fold paralyses and their surgical and voice therapy management. While unilateral vocal fold paralysis contributes to some compromise of the open airway, bilateral abductor paralysis produces a life-threatening obstacle to air passage, requiring immediate surgical intervention. The procedures for management of vocal fold paralysis are presented in Chapter 4 and are not repeated here.

Asthma

In asthma, the patient experiences a narrowing of airway tubes, particularly in the bronchi and bronchioles, which limits the free passage of air. Restrictions in the airway can be caused by the external smooth muscles going into spasm, causing a narrowing of the opening (Berkow, Beers, and Fletcher, 1997). The inner lining of mucosa tissue becomes compressed and inflamed, resulting in mucosal swelling and irritation, causing some production of mucus (which further obstructs the passageway). The patient struggles to take in a breath. The asthmatic spasms can be triggered by such stimuli as pollens, dust mites, animal dander, cold air, smoke, and exercise. The asthmatic symptoms may be chronic (they come and go) or part of a sudden and severe reaction that may require immediate medical intervention.

The speech–language pathologist does not usually encounter the patient during severe respiratory obstruction. Rather, most people with asthma are free of symptoms most of the time, experiencing occasional bouts of wheezing and shortness of breath. Depending on the frequency and severity of respiratory struggle, some patients experience hoarseness and breakdown in normal voicing prosody. Such patients may seek the help of the voice clinician.

The speech–language pathologist must first differentiate true subglottal asthma from parodoxical vocal fold movement. In the asthmatic patient, the primary management step is treating the spasms and inflammation that interrupt the patient's natural breathing. Oral corticosteroids appear to be the most effective treatment for asthma symptoms and airway inflammation; Djukanovic and colleagues (1997) concluded that "a moderate dose of oral corticosteroids leads to a marked reduction in airway inflammation . . . resulting in reduced airway hyperresponsiveness" (p. 831). Another form of steroid application is the use of aerosolized albuterol (Strauss et al., 1997), which seems to reduce airway inflammation experienced by the asthmatic patient. Reduction of airway inflammation appears primary for increasing airway dilation, allowing a greater passage of air into and out of the lungs.

When respiratory symptoms are under some control, the voice clinician may help the patient develop and use a functional voice. Phonation can often be improved by reducing the number of syllables the patient says on one breath. After a baseline measurement is taken, the patient should then be instructed to cut the total number in half. For example, if a patient says 20 syllables on one expiration, the patient should be instructed to limit utterances to half that number, or 10 syllables per breath. This seems to prevent vocal fold squeezing, which makes the last words of the phrase or sentence sound tight or dysphonic. Help the person to develop methods of renewing breath while speaking. Good posture with the head not tilted upward or downward, the open-mouth approach, vocal hygiene, and the yawn–sigh approach have all been found helpful for the asthmatic patient who wishes to improve vocal efficiency.

Emphysema

Among various chronic pulmonary diseases experienced by the adult population, emphysema is the most common. Emphysema is a type of chronic obstructive pulmonary disease involving damage to the air sacs (alveoli) in the lungs. As a result, the body does not get the oxygen it needs. The primary cause of emphysema is smoking or from continuous exposure to smoke-laden dust. The continuous smoke exposure in the lungs causes the alveolar walls to lose their elasticity, collapsing on pulmonary expiration (Berkow, Beers, and Fletcher, 1997). This collapse of the alveoli in turn causes the bronchioles (the airway conduits to and from the alveoli) to collapse. The result of this alveoli–bronchiole collapse is difficulty in emptying the lung during expiration (Sataloff, 1997a). Consequently, the high residual air volumes preclude taking in adequate oxygen renewal on inspiration. The patient with moderate to severe emphysema struggles to get sufficient breath to sustain his or her life. Voice abnormality is of secondary concern.

Up to 30 million people in the United States suffer from an emphysema-related illness, making it the fourth largest cause of mortality in the United States (NEF,

2007). Because the primary cause of emphysema is cigarette smoking, the first mandatory treatment step is to stop smoking. Mild emphysema can begin to show after only five or seven years of continuous, heavy smoking. It is the mildly involved patient, often a professional user of voice, who often seeks clinical help from a speech–language pathologist for a voice problem.

Voice management can only begin after the patient stops smoking. Formal respiratory therapy for these patients is better left in the hands of the respiratory therapist or other pulmonary specialists. For example, the patient might be prescribed with bronchodilators, inhaled steroids, or even supplemental oxygen. The voice clinician often begins intervention by taking voice measurements specific to air volume and available pressures for voicing, measures of duration, and sound pressure level of the voice. Observation of the patient during speaking, oral reading, and singing tasks may also reveal some unnecessary postural–skeletal behaviors the patient is using to maintain breathing, movements that may be inefficient and counterproductive to good voice control.

Some directed practice in diaphragmatic–abdominal breathing in the sitting or standing (vertical) position may be useful, as well as practice in counting syllables per utterance in an attempt to become more aware of when to renew breath. Shortening the length of phonation can help the patient have more control over voice loudness. Using a loop-feedback instrument like the Facilitator can provide direct training with feedback in breath renewal and its direct effect on voice loudness. The emphysema patient can sometimes improve voice quality by speaking at a slightly higher voice pitch. Other facilitating approaches might be tried in the search for a stronger functional voice, such as focus, glottal attack changes, masking, and pitch inflections.

Faulty Breath Control

Many children and adults appear in the clinic with faulty breath control, either caused by some organic disease or from functional misuse, or both. That is, there may be a functional overlay to an organic respiratory disease that can be directly treated, improving overall respiratory function as well as providing better breath support for voice. There are an endless number of respiratory diseases, most of which may have some impact on voice. The speech–language pathologist in working with voice patients soon learns to consult with physicians and therapists who work with patients with respiratory illnesses, as well as becoming familiar with journals such as *American Journal of Respiratory and Critical Care Medicine* or the Voice Foundation's *Journal of Voice* or reference books like *Textbook of Respiratory Medicine* (Murray and Nadel, 1994) or *Professional Voice: The Science and Art of Clinical Care* (Sataloff, 1997b). Such reference sources not only provide information about the medical treatment of various respiratory diseases, but often contain detailed references about possible management and voice therapy for these patients.

What we do with voice problems from respiratory illnesses must be consistent with the limitations imposed by various respiratory diseases and the treatments the patient may be receiving from other professionals. The clinician should not be preoccupied with the presenting disease problem, but face the patient more generically,

as a person with a voice disorder that shows itself in various pitch–loudness quality dimensions. In fact, faulty breath control may show itself more as a functional problem than as an organic one. For most patients, the voice clinician should assess respiratory–voice function following many of the evaluation procedures presented in Chapter 6. The voice evaluation should supplement any other respiratory assessment information. We use the management and therapy suggestions developed in the facilitating approach called Respiration Training for developing better breath support for voice in patients with faulty breath control.

Paradoxical Vocal Fold Movement

Paradoxical vocal fold movement (PVFM) is described by Blager (2006) as a nonorganic disorder of the upper airway with both true and false vocal folds exhibiting paradoxical function of closure on inspiration, expiration, or a combination of both. Also seen in the literature of vocal cord dysfunction (VCD), PVFM is becoming increasingly recognized in the medical community as a disorder to consider when symptoms of respiratory distress do not respond to treatment for asthma. Case (2002) presents an excellent description and photograph of the larynx during a PVFM inspiration, showing the membranous portion of the folds adducted on inspiration with a posterior triangular glottal chink. The relative smallness of the glottal chink does not permit enough open space for a normal inspiration. Trudeau (1998) suggested three possible etiologies of PVFM: psychogenic, as in conversion reaction; visceral, related to irritation from laryngopharyngeal reflux (LPR) and/or upper airway sensitivity; and/or neurological, a form of laryngeal dystonia. These categories need not be mutually exclusive.

Strenuous exercise is also often identified as a "trigger" of PVFM symptoms. It often masquerades as asthma in young athletes (Sullivan, Heywood, and Beukelman, 2001), with the prevalence as high as 5% in Olympic-level athletes (Rundell and Spiering, 2003). Therefore, it is helpful to monitor the patient during physical activity with "flow-volume loop testing" (Gallivan, Hoffman, and Gallivan, 1996). However, the patient is usually asymptomatic during time of evaluation, so a good case history and interview is mandatory. With respect to the asymptomatic patient, Guss and Mirza (2006) have suggested that PVFM can be elicited and observed with methacholine challenge testing (MCT)—that is, an aerosol that stimulates bronchoconstriction.

While most management regimens for PVFM employ voice therapy and intensive use of videoendoscopic biofeedback, Altman, Mirza, Ruiz, and Sataloff (2000) offer the use of botulinum toxin and video feedback as viable treatment options for the problem. However, the long-range efficacy of using botulinum toxin for the treatment of PVFM is not clearly determined.

Trudeau (1998), Blager (1995), Von Berg, Watterson, and Fudge (1999), Mathers-Schmidt (2001), Case (2002), and Murry, Tabaee, Owczarzak, and Aviv (2006) report good success in their respective laryngeal control programs that minimize the airway obstruction experienced by the PVFM patient. Their programs place emphasis on helping the patient to become aware of aberrant and normal vocal fold positioning during both inspiration and expiration. Some of these programs

use video feedback. The present authors use extensive videoendoscopy of correct and abnormal vocal fold postures for both phonation and quiet respiration that the PVFM patient can both observe and produce. Patients become aware of how to produce vocal fold configurations in their own larynx, showing them what to do to "open the airway when you take in a breath." The authors have found the use of the yawn–sigh a useful technique for opening the vocal folds and creating a more open airway. Other therapy procedures described by Trudeau (1998) include nasal inspiration, working on /s/ duration (not to maximum levels), and the use of diaphragmatic–abdominal breathing.

Tracheostomy

A tracheostomy, or external opening into the trachea, may be necessary when an individual experiences respiratory difficulties due to an obstruction of the upper airway, has problems with pulmonary toilet (managing secretions), or requires mechanical ventilation to maintain adequate respiration. Tracheostomy fundamentally alters the physiology of voice and swallow because the stoma is below the level of the larynx, thereby bypassing the upper airway. Decisions regarding the type and size of the tracheostomy tube will be made by the otolaryngologist, based on the individual's diagnosis, physical status, and medical needs. The speech–language pathologist is also a core member of the evaluation team, with clearly established roles and responsibilities (Kazandijian and Dikeman, 2008). Depending on the type of tracheostomy tube, the individual may or may not be able to use a tracheostomy speaking valve, which is a one-way removable valve attached to the open end of the tracheostomy tube. Specific indications and therapy for children and adults with tracheostomy tubes are discussed by Mason (1993) and Harvey-Woodnorth (2004). In addition to providing direct services, speech–language pathologists also are responsible for patient and family counseling and investigation of support services. There are several organizations that provide support to specific tracheostomy- and ventilator-dependent populations, such as the ALS Association, Communication Independence for the Neurologically Impaired, Guillain Barre Syndrome/CIDP Foundation International, Muscular Dystrophy Association, and the National Spinal Cord Injury Association. There is also the Christopher Reeve Paralysis Foundation and the International Ventilator Users network.

MANAGEMENT–VOICE THERAPY FOLLOWING LARYNGEAL CANCER

In addition to being a possible life-threatening condition, head and neck cancer strikes at some of the most basic human functions, including breathing, eating, and verbal communication. Laryngeal cancer accounts for approximately 1 to 2% of all cancers and 20% of all head and neck cancers (American Cancer Society, 2003). Laryngeal cancer normally occurs at one of or a combination of three locations, the supraglottis, the subglottis, and the glottis. For detailed information on the

location and staging of cancer, see *Manual for Stages of Cancer* (American Joint Committee for Cancer Staging and End-Results Reporting, 1998).

The first consideration after a diagnosis of laryngeal cancer is how to best cure the disease and preserve the patient's life. After the best treatment of the disease is selected, one can turn attention to the best means of restoring the voice following cancer treatment. Treatment of laryngeal cancer is generally by means of radiation, surgery, chemotherapy, or combinations of these modes of treatment. The selection of method or methods will be made by the physician (oncologist or laryngologist) and the patient based on the type, location, and extent of the disease process. A discussion of these considerations is presented by Hall and Merricourt (1995) and Keith and Darley (1994). There is more than one type of cancer and not all respond in the same way to a given mode of treatment.

Each cancer treatment mode—radiation therapy (XRT), surgery, and chemotherapy—presents some complications to the voice. For example, irradiation can cause swelling of the mucosa in the early stages of treatment, followed by dryness and stiffness of the vocal fold cover weeks and even months after treatment. The long-term effects of radiation therapy involve the fibrosis of soft tissue, which limits the normal range of muscle motion (Leonard and Kendall, 1997).

When surgery is among the treatment options, the extent and location of the tumor will dictate the extent of surgery. If the tumor crosses the midline, then total (near total or subtotal) laryngectomy may be indicated; if the tumor is located only on one side of the larynx, then hemilaryngectomy or other partial laryngectomy may be an option. Surgery can leave a tissue deficit where a tumor was excised, and stiffness due to scarring may follow healing. The tissue deficit also may leave a gap in the glottal area when the folds are approximated. This gap may cause air wastage and a breathy vocal quality and may result in inadequate vocal loudness and short phonation times. In addition, the gap in tissue and the stiffness of the surrounding tissue may lead to irregular vocal fold vibration due to impaired mucosal wave motion. Even very superficial surgical intervention, such as stripping the vocal fold, can result in significant changes in vocal fold vibration. In fact, the stripping of a vocal fold is never a superficial procedure, as the postsurgical effect is almost always a stiffened vocal fold cover that results in dysphonia. However, the treatment of the disease is the first consideration.

Finally, many individuals experience moderate to severe side effects with radiation or chemotherapy intervention. In sum, dryness, inadequate tissue mass, irregular vocal fold edges, and stiffness can all make vibration of the vocal fold cover extremely difficult or impossible. This often will render the voice abnormal in one or more vocal parameters.

The picture of a larynx in Figure 8.2 shows a lack of tissue mass due to surgery for removal of a vocal fold cancer. There is a resultant gap between the vocal folds even in full adduction. The voice is breathy, reduced in loudness, and rough in quality. The breathy quality results from the air wastage through the glottal gap, while the reduced loudness level is due to inadequate medial compression required for louder voice production. The rough vocal quality is due to two factors: unequal mass between the right and left vocal folds and, thus, an

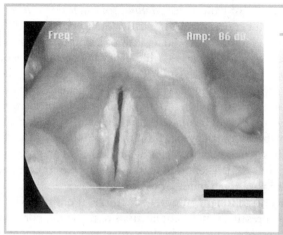

FIGURE 8.2

Lack of tissue mass in right vocal fold after surgical removal of laryngeal cancer.

irregular vocal fold vibrator pattern and second, an attempt to compensate for the excessive glottal gap by hyperactivity of the false vocal folds, which weight the vocal folds unequally. In voice therapy for this patient, we needed to first eliminate the excessive vocal effort, thus reducing the false fold activity, which was accomplished by employing inhalation phonation, retracting the false folds (discussed in Chapter 7). We gradually shifted from inhalation to exhalation phonation using the /i/ vowel because it is produced with the root of the tongue elevated and out of the hypopharynx. The next step in voice therapy was to use an upward pitch shift to slightly increase vocal fold tension and gain slightly better approximation (reducing the glottal gap) of the postsurgical vocal folds. The upward pitch could be only slight due to some vocal fold scarring; however, the dynamic segment of vocal folds postsurgery often respond more favorably (vibrate better) with slight adjustments in pitch (usually upward). A shift of 20 to 25 Hz was desirable in this case. The improved vocal fold approximation from increased vocal fold tension during pitch shift increased vocal loudness. Subglottic air pressure was increased slightly as well. This case demonstrates how the treatment (surgery) for cancer produced a dysphonia as a byproduct of treatment for the disease. Voice therapy was based on achieving the necessary vocal adjustments using facilitation techniques that would alter the effects of postsurgical anatomy and physiology of the larynx and also counter the inappropriate compensatory behaviors the patient had developed.

The second case addresses voice therapy for stiffness of the vocal fold cover due to fibrotic changes secondary to radiotherapy. For this case, we instructed the patient to shift his pitch downward to take advantage of the greater mucosal wave that occurs in lower pitches and also decreased subglottic air pressure so the folds were not overdriven. We successfully used this therapy approach in a 46-year-old patient who had irradiation treatment for a superficial cancer of the vocal fold cover, bilaterally. He was able to return to teaching with a much improved voice that would last throughout the teaching day.

A third case illustrates another role of the speech pathologist in the follow-up and management of patients being treated for laryngeal cancer. A 26-year-old female was seen for evaluation of voice following surgical removal of superficial squamous cell cancer. Of interest, the patient was a nonsmoking vegetarian who did not use alcohol and was also a marathon runner. She was in excellent physical shape but nevertheless got cancer of the larynx. The cancer returned three times in less than two years and was removed each time. The decision of a team of ENT physicians was to continue to monitor the return of the cancer and remove it before it became deeply embedded in the vocal folds. The speech pathology clinic assigned by the treatment team was to evaluate the patient every four to six months along with evaluations by the ENT team. The speech pathologist provided videostroboscopic monitoring of the larynx and acoustic evaluation of the voice as a means of tracking the cancer regrowth. Figure 8.3 is a picture of the larynx of this young adult female patient. In addition, the speech pathologist provided ongoing voice management for optimal use of the postsurgical larynx and to eliminate vocal abuse or hyperfunction, which besides making the voice poorer in quality can contribute to edema, a condition that can make obtaining an accurate status of the cancer more difficult. While this was a very unusual case, the monitoring role of the speech pathologist was not unusual and has been applied in cases of contact ulcer, papilloma, polyps, and polypoid cord degeneration.

Finally, we cannot overrate the important role of endoscopy in the case of differentially diagnosing laryngeal cancer. For example, a 72-year-old gentleman was referred to our clinic for voice therapy to treat hypophonia as a result of Parkinson's disease. Because this patient had been diagnosed with PD years before, he was referred to our clinic without an imaging study of the larynx. Instead of revealing bowed vocal folds bilaterally, rigid endoscopy at our clinic revealed a unilateral space-occupying lesion that was whitish and irregular at the edges. A referral to an otolaryngologist and subsequent biopsy rendered a diagnosis of T1 glottic cancer; this patient was successfully treated with laser surgery and radiation.

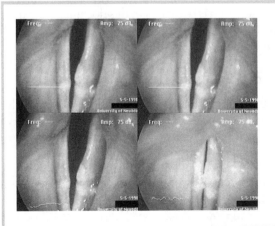

FIGURE **8.3**

Squamous Cell Carcinoma

Four views of the larynx of a 26-year-old female with recurring squamous cell carcinoma, followed over a two-year period.

Facilitating Techniques

Our clinical experience with postsurgical and postradiotherapy treatment dysphonias has demonstrated some success using the following techniques from Chapter 7:

FA.14
FA.19
FA.11
FA.17
FA.12
FA.2
FA.23

1. Inhalation phonation using the vowels /i/, /u/, and /o/
2. Pitch shifts upward and downward based on patient's vocal response
3. Glottal fry if vocal fold stiffness is not too great
4. Nasal/glide stimulation
5. Head turned to the side and lateral digital pressure to the thyroid cartilage
6. Loudness changes, usually reduced
7. Tongue protrusion /i/
8. Glottal fry to tone

LARYNGECTOMY

The area of laryngeal speech and voice rehabilitation after laryngectomy is so vast as to require a multidisciplinary team approach. Medical, nursing, speech–language pathology, audiology, psychology, dietary, and other professionals should be involved in the rehabilitative effort. The anatomic and physiologic changes involved in a total laryngectomy are well described in the literature (Blom, Singer, and Hamaker, 1998; Bohnencamp, 2008; Keith and Darley, 1994). In sum, the laryngeal and hypopharyngeal cartilages are removed along with the hyoid bone, all extrinsic and intrinsic muscles of the larynx, and the upper rings of the trachea. The uppermost portion of the trachea is brought forward and fit flush with the neck. An external stoma (mouth) is made, which will now permanently serve as the patient's new airway. The International Classification of Functioning, Disability and Health (ICF) provides a method of described human function and disability. The ICF has been applied to the laryngectomee (Eadie, 2003). The role and scope of the SLP in laryngectomy rehabilitation is described in this document. Finally, it should be noted that conservation (subtotal laryngectomy) surgery is becoming more common and presents a unique challenge to the voice pathologist and the patient.

Counseling and Communication Options

Because laryngectomy alters respiration, swallowing, and speech, it is essential that the patient understand the concept of laryngectomy and details about the surgery and speech rehabilitation. Therefore, a presurgical counseling session is recommended with the patient and his or her family (Cady, 2002; McColl, Hooper, and Von Berg, 2006). The SLP should illustrate and describe the changes that occur in the speech mechanism as a result of laryngectomy. Written information, illustrations, and films should be provided about various alaryngeal communication options. This information may be accessed through the Internet from either the American Speech-Language-Hearing Association or the International Association of Laryngectomees (IAL), a nonprofit voluntary support organization. The booklet *Self-Help for the Laryngectomee* (Lauder, 2000) can also be reviewed with the patient. The SLP should also demonstrate electrolarynges and address patient concerns and questions.

Naturally, the laryngectomee's primary concern is his or her immediate health prognosis. We address these concerns by explaining that surgical and ancillary intervention are state of the art and that head and neck cancers are among the more curable cancers. A checklist for pre- and postoperative consultation is found in Keith and Darley (1994, pp. 144–145).

There are three general communication options for the laryngectomee, none of which is mutually exclusive. In esophageal speech (ES), air is "inhaled" into the pharyngoesophageal (PE) segment and then expelled, setting the tissue of the PE segment into vibration for a voice source. The second option is the electrolarynx (EL), which introduces sound for voice through an instrument externally placed against the throat or oral structures, or a fitted prosthetic electrolarynx inserted into the mouth while speaking. The third option is tracheoesophageal (TE) voice restoration surgery, whereby an opening or puncture is made through the posterior wall of the trachea, extending through the anterior wall of the esophagus. A prosthesis inserted into the puncture shunts pulmonary air into the esophagus, causing the upper esophageal sphincter and surrounding tissues to vibrate. This creates the sound that can be used for TE speech. The reported rate of surgical complications for tracheoesophageal puncture and prosthesis is very low (Malik, Bruce, and Cherry, 2007).

Numerous studies have reviewed patterns of vocal rehabilitation preferences and use among laryngectomees. A study by Hillman and colleagues (1998) revealed that a small percentage of laryngectomees developed usable esophageal speech (6%) or remained nonvocal (8%). The predominant method of choice was an electrolarynx (55%), while 31% opted for TE speech. This finding is supported by Liu and Ng (2007), who report that EL is the most commonly adopted alaryngeal phonation. These patterns of use are quite different from findings of Ward and colleagues. (2003), who followed 55 total laryngectomy patients over a five-year period. Although an EL was introduced as the initial communication mode directly after surgery, 74% of the patients developed TE speech as their primary mode of communication. Compared with EL users, TE speakers reported significantly lower levels of disability, handicap, and distress. Esophageal speech was not an option in this study. Researchers in Japan (Koike et al., 2002) reported outcomes of speech therapy for 65 laryngectomees who were offered esophageal speech and artificial larynx options only. Forty-two percent of the patients acquired practical esophageal speech and 91% acquired both esophageal and electrolarynx speech.

On the flip side, 151 experienced SLPs ranked their preference for voice rehabilitation methods for laryngectomy patients. TE voice was the most preferred method and the EL was the least preferred (Culton and Gerwin, 1998). Finally, laryngectomy patients were asked to rate levels of satisfaction with their method of alaryngeal communication (Clements et al., 1997). Patients were divided into four groups by method of communication: tablet writers, esophageal speech, electrolarynx, and TE speech. Compared with the other groups, the TE speakers expressed more satisfaction with their speech quality, ability to communicate over the phone, and ability to interact with others. Similar to the Ward and colleagues study (2003), TE speakers also rated their overall quality of life higher. These findings are of interest, because, unlike previous studies focusing on the intelligibility of speech judged by listeners (Doyle, Danhauer, and Reed, 1988; Max, DeBruyn, and Steurs, 1997; Sedory, Hamlet, and Conner, 1989), this study polled patients on their own perceptions of speech. The remaining sections in this chapter address these three communication modes for the postlaryngectomy patient.

The Electrolarynx

We frequently encourage the use of an artificial larynx during the first few days following surgery. There are two different types of EL: the neck type and the intraoral type. When healing is still incomplete and swelling may be significant, we may introduce the patient to an intraoral EL. With this option, the intraoral tube transmits the sound into the mouth directly. The intraoral EL does not require pressure to the neck like other hand-held ELs and thus works when fistulae or swelling are problems. Some neck-type ELs may be converted to intraoral devices. EL devices and their descriptions are available from a variety of sources, notably the International Association of Laryngectomees website. Those SLPs and clients who have experience with ELs acknowledge that ELs are famous for producing a sound source that is monotonic and robotic sounding. For example, several commercially available ELs, such as the Nu-Voice, Romet, Amplicode, and Cooper-Rand, do not have pitch adjustment options. The Servox only features two standard pitch levels. However, new advances in adaptive filtering and algorithms are showing that EL users may soon be able to enjoy a more varied pitch range and lower additive noise than currently associated with ELs (Liu and Ng, 2007). Even if the laryngectomee uses TE speech, an electrolarynx is a good alternate mode of phonation should the other mode fail or the external environmental factors (e.g., background noise) dictate a shift to another mode of speech.

Traditional Esophageal Speech

While the development of TE speech has made the use of esophageal speech less frequent, the SLP should know something about this form of speech and how to teach it if the need arises. Many of the principles for developing esophageal speech can be applied to other types of alaryngeal speech—that is, progression in use of loudness and pitch and consonant selection. At the very least one needs to know where to find information on the teaching of traditional esophageal speech (Boone, McFarlane, and Von Berg, 2005; Case, 2002).

In brief, two methods of teaching esophageal speech may be employed: injection and inhalation. We usually begin with the injection method, which is the easiest to teach and is quite compatible with the articulation practice the patient may have used with the electrolarynx. Both methods (injection and inhalation) employ the same basic principle of compressing air within the oropharynx and injecting this denser air into the more rarefied (less dense) space of the esophagus. Denser air within a body moves in the direction of the less dense body of air whenever the two bodies are coupled. Some of the compressed air within the oral cavity undoubtedly escapes through the lips, some through the velopharyngeal port, and some (particularly if the esophagus is open) into the esophagus. Both methods for esophageal voice bring compressed air into the esophagus; once the air is in the esophagus, external forces compress the air within it and expel it. Hopefully, the esophageal expulsion sets up a vibration of the pharyngoesophageal (PE) segment and the patient experiences an eructation or "voice." Certain consonants appear to have a facilitating effect in producing good esophageal voice. Individuals may have their own favorite facilitating sounds, but more often than not these are plosive consonants (/p/, /b/, /t/, /d/, /k/, and /g/) or affricatives containing plosives (/ʧ/ or /ʤ/).

Tracheoesophageal Puncture Shunt (TEP)

Today, many laryngectomees are candidates for the tracheoesophageal puncture (TEP) and the prosthetic approach to alaryngeal speech rehabilitation. In many patients the TE puncture will be performed at the same time as the total laryngectomy (Hamaker and Hamaker, 1995; Malik et al., 2007). Also, a cricopharyngeal myotomy (weakening the PE segment by surgically cutting the muscle fibers) often will be performed at the time of laryngectomy to create a PE (pharyngoesophageal) segment that will not present excessive resistance to the outward flow of air during phonation and will allow for adequate vibration of the PE segment during alaryngeal voice production.

A number of researchers have described candidacy requirements for successful TE speech. First, the patient must have adequate pulmonary support to shunt air from the lungs and trachea to the esophagus. Therefore, individuals with lung cancer, asthma, chronic obstructive pulmonary disease, or other severe lung disease may not be appropriate candidates for this mode. Second, the patient must possess the necessary cognitive and sensorimotor skills to occlude the stoma for speech (or manipulate a tracheostoma valve) and to remove and clean the prosthesis (Bosone, 1994). Finally, the patient must have a PE segment that vibrates adequately to generate a sound source for speech. This determination of the adequacy of the PE source is performed via insufflation testing, a diagnostic procedure that transfers air from the stoma site to below the PE segment through a transnasally placed catheter. If the PE segment does not adequately vibrate via insufflation testing, alternative intervention techniques may be applied. Techniques currently include Botox injections, myotomy, and pharyngeal plexus neurectomy. For details of these techniques, see ASHA (2004a).

If the TE prosthesis has not been inserted at the time of the primary or secondary puncture, the patient will be ready for prosthesis insertion five to seven days after fistula creation. It is important to understand that there are two major types of prostheses: those that the patient can insert and manipulate and those that are inserted and removed by the physician or the SLP (indwelling). Although a variety of prostheses are available, they have in common a silicone tube, a one-way valve, and a tracheal flange (Keith and Darley, 1994). The fistula is dilated and the prosthesis is inserted. A good description and pictures of these procedures are provided by Blom (1995) and in McFarlane and Watterson (1995b). The fitting of the correct length of the prosthesis is critical for the best TE voice result. A prosthesis that is too short may be expelled during forceful coughing. One that is too long will make contact with the posterior esophageal wall, thus interfering with voice production and causing a leak due to malfunction of the one-way valve or fistula enlargement. The correct length is determined by placing the measuring device into the stoma and through the punctured fistula. This will allow one to gauge the distance from the posterior wall of the trachea to the posterior wall of the esophagus. When the correct prosthesis is selected the TE puncture fistula must be dilated with the dilator. Using an inserting device and a gel cap for an indwelling prosthesis in this case, constant firm pressure is applied until the prosthesis slips into place. The gel cap eases the insertion of the prosthesis by reducing friction and providing lubrication for the surrounding skin. The stoma is then occluded by the thumb or the finger and voice production is tested. If the prosthesis is in place and the back wall of the esophagus is not in contact with the prosthesis, the air will be shunted into the esophagus and the PE segment will be set into vibration.

The patient who has a TE shunt or puncture will generally be able to develop good esophageal voice more quickly than the patient with a conventional laryngectomy. On expiration, by shutting off the open stoma with a finger or by using a one-way stoma valve, the patient is able to divert tracheal air directly into the esophagus. Being able to do this negates the need for teaching the patient to trap air in the esophagus by either the injection or inhalation methods. In addition, the TE speaker has a much larger air reservoir with which to speak (up to 3000 cc of pulmonary air versus approximately 80 to 100 cc of air trapped in the top of the esophagus).

The patient may also wish to wear a one-way valve fastened over the stoma. This valve permits air to come in from the outside on inspiration, but shuts off on expiration, allowing air to travel through the shunt into the esophagus (Lewin et al., 2000). Fujimoto, Madison, and Larrigan (1991) looked at the effect of the valve on developing good voice as opposed to using finger closure of the stoma, finding that there were no real differences in quality of voice between the two methods. The patient who must use his or her hands in work might profit from wearing the stoma valve; otherwise, occluding the open stoma when one wants to speak might be best achieved by using one's finger to close off the stoma. It does appear, however, that research favors the low-pressure prosthesis over the duckbill prosthesis for developing the best speaking voice (Pauloski et al., 1989).

Anyone who is attempting to assist a patient to develop TE speech should become thoroughly familiar with the devices, procedures, and materials involved. This information is constantly being updated (ASHA, 2004a). Finally, the patient with a new laryngectomy faces a number of social obstacles. Research by Blood,

Luther, and Stemple (1992) found that 73% of 41 laryngectomy patients showed good adjustment to their problem. Fear of cancer reoccurrence and some loss of self-esteem are among problems the patients report. The speech–language pathologist working with the laryngectomee must provide some counseling work and social guidance for the patient (Cady, 2002). The patient needs exposure to other laryngectomy patients, participation in laryngectomy clubs, such as the IAL and WebWhispers Nu-Voice Club, and encouragement to participate again in life activities experienced before the operation. Successful voice and speech rehabilitation after laryngectomy is highly related to the patient's overall life adjustment, coping skills, and general well-being (Schuster et al., 2003).

SUMMARY

In Chapter 8 we have addressed a variety of special voice considerations and their management. Aging voice will become more relevant as the U.S. population ages, and it is important to know the prevalence, risk factors, and psychosocial consequences of voice changes for this particular cohort. Equally important to the SLP's knowledge base are voice considerations of the deaf and hard of hearing, pediatric, professional voice, and transgender populations. Because respiratory support and coordination are integral to vocal quality, pitch, and intensity, the clinician should appreciate the etiologies and approaches to respiratory-based voice problems. Included in this section are techniques and references devoted to laryngeal control programs for those clients presenting with paradoxical vocal fold movement. The final section is devoted to the SLP's role in the management of voice for cases of tracheostomy and laryngeal cancer. Readers learn that there are three general communication options for the new laryngectomee, and that the SLP should be able to provide resources and counseling for all three options.

Thought Questions

1. Why is the aging voice so heterogeneous?
2. Which variables define a professional voice user? Which special demands are placed on the professional user's voice?
3. Describe three intervention regimens for individuals with paradoxical vocal fold movement.
4. Investigate and report on one organization that assists tracheostomy and ventilator-dependent populations.
5. Identify the three primary treatment options for laryngeal cancer. Discuss the vocal changes that may occur subsequent to these interventions.
6. Cite two advantages and two disadvantages each for the electrolarynx, esophageal speech, and tracheoesophageal speech.

chapter

Therapy for Resonance Disorders

LEARNING OBJECTIVES

- Differentiate the terms "hypernasality," "hyponasality," and "assimilative nasality"
- List the clinical probes that can be used to assess hypernasality
- Define the term "stimulability testing"
- Discuss the role of oral examination in determining velopharyngeal function
- List the advantages and disadvantages of instrumental assessment of velopharyngeal function

In this text the disorders of resonance are treated separately from the disorders of voice that result from the larynx being misused or from laryngeal lesions. While many of the neurological disorders discussed in Chapter 4 have a hypernasal component or resonance component, these are treated separately in that chapter. The resonance disorders of hypernasality, hyponasality, assimilative nasality, and the oral–pharyngeal resonance disorders of stridency, thin voice quality, and cul-de-sac voice will be addressed in this chapter.

The most common resonance disorder is hypernasality (excessive nasal resonance), which can be an early sign of a neurological disease or can be the result of a congenital disorder such as cleft palate or a submucous cleft of the velum. It can also result from a surgical treatment that disturbs the anatomy and/or physiology of the resonance system. The cause of hypernasality must be determined as a prelude to successful treatment. Hyponasality can be caused by a number of obstructions, such as nasal polyps, allergies, or hypertrophied adenoids. Another nasalance problem, assimilative nasality, must be distinguished from either hypernasality or hyponasality. Speech–language pathologists play a primary role in the diagnosis and treatment of various nasality problems.

Resonance is selective amplification and filtering of the complex overtone structure by the cavities of the vocal tract after the tone has been produced by the vibration of the vocal folds. Stated another way, vocal resonance is the perceptual increase in loudness of the laryngeal tone due to the concentration and reflection of soundwaves by the oral, pharyngeal, and nasal cavities during voice production. The vocal folds provide the source of vibration that gives rise to the complex sound waves. These periodic vibrations, characteristic of the normal voice, are filtered in the supraglottal space of the pharyngeal, oral, and nasal cavities, or the upper airway. Our discussion of resonance in Chapter 2 showed that the F-shaped upper airway amplifies and filters the sounds coming into it from the larynx, depending on the frequency of the sound waves and the shape and size of the particular cavity. The pharyngeal cavities constantly change their horizontal and vertical dimensions by active movement of muscles, which in turn alters the overall configuration (Kent and Read, 2002; Pershall and Boone, 1986; Watterson and McFarlane, 1990). The open coupling between the pharyngeal cavity and the oral cavity (particularly when the velopharyngeal mechanism is closed) enables the traveling sound wave to be further filtered by the continuous modifications of oral cavity size that occur during speech by the movements of the tongue and jaw. What emerges as voice resonance is the fundamental frequency (laryngeal vibration) modified by the natural resonant frequencies occurring at the various supraglottal sites (above the vocal folds) within the pharynx and through the oral cavity. When the velopharyngeal port is open, the pharyngeal–oral coupling with the nasal cavity is then possible so that sound waves are further absorbed and filtered as they pass through the chambers of the nasal cavity, as for the production of /m/, /n/, and /ŋ/ in English. However, for the remaining sounds of English, the velopharyngeal (VP) port is closed, or nearly so, and the impedance is high for the transmission of sound waves into the nasal cavities (Peterson-Falzone, Hardin-Jones, and Karnell, 2001).

NASAL RESONANCE PROBLEMS

Under the broad heading of nasal resonance problems fall three types of disorders: hypernasality, hyponasality, and assimilative nasality. Although individuals listening to speakers with these problems might only be able to say, "The voices all sound nasal," distinct differences among the three types call for differential diagnosis and management and different voice therapy approaches. As a prelude to our discussion of separate approaches, let us define the three terms.

Hypernasality

Hypernasality is an excessively undesirable amount of perceived nasal cavity resonance during the phonation of normally nonnasal vowels and nonnasal voiced consonants. Voiced consonants and vowel production in the English language are primarily characterized by oral resonance with only slightly nasalized components being acceptable. If the oral and nasal cavities are coupled to one another by lack of velopharyngeal closure (for whatever reason), the periodic sound waves carrying laryngeal vibration will receive heavy resonance within the nasal cavity. Velopharyngeal dysfunction (VPD) is the term for inappropriate transmission of the sound wave into the nasal cavities. VPD may be caused by impaired motion of the VP mechanism (incompetence), a tissue deficiency (insufficiency), or a mixture of both (inadequacy) (Marsh, 2004). The speech characteristics of VPD are inappropriate nasal air emission, reduced intraoral air pressure, and excessive nasal resonance or hypernasality (Smith & Kuehn, 2007).

Hyponasality

Hyponasality is reduced nasal resonance for the three nasalized phonemes /m/, /n/, and /ŋ/. Usually the result of anatomical obstructions within the nasal cavity, hyponasality could be categorized as an articulatory substitution disorder for which the nasal consonants are usually perceived as their voiced, nonnasal cognates (/b/, /d/, /g/). Hyponasality may be associated with abnormally large adenoids and tonsils, a deviated septum, an obstructed nares, choanal atresia (bony or membranous occlusion of the passageway between nose and pharynx), nasal cavity turbinate swelling, or allergic rhinitis. In a study by Andreassen and colleagues (1994), 14 children were seen prior to adenoidectomy and at intervals of one, three, and six months following surgery. Aerodynamic, acoustic, and perceptual measures were obtained at each visit, It was reported (p. 263) that there was a significant reduction in nasal airway resistance, coupled with a significant increase in nasalance values, following surgery. Perception of hyponasality did not change significantly, however.

Assimilative Nasality

In assimilative nasality, the speaker's vowels or voiced consonants appear nasal when adjacent to the three nasal consonants. The velopharyngeal port is opened too soon and remains open too long, so that vowel or voiced consonant resonance preceding and following nasal consonant resonance is also nasalized. Dworkin, Marunik, and Krouse (2004) report that this type of nasality may be a result of overexposure to faulty speech models or exaggerated regional dialect patterns that may normally have subtle nasal (twang) characteristics. This type of voice disorder is considered functional, and speech and voice intervention is warranted.

Normal English consonants are produced with high intraoral pressures (3 to 8 cm H_2O) with essentially no nasal airflow except for the three nasal consonants, which have low intraoral pressures (0.5 to 1.5 cm H_2O) and high rates of nasal airflow (100 to 300 cc/sec), as reported by Mason and Warren (1980). Aerodynamic studies of cleft palate speakers and speakers with problems of excessive nasality have provided some needed quantification to help differentiate patients with excessive nasal resonance from patients lacking sufficient nasal resonance (Warren, 1979). From his studies of air pressures and airflow patterns, Warren has estimated the size of the velopharyngeal (VP) port for various speaking activities. Although most normal speakers demonstrate tight velopharyngeal closure with no air leakage, speakers with VP openings of 5 mm or less may still have voice quality that is perceived by listeners as normal (Mason and Warren, 1980). Patients with nasal voices who produce high nasal airflow rates are *perceived* (we stress *perceived* because hypernasality is a perceptual phenomenon that can only occur on voiced sounds) as having hypernasality, whereas hyponasality is perceived as a speaker with a cold or stuffed up nose and is accompanied by low nasal airflows, due to an occluded nasal passage (e.g., nasal polyps or swollen turbinates) or a closed VP mechanism. Probably no area of voice therapy is more neglected or more confusing than therapy for nasal resonance problems.

Historically, the implication in the early literature was that most problems of nasality (usually hypernasality) could be successfully treated by voice therapy, that is, by ear training, or by blowing exercises (Kantner, 1947), or by the exercises for the velum suggested by Buller (1942), or by the treatment Williamson (1945) used for 72 cases of hypernasality, which put some emphasis on relaxing the entire vocal tract. Most of these early approaches were developed for functional, or learned, hypernasality, but were later applied by various clinicians to organically based problems of VP dysfunction and cleft palate. For most of these structural problems and most neurological disorders, however, such approaches as blowing and relaxation were ineffective. As discussed earlier, if the velum presents with tissue deficiency or weak, irregular, or reduced range of movement, behavioral therapy *alone* will not normalize velopharyngeal anatomy and function. Realistic management and therapy for any problem in nasal resonance, therefore, requires that the patient have a thorough differential evaluation, including detailed examination of the VP mechanism, aerodynamic studies, functional speech–voice testing, a detailed acoustical and perceptual analysis of voice, and videoendoscopic studies (Dworkin et al., 2004; McFarlane, 1990; Watterson and McFarlane, 1990).

Evaluation of Nasal Resonance Disorders

There are more similarities than differences between patients with resonance disorders and those with phonation disorders. For this reason, the evaluational procedures outlined in Chapter 6 are equally relevant here. In addition to obtaining the necessary medical data (such as what treatment has already been provided), clinicians must pursue case history information (description of the problem and its cause, description of daily voice use, variations of the problem, onset and duration of the problem, and so on). Clinicians must observe closely how well the patients seem to function in the clinic and during out-of-clinic situations. Considering how subjective our judgments of resonance disorders are, it is crucial that clinicians know how their patients perceive their own voices. A mild resonance problem, for example, can be perceived by a patient and/or others as severe, but a severe resonance problem, at times, may be ignored. Speakers with resonance disorders are perceived more negatively by listeners than normal speakers (Lallh and Rochet, 2000). Listeners report more anxiety when listening to hypernasal speakers than when listening to speakers with normal resonance (McKinnon et al., 1986). Resonance disordered speakers are also considered less attractive, less pleasant, and more cruel than normal speakers (Blood et al., 1979). Blood and Hyman (1977) also found that children were less likely to want to talk to a child with hypernasality or to say that they liked a child with hypernasal speech.

Auditory–Perceptual Analysis.   An obvious way to begin the evaluation of someone with a nasal resonance disorder is to listen carefully to his or her voice during spontaneous conversation. This can provide a gross indication of what the problem may be (assimilative nasality, hypernasality, or hyponasality). The perceptual aspect of nasal resonance disorders is extremely important. It is, however, difficult to make a clinical judgment about nasality by listening to someone as he or she speaks; in fact, such a judgment is likely to be wrong (Bradford, Brooks, and Shelton, 1964; Hayden and Klimacka, 2000). Although the casual judgment that "something is nasal about the speech" is usually correct, few examiners can quickly and reliably differentiate the type of nasality (hypernasality, assimilative nasality, hyponasality) on the basis of such a conversational sample alone (Lohmander and Olssen, 2004). Perceptual judgments are more accurate if made on the basis of recorded samples of a patient's conversational speech, his or her vowels in isolation, and his or her sentences (some with only oral phonemes and some loaded with nasal phonemes). Loading sentences with nasal phonemes is helpful for making judgments of hyponasal speech. The recorded sample allows the clinician repeated playback. Focusing on a specific parameter (loudness, pitch, quality, hypernasal versus hyponasal) on each playback may increase the clinician's objectivity. Furthermore, it appears that the reliability of perceptual judgments of nasality is influenced by listener experience and training. In a study by Lewis, Watterson, and Houghton (2003) agreement of nasality ratings was examined across four groups of listeners: naive listeners, graduate students in speech–language pathology, experienced speech–language pathologists, and experienced craniofacial surgeons. Each listened to recorded speech samples ranging from normal to severely hypernasal. Results revealed that agreement levels for nasality ratings were highest for the speech–language pathologists, followed by the surgeons. In addition to being the most reliable, these two groups of raters also tended to rate the speech samples as less severe than their less-experienced counterparts.

We have found that asking patients to repeat or read aloud passages free of nasal consonants, such as "Betty takes Bob to the show" (Boone, 1993), or passages loaded with nasal consonants, such as "Many men in the moon" (Boone, 1993), helps us differentiate hypernasality, hyponasality, and assimilative nasality from one another. It is important to note that hypernasality occurs only on vowels, semivowels, and voiced consonants. Using phrases loaded with nasal consonants is only to demonstrate hyponasality. The absence of normal nasal resonance on these nasally loaded phrases is diagnostic of hyponasality.

We have also found that if we use the following simple screening procedures, we get a good, quick clinical classification of the type of resonance disorder present. These quick tests are simple and require no instruments to perform.

First, we have the patient say these two sentences while gently pinching the nares: "My name means money" and "Mary made lemon jam." If these sound "plugged" both when the nares are pinched and when the nares are released, the problem is hyponasality. In other words, if there is no difference between the nose-held and nose-released conditions, the problem is hyponasality. If there is a big difference between the nose-held and nose-released conditions, then the problem is likely hypernasality.

Another simple clinical technique is called the "snap release /s/." We have the patient sustain a loud /s/ while the nares are pinched and quickly released. If a "snap" is heard on releasing the nares, this means the VP mechanism is partially open and the problem is probably hypernasality. The actual "snap" is nasal air emission but gives a clue of the status of the VP mechanism. While hypernasality is a phenomenon of voiced sounds only, this technique is using a nonvoiced sound /s/ to test the adequacy of closure of the VP mechanism. This is done because there is more intra-oral breath pressure required for a voiceless consonant, /s/, than a voiced consonant.

Next, we have the patient say, "This horse eats grass" and "I see the teacher at church." If we hear any "snorting" back in the pharynx, we can assume that it is probably due to inadequate closure of the velopharyngeal port and that the problem with this speaker's voice is hypernasality. We next ask the patient to say, "Maybe baby, maybe baby." If there is no difference between the /m/ in *maybe* and the /b/ in *baby* and both sound like *maybe*, the problem is hypernasality; however, if both words sound like *baby* the problem is hyponasality. Finally, we ask the patient to sustain the /i/ and the /u/ vowels, while we gently flutter the nose (nasal flutter test) by rapidly pinching and releasing the nares with the thumb and forefinger. If we hear a pulsing change in the acoustic signal, the problem is hypernasality.

Beyond these clinical techniques, we recommend a few additional strategies to assess nasal air emission and hypernasality using some relatively inexpensive but effective instruments. Place a fogging mirror under a naris and instruct the client to repeat a nonnasal sentence, such as, "Buy baby a bib." Ensure that the mirror is deflected away from the naris when the client is quietly breathing and at the ends of productions. The mirror will fog if the velopharyngeal mechanism is open during nonnasal productions. The mirror is also effective for detecting nasal energy during sustained nonnasal phonemes, such as /s/.

Another effective technique is a listening tube, or what we call an "octopus." By fitting nasal olives at the ends of hollow rubber tubing, the clinician is able to detect "puffs" of nasal emission or hypernasality by placing the olive at one of the patient's nares and the other at the clinician's ear. Finally, with the See-Scape (PRO-ED), a small Styrofoam disk encased in a clear plastic tube "floats" when a patient demonstrates nasal airflow. The airflow is detected in much the same manner as the listening tube. If the patient exhibits nasal energy during nonnasal sentences, the float rises from the bottom toward the top of the tube. These three techniques, while diagnostic, also serve as therapy techniques for individuals with excessive nasal emission or nasal resonance.

Hoarseness.   Individuals with hypernasality also are at increased risk for hoarseness associated with vocal hyperfunction. Although the reported prevalence of voice deviations in persons with cleft palate varies widely, they appear to be more frequent than in persons without clefts (Kuehn and Moller, 2000). For example, in a recent study by Hocevar-Boltezar, Jarc, and Kozelj (2006) dysphonia was detected in 12.5% of children with cleft palate and in 12.3% of children with unilateral cleft lip and palate. In 9.2% of all cleft children, the functional voice disorder caused a hoarse voice. Furthermore, two-thirds of cleft children with functional dysphonia had protracted hearing loss. The most frequent perceived deviations are hoarseness, unusual habitual pitch, breathiness, harshness, and reduced loudness. The most common anatomic finding related to voice deviations is vocal nodules. In light of this, the clinician must not only make judgments about resonance but must also listen closely to and make observations about the voice.

Stimulability Testing.   Although stimulability testing was designed for use with problems of articulation, it is also effective with problems of voice. The basic purpose of stimulability testing, as first described by Milisen (1957), was to see how well the patient can correctly produce an errored sound when he or she is repeatedly presented with the correct sound through both auditory and visual stimuli. One way of distinguishing between true problems of velopharyngeal inadequacy (the mechanism is incapable of adequate closure) and functional velopharyngeal inadequacy (the mechanism has the capability of closure) is to determine whether the patient can produce oral resonance under stimulability conditions (Morris and Smith, 1962). Obviously, the patient's success in producing oral resonance would be a strong indication that velopharyngeal closure is possible. Shelton, Hahn, and Morris (1968) have observed:

> If repeated stimulation consistently results in consonant productions, which are distorted by nasal emission and vowels which are unpleasantly nasal, the inference can be drawn, at least tentatively, that the individual is not able to change his speaking behavior because of velopharyngeal incompetence. (p. 236)

Success in producing oral resonance under conditions of stimulability would be a good indicator for voice therapy. It is also a favorable prognostic sign.

Another simple stimulability test is to hold the patient's velum up with a tongue depressor while fluttering the nose during the patient's production of a sustained /i/ vowel. Next, remove the tongue depressor and repeat the process listening for a difference in resonance. If the difference is dramatic the patient will likely not be able to benefit from voice–speech therapy alone but will require a palatal lift, speech obturator, or surgical management. Watterson and McFarlane (1990) describe five classes of velopharyngeal function based on videoendoscopic observations during speech testing: (1) normal VP function, (2) consistent VPI (velopharyngeal incompetency), (3) task-specific VPI, (4) irregular VPI, and (5) abnormal resonance without VPI.

Articulation Testing.   Articulatory proficiency can provide a good index of a patient's velopharyngeal closure. *Nasal emission*, the escape of air through the nose, is a common articulation error on plosive and fricative phonemes among subjects with velopharyngeal dysfunction (VPD). Even though a patient may have his or her articulators in the correct position in relation to the lingual–alveolar–labial contacts the error occurs because increased oral pressure escapes nasally through the VP port. The presence or absence of nasal emission, therefore, is an important diagnostic sign of velopharyngeal adequacy. It is important in articulation testing to distinguish between errors that result from faulty articulatory positioning and errors related to dysfunction of the velopharyngeal structure.

An excellent articulation test for assessing competency of velopharyngeal closure is found in the 43 special test items from the Templin-Darley Tests of Articulation (Templin and Darley, 1980), known as the Iowa Pressure Articulation Test (IPAT). This test is particularly sensitive for identifying the presence of nasal emission during the production of certain consonants. However, any standardized articulation test is useful for determining phonemes that are distorted because of inadequate velopharyngeal closure. The clinician must closely assess the identified errors to determine if lingual placements are accurate to make the target phoneme correctly. Many younger children with velopharyngeal problems exhibit sound substitutions and omission errors (compensatory articulation) in addition to the nasal emission and nasal snort distortions. Older children and adults with nasal emission problems may well have correct articulatory lingual placements, and their distortions are a product of posterior nasal escape of the airstream. Following successful pharyngeal flap surgery or the proper fitting of an appliance, nasal emission and compensation errors sometime continue until they are addressed through speech remediation. General intervention strategies for compensatory articulation have been reported by Trost-Cardamone (1990) and Kummer and Lee (1996).

The 16 so-called pressure consonants provide the best test of the adequacy of the velopharyngeal mechanism. These pressure consonants—/p, b, k, g, t, d, f, v, s, z, ʃ, ʒ, ʤ, ʧ, ð, θ/—should be included in any testing of the adequacy of the velopharyngeal port mechanism, because these sounds require the greatest degree of VP closure and greatest intraoral air pressure. On the other end of the spectrum, hyponasality in its purest and most overt form would be exhibited on an articulation test with these oral substitutions for the nasal phonemes: /b/m/, /d/n/, and /g/ŋ/. The sentence "My name means money" would be produced, for example, as "By dabe beads buddy."

Assimilative nasality would be observable only for vowels or voiced consonants in words containing nasal phonemes.

The Oral Examination

The oral examination provides a limited amount of information about the strength, range of motion, and degree of velopharyngeal function because the anatomic point of closure is superior to the lower border of the velum. That is, the clinician cannot actually see the nature of velar and pharyngeal function simply by viewing the mechanism through the oral cavity. For example, poor uvular-tip contact with the posterior pharyngeal wall does not indicate a lack of closure more superiorly in the pharynx, where closure may actually occur. Conversely, the contact of the uvula to the posterior pharyngeal wall is not necessarily an indication of adequate VP function. A markedly short, sluggish, or flaccid palate can certainly be noted on direct inspection of the oral cavity, and such a notation is a diagnostically important indicator for further evaluation of VP function. However, to truly determine the degree, speed, accuracy, and range of motion of the velopharynx, direct observation of the entire system is necessary.

By direct visualization, the clinician can make a gross observation of the relationship of the velum to the pharynx, note the relative size of the tongue, make a judgment about maxillary–mandibular occlusion, view the height and width of the palatal arch, survey the general condition of mucosa, faucial arches, and dentition, and determine if there are any clefts or open fistulas or evidence of submucous cleft. Oral inspection of the tongue is critical because some problems of functional nasality may be related to inappropriate size of tongue in relation to the oral cavity, poor tongue carriage, or irregular tongue movement due to an upper or lower motor neuron lesion.

The clinician should make a thorough search for any openings of the hard or soft palate that might contribute to an articulation distortion or to some problem of nasal resonance. Some patients have small openings (fistulas) or lack of fusion around the border of the premaxilla, particularly in the area of the alveolar ridge. In some individuals such fistulas may produce airstream noises, creating articulatory distortion (by loss of intraoral air pressure), but almost never will such isolated openings this far forward on the maxilla produce nasal resonance.

The absence or presence of soft-palate and hard-palate clefts should be noted; if such clefts have been previously corrected surgically, the degree of closure should be noted. In the case of a bony-palate defect, for example, sometimes the bony opening has been covered by a thin layer of mucosal tissue, not thick enough to prevent oral cavity sound waves from traveling into the nasal cavity. This same observation applies to the occasional submucosal cleft at the midline of the junction of the hard and soft palates. The major signs of a submucosal cleft are bifid or split uvula, inverted A-shape defect in the velum, lack of a palpable posterior nasal spine, or a thin soft palate (which may appear darker in color) in the midline portion. Any other structural deviations—of dentition, occlusion, labial competence, and so on—should be noted and considered with regard to their possible effects on speech production and nasal resonance.

Laboratory Instrumentation

Many instruments available today can help the clinician evaluate various aspects of nasal resonance. These instruments can also be valuable in the process of managing the patient with a nasalization problem. We consider separately instruments that provide aerodynamic data, acoustic information, radiographic visualization, and visual probe information.

Aerodynamic Instruments. Pressure transducers and pneumotachometers are instruments of choice for measuring the relative air pressures and airflows emitted simultaneously from the nasal and oral cavities during speech (Andreassen, Smith, and Guyette, 1992; Leeper, Tissington, and Munhall, 1998). There are other instruments that measure pressure and flow. As mentioned in Chapter 6, the Phonatory Function Analyzer is a good instrument for airflow measures and can be used with a tube in the mouth or with a face mask. The Phonatory Aerodynamic System (KayPENTAX) is a new device that combines airflow and air pressure measurement capabilities. Pressure and flow data are measured from the two channels simultaneously, which permits relative comparisons. Normal speakers, except during the production of nasal consonants, exhibit relatively no nasal pressure or flow (Smith, Guyette, Patil, and Brannan, 2003; Smith, Patil, Guyette, Brannan, and Cohen, 2004). Speakers with nasality problems show deviations in the relative amount of nasal and oral flows (Mason and Warren, 1980; Smith and Guyette, 1996). The aerodynamic procedures basically provide the clinician information about possible leakage through the nose when the velopharyngeal mechanism should be closed. Manometers have also been useful for measuring relative nasal–oral airflows. Manometers measure the amount of pressure of the emitted airstream and do not measure resonance per se; as we have mentioned resonance is a perceptual event. Manometers are discussed in Chapter 6.

Acoustics. The Nasometer (KayPENTAX Corp.) is a noninvasive computer-based system developed by Fletcher (1978) to measure the relative amount of oral-to-nasal acoustic energy in an individual's speech. An adaptation of the original Tonar II (Fletcher, 1972), the Nasometer collects oral and nasal sound intensity using two microphones located on either side of a nasal separator. The sound separator rests against the upper lip of the subject and is held in place by headgear (see Figure 9.1). The Nasometer computer digitizes, filters, and then compares the separated signals in a ratio. The product, called *nasalance*, increases as nasal intensity increases relative to oral intensity. In addition to providing nasalance data, the Nasometer provides visual feedback on a computer screen for the patient that allows the clinician to set a predetermined level of acceptable nasalance. This feature adds another feedback dimension in real time to the client when attempting to alter oral–nasal ratios.

Three passages are commonly used to obtain nasalance scores (Fletcher, Adams, and McCutcheon, 1989): the Zoo Passage, which contains no nasal phonemes, the Rainbow Passage, which contains 11% nasal phonemes, and the Nasal Sentences, which contain approximately 35% nasal phonemes. Fletcher and colleagues (1989) obtained nasalance scores from 117 children with no history of resonance disorders. The mean nasalance scores for each stimulus were significantly different from the others, indicating that nasalance scores are sensitive to the proportion of nasal phonemes in each speech sample.

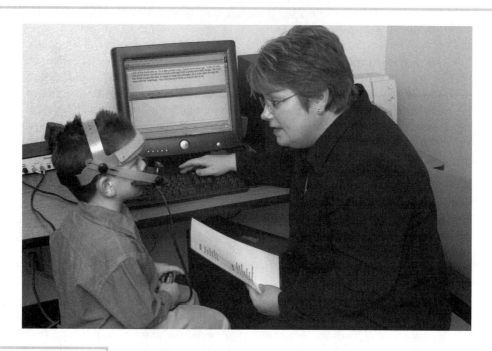

FIGURE **9.1**

A four-year-old boy wears the oral–nasal dual microphones for determining his oral–nasal ratio on the Nasometer.

Using the Nasometer in a study of 20 children with normal VP function and 20 children at risk for velopharyngeal insufficiency, Watterson, Hinton, and McFarlane (1996) constructed and tested two novel stimuli for obtaining nasalance measures from young children in an attempt to establish a cutoff score between normal and excessive nasalance. The new passages constructed and studied were the Turtle Passage and the Mouse Passage. The Turtle Passage contained no normally nasal consonants while the Mouse Passage contained about 11% nasal consonants. They concluded: "Clinicians should have least confidence in nasalance scores for patients who are borderline normal. Because borderline normal patients are difficult to classify, however, absolute nasalance cutoff scores may never be a reality" (p. 72). Watterson, Lewis, and Deutsch (1998) used the Nasometer to study nasalance and nasality in low- and high-pressure speech. From their study of 20 children with managed clefts and 5 children without clefts, they concluded: "Sensitivity and specificity scores indicated that the Nasometer was reasonably accurate in distinguishing between normal and hypernasal speech samples."

The NasalView (Tiger Electronics Inc.) is a more recent computer-based system that measures oral–nasal resonance. Lewis and Watterson (2003) compared nasalance scores from the Nasometer and NasalView from five sentences produced by 50 elementary school children with no history of resonance disorders. They found that the speech stimuli weighted with different vowel types were differentially affected by the different acoustic filtering used in the Nasometer and the NasalView. They suggested that the two instruments provide different information and that scores are not interchangeable.

The OroNasal System (Glottal Enterprises Inc.) is also a relatively new computer-based system that measures oral–nasal resonance. Bressman (2005) compared nasalance scores from the Nasometer, NasalView, and OroNasal System for the Rainbow, Zoo, and Nasal Sentences passages produced by 76 adults with no history of resonance disorders. Bressman found that each instrument reported different nasalance scores for each passage, suggesting that the three instruments are not interchangeable.

Spectrography.   It has been demonstrated spectrographically that speakers with increased nasalization demonstrate more prominent third formants with an increase in formant bandwidth, accompanied by a rise in fundamental frequency. In his acoustic study of nasality using the spectrograph, Dickson (1962) concluded that there was no way to "differentiate nasality in cleft palate and non–cleft palate individuals either in terms of their acoustic spectra or the variability of the nasality judgments" (p. 111). It is doubtful that the visual readout provided by the spectrograph can provide the clinician with any more information about the type of nasality he or she hears than does listening carefully to the same samples. The spectrograph and Computerized Speech Lab (CSL) can help identify the aperiodic noise of nasal emission, but differentiating between spectrograms of speakers with hypernasality and those with hyponasality or assimilative nasality is most difficult. As clinicians learn to use the spectral analyses the spectrograph and CSL can provide, however, these instruments may well become most useful tools for studying various parameters of nasality. The CSL, which was discussed in Chapter 6, may be seen in Figure 6.13 (p. 167).

Radiographic Instruments.   Radiography permits the imaging of internal body parts. Radiographic studies of the velopharyngeal mechanism during speech provide ready information about structural and physiological limitations of the mechanism in those patients who demonstrate velopharyngeal incompetence. For example, through a lateral-view film we can determine the relative amount of velopharyngeal opening during speech, the length of the velum and relative movements of the velum, and the posterior pharyngeal and lateral walls (Johns, Rohrich, and Awada, 2003). However, there are limitations to the use of lateral views attempting to view closure, because lateral wall movement of the pharynx, which may contribute heavily to velopharyngeal closure, cannot be visualized. Sometimes the patient is asked to swallow barium and, as the barium passes through the pharynx, measurements are made of the relative pharyngeal opening as it relates to the velopharyngeal closing mechanism (Skolnick, Glaser, and McWilliams, 1980). The most useful radiographic views of velopharyngeal closure require the patient to make some speech utterances, including phrases and sentences that include pressure consonants. The speech–language pathologist needs to work closely with the radiologist, presenting the speech tasks as the films are made and "reading" the films when they are completed. Sometimes a radiographic display can demonstrate a problem in velopharyngeal closure that cannot be detected by any other method except for nasovideoendoscopy.

Visual Probe Instruments.   Shelton and Trier (1976) have written that direct measures of velopharyngeal competence through the use of "endoscopes, nasopharyngoscopes, and ultrasound apparatus" offer some advantages in making treatment decisions. The oral endoscope (Zwitman, Gyepes, and Ward, 1976) has been a useful instrument for determining the degree and type of velopharyngeal closure, as shown in Figure 9.2. The body of the oral endoscope is extended above the tongue within the oral cavity so that the lighted tip and viewing window lie just below the uvula and within the oropharyngeal opening. By turning the viewing window up toward the velopharyngeal area, the velum, the lateral pharyngeal walls, and the posterior pharynx may be visualized. Two views of varying degrees of velopharyngeal closure in the same subject are shown in Figure 9.2. One important disadvantage of the oral endoscope is that one can only observe vowel or limited consonant and vowel combinations such as /pa/ or /ba/. This is due to the unnatural introduction of the oral endoscope into the oral cavity and its effect on articulation and connected speech (McFarlane, 1990).

For many of us who work in the area of cleft palate or who work with those who have velopharyngeal inadequacy due to structural defects (such as postcancer surgery) or neurological defect (such as one of the dysarthrias, discussed in Chapter 4) the use of nasovideoendoscopy of the VP mechanism has become the "gold standard." For example, with a nasal fiberoptic endoscope, which places a small flexible scope through the nose and down into the pharynx, the clinician can see velopharyngeal closure from above the closure site (Lam et al., 2006; Watterson and McFarlane, 1990) and the dynamics of VP function can be studied. The primary advantage of the flexible endoscope is that it is not invasive to the oral cavity and consequently does not impede tongue, lip, or jaw movements during dynamic articulation (a limitation of the oral endoscope). The oral and nasal endoscopic probes are effective instruments for assessing velopharyngeal competence in patients with nasal resonance problems, because they offer direct observation of velar length and movement, degree of lateral and posterior pharyngeal wall movement, and the kind of velopharyngeal closure the patient is using. Perhaps most importantly, this examination allows the clinician and the patient to see the various types and degrees of velopharyngeal closure during a variety of phonetic contexts (Boone and McFarlane, 1994; McFarlane, 1990).

Watterson and McFarlane (1990) discuss in detail the use of transnasal videoendoscopy of the velopharyngeal port mechanism. They discuss the use of sustained vowels, sustained consonants, single words and sentences, and phrases as speech stimuli in speech testing for VP competency. The use of high vowels such as /i/ and /u/ as well as stops (/p/k/t/), fricatives, and affricates allows the examiner

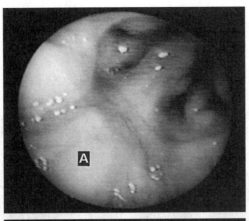

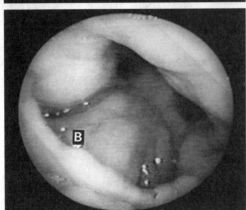

FIGURE **9.2**

Velopharyngeal Closure

This oral videoendoscopic view of velopharyngeal closure is taken with a rigid endoscope placed intraorally and flipped up to view the velopharynx instead of the hypopharynx. Note in view A one can see the nasal septum and turbinates, and in view B the velum (top right corner) has closed and now obstructs the view of the septum and turbinates. The bulging of Passavant's Pad is located at B on the posterior pharyngeal wall.

to make important statements about the ability of the VP mechanism to successfully manage complex speech tasks. The information gained by using such stimuli will guide therapy and management decisions. For example, it is important to know whether the patient consistently experiences nasal air escape on a particular phoneme, such as /s/, or if there is only a breakdown of VP function at the phrase level or when the /s/ is in the context of a blend.

As McFarlane (1990) and Boone and McFarlane (1994) have indicated, even children can be examined with naso- or orovideoendoscopy without the use of any topical anesthetics. Figure 9.3 shows a patient being examined with rigid endoscopy and Figure 9.4 shows a child being examined with nasoendoscopy without the aid of topical anesthesia. Indeed, in a prospective double-blind study, Leder and colleagues (1997) concluded that "speech–language pathologists can perform independent and comfortable transnasal endoscopy without administration of any substance to the nasal mucosa" (p. 1352).

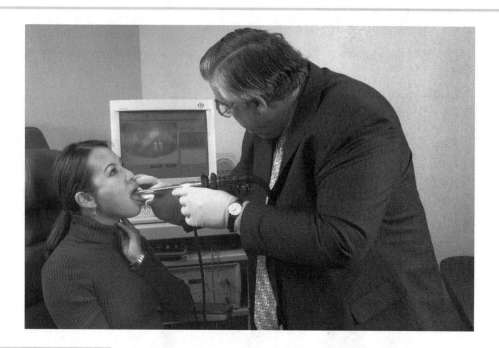

FIGURE **9.3**

Oral Videoendoscopy

This patient is examined by oral videoendoscopy. Children and adults are routinely evaluated in this manner without the use of any topical anesthetic.

Distinct variations in patterns of velopharyngeal closure have been demonstrated by Armour, Fischbach, Klaiman, and Fisher (2005) and Zwitman (1990). Some subjects have only velar movement without associated pharyngeal wall movement, some subjects primarily have lateral and posterior pharyngeal wall constriction, and some subjects achieve closure by a combination of velar and pharyngeal movements. Watterson and McFarlane (1990) have described five useful classes of VP function and provide a basis for making recommendations for clinical treatment.

Treatment of Nasal Resonance Disorders

Hypernasality.   The presence of excessive nasal resonance (hypernasality) is relatively dependent on the judgment of the listener. That is, some languages and regional dialects require heavy nasal resonance and therefore consider pronounced nasalization of vowels to be normal. Others, however, such as general U.S. English, tolerate little nasal resonance beyond the three nasal consonants. Thus, a native New

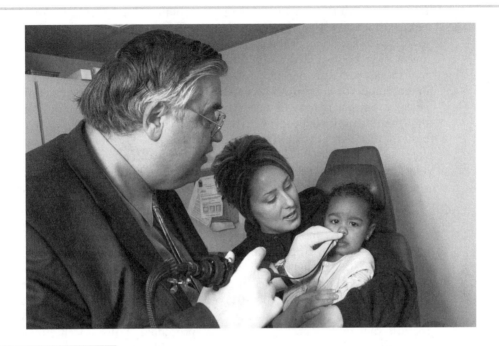

FIGURE **9.4**

Nasoendoscopy of a Child with a Voice Disorder

Englander with a nasal "twang" exhibits normal voice resonance in Portland, Maine, but when he or she travels to New Knoxville, Ohio, the people there may perceive his or her voice as excessively nasal. Variations do exist in the degree of nasality among the voices of the people in Ohio, of course, but a certain amount of resonance variability can exist among any particular population without anyone being bothered by it. If, however, a particular voice in Ohio (or any other place) stands out as "excessively nasal," then that voice will be considered to have a resonance disorder. The judgment of hypernasality, then, is as dependent on the speech–language milieu of the speaker and his or her listeners as it is on the actual performance of the speaker.

The speaker who is judged to be hypernasal increases the nasalization of his or her vowels by failing to close his or her velopharyngeal port, which may be related to structural–organic defects or may have a functional etiology. Hypernasality frequently accompanies unrepaired cleft palate or a short palate. Among other organic causes of the disorder are surgical trauma (e.g., postadenoidectomy), accidental injury to the soft palate, and impaired innervation of the soft palate as a result of poliomyelitis or some other form of upper or lower motor neuron disease. Sometimes temporary hypernasality may follow surgical removal of the adenoids and tonsils as the patient attempts to minimize the pain by not moving his or her velopharyngeal mechanism. But when hypernasality persists for two or three months or more following adenoidectomy or tonsillectomy, the adequacy of the velopharyngeal mechanism must be suspected and evaluated (Robb, 2007). Some people speak with hypernasal resonance for purely functional reasons, perhaps to maintain a lingering internal model of a previously acceptable form of resonance or perhaps to imitate the voice of someone they admire (such as a famous political figure or performer). Although the majority of people with hypernasal voices probably have some structural basis for their lack of velopharyngeal competence, the ease of imitating a hypernasal voice tells us that it could be relatively easy to become hypernasal with perfectly adequate and normal velopharyngeal anatomy and physiology. Hypernasality is one voice problem in which the distinction must be made between organic and functional causes, as the treatment recommended is quite specific to the diagnosis.

If there are any indications of physical inadequacy of velopharyngeal closure, the primary role of the speech pathologist is to refer the patient to a specialist who can provide the needed physical management—a plastic surgeon, say, or a prosthodontist. The speech–language pathologist will make the determination of the mechanism's adequacy for speech purposes and together the patient and other professionals will determine the best corrective approach. If surgery is selected, the speech pathologist will share the results of the speech–voice evaluation to aid with the selection of an appropriate surgical procedure. Postsurgically, the speech–language pathologist will evaluate the repaired VP mechanism to determine its adequacy for speech–language production. If dental appliances are to be selected, the speech–language pathologist will suggest the type of appliance, lift, or prosthesis with a bulb, and the SLP will assist with the design and fitting of the appliance. If a prosthetic form of management is used, then the speech pathologist will be involved in the initial fabrication and fitting of the velar lift or obturator. Subsequent modifications of these devices will be directed by the speech pathologist, based on the results of speech testing and the patient's response to clinical speech stimulation.

There is very little evidence that voice therapy to improve resonance has any positive effect in the presence of physical inadequacy. In fact, there is some indication that voice therapy to improve the oral resonance of patients with palatal insufficiency (those who lack the physical equipment to produce closure) will usually not only fail, but will also be interpreted by the patient as his or her own fault—as a defeat indicating low personal worth—and thus will take an obvious toll on the patient's self-image. An example of the ineffectiveness of speech therapy in the presence of a severe inadequacy of velopharyngeal closure is provided by this case of a teenage girl with VPD who had received speech therapy for both articulation and resonance for a period of seven years:

Barbara, age 14, had received seven years of group and individual speech therapy in the public schools and in a community speech and hearing clinic for "a severe articulation defect characterized by sibilant distortion and for a severely nasal voice." Barbara's mother became upset because of Barbara's continued lack of progress and her tendency to withdraw from social contact with her peers, which, the mother felt, was related to her embarrassment over her continued poor speech. Barbara was evaluated by a comprehensive cleft palate team, which, after reviewing her history, found that her nasality dated from a severe bout of influenza when she was six years old. The influenza had been followed immediately by a deterioration of speech. Subsequent speech therapy records were incomplete, although the mother reported that the therapy had included extensive blowing drills, tongue–palate exercises, and articulation work. Physical examination of the velar mechanism found that Barbara had good tongue and pharyngeal movements but bilateral paralysis of the soft palate; even on gag reflex stimulation, only a "flicker" of palatal movement was observed. Lateral cinefluorographic films confirmed the relatively complete absence of velar movement. The examining speech pathologist found that Barbara had normal articulation placement of the tongue for all speech sounds, despite severe nasal emission of airflow for fricative and affricate phonemes. Low back vowels were relatively oral in resonance, whereas middle and high vowels became increasingly nasal. It was the consensus of the evaluation team that, with her structural inadequacy, Barbara was (and had been) a poor candidate for speech therapy. It was recommended that she receive a pharyngeal flap and be evaluated again several weeks after the operation. The surgery was successful and had an amazingly positive effect on Barbara's speech. Although hypernasality disappeared, some slight nasal emission remained. Barbara was subsequently enrolled in individual speech therapy, where she experienced total success in developing normal fricative–affricate production.

Such a case dramatically shows the futility of continued speech therapy when real structural inadequacy exists. Without the operation, Barbara could have received speech therapy for the rest of her life, with no effect whatsoever on her speech. If velopharyngeal insufficiency is found, there are two primary alternatives for treatment, surgical or dental. When structural adequacy is achieved, remediation services of the speech–language pathologist can produce further changes in the patient's speech and resonance.

Surgical Treatment for Hypernasality. The evaluation of the oral and VP mechanism may reveal the existence of such structural inadequacies as open fistulas, open bony and soft tissue clefts, submucosal clefts, and short or relatively immobile soft palates. The plastic surgeon is usually the medical specialist most experienced in making decisions about when and if surgical closure of palatal openings is required, based on the recommendation of the speech–language pathologist. The speech pathologist is best able to assess the adequacy of the velopharyngeal port mechanism during speech. Usually, the major reason (often the only reason) for surgical or prosthetic treatment in these patients is to improve speech, but swallowing also almost always improves.

A plastic surgeon wrote, "The surgeon requires the involvement of the speech pathologist in diagnosis as well as therapy" (Grace, 1984, p. 152). This includes preoperative testing, pressure and flow measurements, and mutual evaluation of radiographic studies. Paralleling the widespread use of direct endoscopic visual observation in medicine, the development of oral and nasoendoscopy has become an indispensable tool for diagnosing many speech disorders. Although nasoendoscopy is used by some plastic surgeons, it is also often used by speech–language pathologists. It should be routinely available in centers managing organically based resonance disorders.

When the diagnostic tests have been completed, the speech pathologist and surgeon must arrive at the plan for management. The speech pathologist should be familiar with available options for anatomic correction and should participate in the decision for surgery. "The surgeon must know the alternative treatments and anticipated results of his operations. The timing of surgery can be a mutual decision" (Grace, 1984, p. 152). For those individuals who have cleft palate, the primary surgical procedure usually involves closing the cleft and still maintaining adequate palatal length. Most patients with cleft palate, however, require multiple secondary surgical procedures at later times, such as rebuilding structures or eliminating earlier surgical scars (Peterson-Falzone, Hardin-Jones, and Karnell, 2001). The typical patient with hypernasality has a velum that is too short for closure or a velum that does not move adequately for closure. Such a patient often profits from a surgically constructed pharyngeal flap (LaRossa et al., 2004).

In this procedure, the surgeon takes a small piece of mucosal tissue from the pharynx and uses it to bridge the excessive velopharyngeal opening, attaching the tissue to the soft palate (LaRossa, 2000). This tissue acts as a substitute structure for an inadequate velum by deflecting both airflow and sound waves into the oral cavity and allowing the walls of the pharynx to close adequately onto the lateral margins of the pharyngeal flap. Bzoch (1989), discussing the physiological and speech results for 40 patients who had received pharyngeal flap surgery, reported that the procedure was most effective in reducing both hypernasality and nasal emission (if present) in most of the subjects. Although pharyngeal flap surgery, or any other form of palatal surgery, must not be considered a panacea for all resonance problems, it often helps align oral–nasal structures in such a way that (allowing open or closed coupling of the nasal and oral cavity), for the first time, speech and voice therapy can be effective.

Regarding the use of surgical methods to correct speech problems, Grace observed:

> Postoperative speech testing is mandatory to objectively evaluate the results of surgery and reassess speech goals. The surgeon may profit from observing a postoperative evaluation, much as the speech pathologist would profit from seeing surgery. All too often there is a tendency for the surgeon to divorce the patient when the surgery is completed, with the expectation that the battle will be won or lost by the speech pathologist. (Grace, 1984, p. 154)

When speaking of surgery in cleft palate patients, Grace went on to say, "In truth, the success of surgery varies widely from patient to patient, and it cannot be assumed that anatomy is restored to normal upon completion of the operation" (p. 154). This reality is reflected in the ongoing exploration for improved surgical techniques, such as sphincter pharyngoplasty (Witt et al., 1999), covering the exposed muscular surface of the flap with nasal mucosa (Stoll et al., 2001), and distraction osteogenesis (Guyette, Polley, Botts, Figueroa, and Smith, 2001; Guyette, Polley, Figueroa, and Smith, 2001).

Dental Treatment of Hypernasality.   Both orthodontists and prosthodontists can play important roles in treating individuals with hypernasality, particularly those with cleft palate. The orthodontist may have to expand the dental arches so that the patient can experience more normal palatal growth and dentition. The prosthodontist, by constructing various prosthetic speech appliances and obturators, may be able to help the patient preserve his or her facial contour and, by filling in various maxillary defects with prostheses, may cover open palatal defects such as fistulas and clefts. The prosthodontist may also be able to build speech-training appliances to provide posterior velopharyngeal closure. In evaluating 21 adults with acquired or congenital palate problems, Arndt, Shelton, and Bradford (1965) found that both groups made significant "articulation and voice gains with obturation." These findings have subsequently been confirmed by Tachimura, Nohara, and Wada (2000) using electromyography and by Konst and colleagues (2003). These researchers found that children with unilateral cleft lip and palate who used a prosthesis during the first year of life followed a more normal path of phonological development between two and three years of age. Many cleft palate subjects are fitted with appliances featuring acrylic bulbs that are fitted into the VP port space. If the bulbs are well positioned near the posterior and lateral pharyngeal walls, there is often a noticeable reduction of both nasality and air escape. Articulation, which is dependent on adequate intraoral air pressure and normal resonance, may be achieved with speech–voice therapy in conjunction with a properly fitted speech appliance such as an obturator or palatal lift. Two lateral views of obturators are shown in Figure 9.5. Figure 9.6 shows a palatal lift prosthesis designed for an adult male with a paralyzed palate following traumatic brain injury in an accident.

When commenting on the role of the speech pathologist in the prosthodontic management of patients with velopharyngeal inadequacy, Ahlstrom (1984), a prosthodontist, stated, "One of the primary diagnostic services that a speech pathologist can offer is the determination of velopharyngeal competence in patients. This helps the prosthodontist in determination of what type of appliance or procedure may be necessary" (p. 150). Many patients with dysarthria, which may include a hypernasality component, have immobile velums and thus lack sufficient velar movement to achieve closure. Such patients, who experience weakened or paralyzed soft palates, might well profit from consulting a prosthodontist about being fitted with a lift appliance to hold the immobile palate in a higher position so that some pharyngeal contact will be possible (Mazaheri, 1979). The palatal lift in Figure 9.6 was made for just such a patient who now has normal resonance with the device. For nasality problems related to velopharyngeal inadequacy, speech pathologists should freely consult both orthodontists and prosthodontists for their ideas on how to achieve adequate functioning of the oral structures (Sell, Mars, and Worrell, 2006).

Voice Therapy for Hypernasality.   Any attempts at voice therapy for hypernasality should be deferred until both the evaluation of the problem and attempts

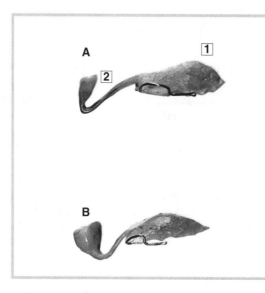

FIGURE **9.5**

Obturators

This photo features two different sizes of obturators. A was made for an adult. (1) is the palatal part, and (2) is the pharyngeal part. B was made for a five-year-old girl with structural (cleft palate) hypernasality with an extremely short velum following surgical repair.

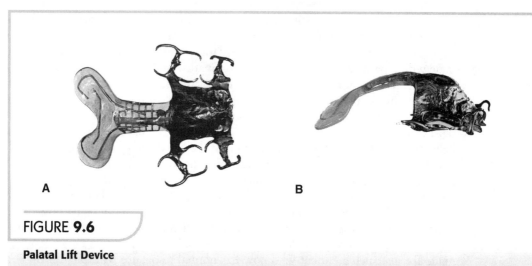

FIGURE **9.6**

Palatal Lift Device

(A) is a superior or top view; (B) is a lateral or side view. This palatal lift was designed for an adult with a neurogenic (dysarthria) problem of hypernasality (velopharyngeal *incompetency*). Note the fluke-shaped lift that elevates the palate. This is quite different from the obturator knob in Figure 9.5, which is designed to occlude part of the velopharyngeal port for velopharyngeal *insufficiency*.

at physical correction (surgical or prosthodontic) have been completed. The primary requirement for developing good oral voice quality is the structural adequacy of the velopharyngeal closing mechanism. Without adequate closure, voice therapy will be futile. However, for individuals who speak with hypernasality for functional reasons, voice therapy can help develop more oral resonance. Added to this group are occasional patients who have had surgical or dental treatment that has left them with only a marginal velopharyngeal closing mechanism; in voice therapy, this mechanism may be trained to work more optimally. Watterson, York, and McFarlane (1994) studied nasalance in the speech of 30 normal young adults and found that, while there was no statistical difference in nasalance scores under three different loudness levels, there was a strong systematic trend for the lowest nasalance scores to occur in the loudest conditions, while the highest nasalance scores occurred under the softest conditions. The implication is to experiment with increased loudness levels in cases of minimal or borderline VPI.

The Nasometer display gives the patient instant feedback information about the peak nasalance level, the target level of oral–nasal ratio, and the moment-to-moment level of nasalance. If the patient is capable of developing greater oral resonance, he or she works incrementally, using the Nasometer feedback system, toward goals of acceptable oral resonance. Various facilitating techniques (described in Chapter 7) may be used successfully with the Nasometer, nasal listening tube, Facilitator loop feedback, See-Scape, nasal mirror, or stethoscope. They can even be used with an audio recorder or the unaided ear. Kuehn (1997) has experimented with the use of continuous positive airway pressure (with sleep apnea equipment) as a possible means to reduce hypernasality. To date, studies of the approach seem to indicate that the levator veli palatini muscle works harder and contracts with more force when presented with positive airway pressure. This seems to be true for both normal people and those with repaired cleft palates.

Some other techniques have been helpful clinically:

1. *Altering tongue position.* A high, forward carriage of the tongue sometimes contributes to nasal resonance. Efforts to develop a lower, more posterior carriage may decrease the perceived nasality.

2. *Change of loudness.* A voice that has been perceived as hypernasal will sometimes be perceived as more normal if some other change in vocalization is made, such as an increase in loudness. By speaking in a louder voice, the patient frequently sounds less hypernasal (Watterson, York, and McFarlane, 1994). One should try both *increased and decreased* loudness levels with each patient to determine which condition best reduces nasality.

3. *Auditory feedback.* If the patient is motivated to reduce his or her hypernasality, a great deal of therapy time should be spent learning to hear the differences between his or her nasal and oral resonances.

4. *Establishing new pitch.* Some patients with hypernasality speak at inappropriately high pitch levels, which contribute to the listener's perception of nasality.

Speaking at the lower end of one's pitch range seems to contribute to greater oral resonance.

5. *Counseling.* No voice therapy should ever be started without first explaining to the patient what the problem seems to be and the general course of therapy that is being planned.

6. *Feedback.* Developing an aural awareness of hypernasality with some oral–pharyngeal awareness of what hypernasality "feels" like is a most helpful therapeutic device.

7. *Open mouth.* Hypernasality is sometimes produced by an overall restriction of the oral opening. In such cases, efforts to develop greater oral openness may reduce the listener's perception of excessive nasality.

8. *Focus.* Although, for some patients, focusing on the facial mask area seems to increase nasality, for other patients, particularly those whose hypernasality is of functional origin, doing so noticeably improves resonance.

9. *Respiration training.* Increased loudness is often achieved by respiration training.

These techniques achieve their results by altering the speech production, for example, by pitch modification, increased or decreased airflow, reduced air pressure on the velopharyngeal port, or enhanced feedback to the patient by using mirror fogging, acoustic changes, or changes in the location of vibratory patterns. We find these methods very successful with patients who have resonance disorders or whose velopharyngeal ports are "borderline adequate" or better. When the velopharyngeal mechanism is less adequate, surgical or prosthetic management is in order prior to initiating voice therapy techniques. When the degree of velopharyngeal mechanism adequacy is seriously in question, a period of intensive trial voice and articulation therapy may determine the need for other management approaches. This trial therapy should be intensive (three sessions per week minimum) but of short duration (six weeks), and it should be conducted with the understanding that it is a trial to determine whether further therapy is indicated or some other management approach is required. Under no circumstances should voice therapy for resonance disorders be continued when success is not forthcoming. Long periods of time without any progress are poor for motivation and the patient's self-image.

Hyponasality. Except for the nasal resonance required for /m/, /n/, and /ŋ/, vowels in U.S. English require only slight nasal resonance. In severe cases lack of nasal resonance produces actual articulatory substitutions for the three nasal phonemes as well as slight alterations of vowels. Hyponasality is characterized by the diversion of sound waves and airflow out through the oral cavity, which permits little or no nasal resonance. As discussed earlier in this chapter, this problem is related to some kind of nasal or nasopharyngeal obstruction, such as excessive adenoidal growth, severe nasopharyngeal infection, as in head colds, large polyps in the nasal cavity, and so on. Some patients who are hypernasal before surgical or prosthetic management emerge from such treatment with complete or highly excessive velopharyngeal obstruction. Perhaps the pharyngeal flap is too broad and permits little or no ventilation of the nasopharynx, or perhaps an obturator bulb fits too tightly (which can be easily reduced) and results in no nasal airflow or nasal resonance. Some kind of obstruction is the usual reason for a hyponasality problem, and the search for it must precede any attempt at voice therapy. We have seen a few cases, however, in which hyponasality was caused by psychological or other functional factors.

Nasal airflow competence can be tested simply as part of an overall resonance evaluation. Ask the patient to take a big breath, close his or her mouth, and exhale through the nose. Then test the airflow through each nostril separately, compressing the naris of one nostril at a time with a finger. If there is any observable decrement in airflow, the nasal passage should be investigated medically. Appropriate medical therapy (medications, reduction of turbinates surgically, septal repair) should precede any voice therapy for hyponasality. Only rarely do patients have markedly hyponasal voices for wholly functional reasons. Even though their hyponasal resonance may originally have had a physical cause, that cause may be no longer present, and the hyponasality may remain as a habit, a "set." One TV newsman with whom we worked had a hyponasal voice quality after many years of suffering from allergies. After moving to a new area of the country where the allergies were no longer a problem, he maintained his hyponasal voice by strength of habit until voice therapy produced a normal voice quality. Occasionally a patient has chosen a hyponasal voice as a model, for whatever reason, and has learned to match its hyponasality with some consistency. We once had a patient who would use a marked hyponasal voice quality when he was challenged at work. Voice therapy was helpful in both these cases.

Voice therapy for increasing nasal resonance might include the following:

1. *Auditory feedback.* Considerable effort must be expended in contrasting for the patient the difference between the nasal and oral production of /m/, /n/, and /ng/. Oral and nasal resonance of vowels can also be presented for listening contrast. The Facilitator mentioned in Chapter 7 can be helpful with this technique.

2. *Counseling.* The resonance requirements for normal English must be explained to the patient, and his or her own lack of nasal resonance, particularly for /m/, /n/, and /ng/, pointed out. If the patient's problem is wholly functional, this explanation is of primary importance.

3. *Feedback.* Emphasis must be given to contrasting what it sounds like and "feels" like to produce oral and nasal resonance. The patient should be encouraged to make exaggerated humming sounds both orally and nasally, concentrating on the "feel" of the two types of productions.

4. *Nasal/glide stimulation.* This technique is one of the most powerful for hyponasality treatment. The phrases listed under this technique in Chapter 7 are very helpful ("Momma made lemon jam," etc.).

5. *Focus.* Direction of the tone into the facial mask is usually successful.

Assimilative Nasality.   The nasalization of vowels and voice consonants immediately before and after nasal consonants is known as *assimilative nasality.*

Performance on stimulability testing will provide a good clue whether such nasal resonance is related to poor velar functioning or is functionally induced. A few neurological disorders, such as bulbar palsy, multiple sclerosis, and spastic dysarthria prevent the patient from moving the velum quickly enough to facilitate the movements required for normal resonance. The velar openings begin too soon and are maintained too long, lagging behind the rapid requirements of normal speech and nasalizing vowels that occur next to nasal phonemes. Any patient who presents with sudden onset of hypernasality or assimilative nasality should be suspected for having a neurological disorder or disease until proven otherwise; referral to a neurologist is in order. Most cases of assimilative nasality, however, are of functional origin, and the patient shows good oral resonance under special conditions of stimulability. Remember that in connected speech, all sounds are interdependent; as one sound is being produced, articulators are positioning for the next sound. This phonemic coarticulation allows for a certain amount of assimilation, even in normal speech. Assimilative nasality, therefore, is another perceptual problem; whether the speaker's nasalization of vowels adjacent to nasal phonemes is excessive or not depends on the perception of the listener. The perception of assimilative nasality is, of course, related to the perception of excessive nasality; a normal, minor amount of nasality in the vowels following nasal phonemes would not be perceived, and increased amounts of nasal resonance would be judged quite differently by different listeners, according to their individual standards and experience. Therapy for assimilative nasality is likewise highly variable. It is, in fact, largely related to the locale (in some areas such resonance is a normal voice pattern), the standards of the speaker or clinician, their motivations, and so on.

The Nasometer is a useful therapy instrument for the patient who wants to reduce his or her assimilative nasality. The clinician and the patient can predetermine oral–nasal ratio goals that favor orality and then work incrementally toward eliminating the assimilative nasal resonance. The listening tube and See-Scape, discussed previously in this chapter, may also be effective feedback strategies. Voice therapy for assimilative nasality is best attempted only by those patients who are strongly motivated to develop more oral resonance. Facilitating approaches (see Chapter 7) might include the following:

1. *Auditory feedback.* Ear training should help patients discriminate between their nasalized vowels and their oral vowels. Patients should listen to recordings of their own oral/consonant/vowel/oral/consonant words as contrasted with their nasal consonant/vowel/nasal consonant words, such as these pairs: *bad–man, bed–men, bead–mean, bub–mum,* and so on. Voice and diction books often contain word pairs matching monosyllabic words using /b/, /d/, and /g/ with those using /m/, /n/, and /ŋ/. Once the patient can hear the differences between oral and nasal cognates, determine whether he or she can produce them.

2. *Counseling.* Because nasal assimilations are difficult to explain verbally, any attempt at explanation should be accompanied by demonstration. The best demonstration is to present the contrast between oral and nasal resonance of vowels that follow or precede the three nasal phonemes.

THERAPY FOR ORAL–PHARYNGEAL
RESONANCE PROBLEMS

Although during speech both the oral and pharyngeal cavities are constantly chang-ing in size and shape, the oral cavity is the most changeable resonance cavity. Speech is possible only because of the capability for variation of such oral structures as the lips, mandible, tongue, and velum. The most dramatic oral movements in speech are those of the tongue, which makes various constrictive–restrictive contacts at dif-ferent sites within the oral cavity to produce consonant articulation. Vowel and diphthong production are possible only because of size–shape adjustments of the oral cavity that require a delicate blend of muscle adjustment of all oral muscle structures. Although many individuals display faulty positioning of oral structures for articulation, and thus articulate "badly," fewer individuals are recognized to have problems positioning their oral structures for resonance. Slight departures in articulatory proficiency are much more easily recognized than are minor problems in voice resonance. Even though an articulation error may be viewed consistently as a problem, faulty oral–pharyngeal resonance is usually accepted as "the way he or she talks," or as a regional dialect. Nasality problems are more likely to be rec-ognized by lay and professional listeners as requiring correction than are oral–pharyngeal resonance departures. Any judgment of resonance is heavily influenced by the appropriateness of pitch, the degree of glottal competence as heard in the pe-riodic quality of phonation, and the degree of accuracy of articulation. Because quality of resonance, then, appears basically to be a subjective experience, the goal in resonance therapy must be to achieve whatever voice "sounds best."

Singing teachers have long been aware of the vital role the tongue plays in in-fluencing the quality of the voice, and they devote considerable instructional and practice time to helping singing students develop optimum carriage of the tongue (Coffin, 1981). Although the postures needed to produce various phonemes will attract the tongue to different anatomic sites within the oral cavity, with noticeable changes of oral resonance, more objective evidence of the role of the tongue in oral resonance may be obtained through spectrographic and videofluorographic analy-sis. In the spectral analyses afforded by the spectrograph, we can study the effects of tongue positioning and the distribution of spectral formants. The second for-mant seems to "travel" the most, changing position up and down the spectrum for various vowel productions. Boone and McFarlane (1993) demonstrate this in their study of the yawn–sigh technique (Chapter 7). The primary oral shaper for production of vowels appears to be the tongue. Decisions about quality of reso-nance (for example, is the voice hypernasal or hyponasal) are, however, almost im-possible to render from the visual inspection of spectrograms. It is most difficult to quantify formant variations and relate them to variations in voice quality.

In describing the difficulty of spectrographic analysis, Moll (1968) has writ-ten that "this presumably more 'objective' measure involves overall judgments which probably are more difficult than those made in judging nasality from ac-tual speech" (p. 99). Visual inspection of the spectrogram is a difficult task, particularly when one attempts to relate formant positioning to judgments of voice quality. As for the videofluorograph, its use for studying tongue, velar, mandibular, and pharyngeal movements, when such movements apply to voice quality, becomes far more effective when a voice track is added. The addition of the speaker's voice not only enables the viewer to match the sound of the voice with the analysis of the speaker's movements, but, more important, provides the viewer with the primary vehicle for determining whether a problem of quality exists. Quality judgments cannot be made from the visual study of oral movements alone, but depend primarily on hearing the sound of the voice. By using both the pitch and intensity readings at the same time on the Visi-Pitch, we have found that the real-time tracings on the Visi-Pitch monitor give useful information specific to better resonance. Often the resonance that sounds better to the ear is represented on the scope as less aperiodic (the frequency readout has less scatter) and more intense (greater amplitude of the intensity curve). The "better-sounding" voice often comes quite unexpectedly as the clinician and the patient use various facilitating approaches in their search for good oral resonance. Once the "good" voice is achieved, the Visi-Pitch offers useful feedback for the patient, often confirming by improvement in the scope tracings the subjective judgments the clinician and patient have made.

Reducing the Strident Voice.   One of the most annoying oral–pharyngeal resonance problems is the strident voice. We use the term *stridency*, which means the unpleasant, shrill, metallic-sounding voice that appears to be related to hypertonicity of the pharyngeal constrictors (walls of the pharynx). Fisher (1975) described the strident voice as having brilliance of high overtones sounding "brassy, tinny, blatant." Physiologically, stridency may be produced by the elevation of the larynx and hypertonicity of the pharyngeal constrictors, which decrease both the length and the width of the pharynx. The surface of the pharynx becomes taut because of the tight pharyngeal constriction. The smaller pharyngeal cavity, coupled with its tighter, reflective mucosal surface, produces the ideal resonating structure for accentuating high-frequency resonance. Stridency may be developed deliberately—for example, by a carnival barker or a store demonstrator for its obvious attention-getting effects—or it may emerge when a person becomes overly tense and constricts the pharynx as part of his or her overall response to stress. A person who has this sort of strident voice—and who wants to correct it—can, in voice therapy, often develop some relaxed oral–pharyngeal behaviors that decrease pharyngeal constriction (increasing the size of the pharynx) and lessen the amount of stridency. Anything that an individual can do to lower the larynx, decrease pharyngeal constriction, and promote general throat relaxation will usually reduce stridency. The following facilitating techniques (described in Chapter 7) are most helpful in greatly reducing stridency:

1. *Inhalation phonation.* This tends to increase the size of the pharynx, relax the walls of the pharynx, and open the laryngeal aditus.

2. *Auditory feedback.* Explore various vocal productions with the patient with the goal of producing a nonstrident voice. When the patient is able to produce good oral resonance, contrast this production with recorded strident vocalizations using loop tape feedback devices and following the various ear-training procedures. The Facilitator can be helpful here.

3. *Establishing new pitch.* The strident voice is frequently accompanied by an inappropriately high voice pitch. Efforts to lower the pitch level often produce a voice that sounds less strident. We have found that a piano keyboard or an inexpensive electric keyboard or the CSL and even the Facilitator are valuable tools in helping patients find and establish a new pitch level or range that produces a much less strident-sounding voice.

4. *Counseling.* Although it is difficult to explain problems of resonance to someone else, sometimes such an explanation is essential if the patient is ever to develop any kind of self-awareness about the problem.

5. *Glottal fry.* The glottal fry produces two beneficial effects. First, the fundamental frequency is somewhat lower following production of the glottal fry; second, the resonating cavity of the laryngeal aditus is enlarged following the production of the glottal fry (especially on ingressive glottal fry). The relaxation of the folds and the opening of the laryngeal aditus effectively reduce strident vocal quality.

6. *Hierarchy analysis.* For the individual whose voice becomes strident whenever he or she is tense, it is important to try to isolate those situations in which his or her nonstridency is maintained.

7. *Open mouth.* Because stridency is generally the product of overconstriction, oral openness is an excellent way to counteract these tight, constrictive tendencies.

8. *Relaxation.* It is difficult to produce strident resonance under conditions of relaxation and freedom from tension. Either general relaxation or a more specific relaxation of the vocal tract is helpful in reducing oral–pharyngeal tightness.

9. *Tongue protrusion /i/.* This increases the length and width of the pharynx (the whole throat cavity).

10. *Yawn–sigh.* Because the yawn–sigh approach produces an openness and relaxation completely opposite to the tightness of pharyngeal constriction, it is perhaps the most effective approach in this list for reducing stridency.

Improving Oral Resonance. Two problems of oral resonance are related to faulty tongue position, a *thin type* of resonance produced by excessively anterior tongue carriage and a *cul-de-sac-type* produced by posterior retraction of the tongue. The thin voice lacks adequate oral resonance, and its user sounds immature and unsure of himself or herself. This problem, which is somewhat common among both men and women, is characterized by a generalized oral constriction with high, anterior carriage of the tongue and only minimal lip–mandibular opening. The user of such a voice appears to be holding back psychologically, either withdrawing from interpersonal contact by demonstrating all the symptoms of withdrawal, or retreating psychologically to a more infantile level of behavior by demonstrating a "babylike" vocal quality. The first type, who withdraws from interpersonal contact, employs his or her thin resonance situationally, particularly when he or she feels most insecure; the second type uses the thin voice, the "baby resonance," more intentionally, in situations in which he or she wants to appear cute, to "get his or her own way," and so on. The following facilitating approaches (described in Chapter 7) have been useful in promoting a more natural adult oral resonance:

1. *Change of loudness.* When the resonance problem is part of a general picture of psychological withdrawal in particular situations, efforts to increase voice loudness are appropriate for overall improvement of resonance.

2. *Digital manipulation.* This is especially helpful when the pitch of the voice is too high or the quality is breathy.

3. *Establishing new pitch.* The thin voice is perceived by listeners to be drastically lacking in authority. Frequently, the pitch is too high. Efforts to lower the voice pitch often have a positive effect on resonance.

4. *Focus.* In Chapter 7, we looked at tongue position and its influence on voice quality. The "babylike" voice may disappear with greater posterior tongue carriage.

5. *Glottal fry.* The larger pharyngeal adjustment produced by glottal fry is generally helpful to produce improved resonance.

6. *Hierarchy analysis.* Symptomatic voice therapy is based on the premise that it is often possible to isolate particular situations in which we function poorly, with maladaptive behavior, and other situations in which we function comparatively well. By isolating the various situations and their modes of behavior, we can often introduce more effective behavior into "bad" situations in place of the maladaptive behavior. For those individuals who use a thin voice in specific situations, particularly during moments of tension, hierarchy analysis may be a necessary preliminary step to eliminate the aberrant vocal quality.

7. *Open mouth.* The restrictive oral tendencies of a thin-voiced speaker may be effectively reduced by developing greater oral openness.

8. *Relaxation.* If the thin vocal quality is highly situational and the obvious result of tension, relaxation approaches may be helpful, particularly when used in combination with hierarchy analysis.

9. *Respiration training.* Sometimes direct work on increasing voice loudness requires some work increasing control of the airflow during expiration.

10. *Visual feedback.* Those patients whose anterior resonance focus is related to situational tensions may use feedback apparatuses to become aware of their varying states of tension. Feedback is best used with relaxation and hierarchy analysis.

11. *Yawn–sigh.* The yawn–sigh approach is an excellent way of developing a more relaxed, posterior tongue carriage.

Patients with a thin voice are often judged by listeners to be immature, young, or lacking in authority. We have provided successful voice therapy to several attorneys, managers, and executives who suffered from thin voice quality, which was ineffective in their work. We helped one attorney improve his voice and his performance in the courtroom and during client conferences by using the open-mouth and glottal fry techniques.

The cul-de-sac voice is found in individuals from various etiologic groups: patients with oral apraxia; cerebral palsied children, particularly the athetoid type, who have a posterior focus to their resonance added to their dysarthria; some patients with bulbar or pseudobulbar-type lesions, who have a pharyngeal focus to their vocal resonance; and deaf children. The cul-de-sac voice, regardless of its initial physical cause, is produced by the deep retraction of the tongue into the oral cavity and hypopharynx, sometimes touching the pharyngeal wall and sometimes not. The body of the tongue literally obstructs the escaping airflow and the periodic sound waves generated from the larynx below. Although such a voice is often found in individuals with neural lesions who cannot control their muscles, and among deaf children and adults, it is also produced situationally by certain individuals for wholly functional reasons. Such posterior resonance is very difficult to correct in patients who have muscle disorders related to various problems of innervation, particularly dysarthric patients. Resonance deviations in the deaf may be changed somewhat in voice therapy, as described in Chapter 8, by dealing with special problems. For individuals who produce cul-de-sac resonance for purely functional reasons (whatever they are), the following facilitating approaches from Chapter 7 are useful:

1. *Auditory feedback.* If, in the search for a better voice, the patient is able to produce a more forward, oral-sounding one, this should be contrasted with his or her cul-de-sac voice by listening to auditory feedback.

2. *Focus.* The forward focus in resonance required to place the voice in the facial mask makes the approach a useful one for patients with a cul-de-sac focus. High front vowels and front-of-the-mouth consonants are particularly good practice sounds to use with the place-the-voice approach.

3. *Glottal fry.* The production of the glottal fry opens the pharynx and the laryngeal aditus, thus enlarging the resonance cavity and adding to the openness of the whole vocal tract. The whole pharynx is relaxed, eliminating the cul-de-sac resonance.

4. *Hierarchy analysis.* If cul-de-sac resonance occurs only in particular situations, perhaps at those times when the individual is tense and under stress, the hierarchy

approach may be useful. If the individual can produce good oral resonance in low-stress situations, he or she should practice using the same resonance at levels of increasing stress, on up the hierarchy.

5. *Nasal/glide stimulation.* This helps to get a forward placement of the tongue and the sound and can be used in conjunction with focus.

6. *Relaxation.* Posterior tongue retraction during moments of stress is often a learned response to tension. The patient who can learn a more relaxed positioning of the overall vocal tract may be able to reduce excessive tongue retraction.

7. *Tongue protrusion /i/.* Because the tongue is extended outside of the mouth and the pitch is elevated, the base of the tongue is pulled forward and out of the oral pharynx, and this is emphasized with the /i/ vowel. This eliminates the retracted tongue position that produces the back quality.

8. *Visual feedback.* Posterior focus of voice resonance may for some patients be situationally related to tension. Feedback is often useful for helping these patients monitor their varying tension states.

SUMMARY

Resonance deviations of the voice are often produced by physical problems of structure or function at various sites within the upper airway. Primary efforts must be given to identifying any structural abnormalities and correcting these problems by dental, medical, or surgical intervention. Speech–language pathologists play an important role in the early evaluation and diagnosis of a resonance problem, as well as in providing needed voice therapy to correct the problem. For both organic and functional resonance problems, specific facilitating approaches are listed to help patients develop better nasal and oral resonance.

Thought Questions

1. Describe the differences between hyper-, hypo-, and assimilative nasality. Why do you think that these resonance disturbances might be considered as "nasal" by a nontrained listener?
2. What are two clinical probes that can be used to assess hypernasality? Explain physiologically what is occurring during these probes.
3. Why is stimulability testing so important?
4. Explain what can be determined regarding velopharyngeal function during an oral examination.
5. Describe the various instrumental assessments of velopharyngeal function. Cite their advantages and disadvantages.
6. What testing can differentiate between hyper- and hyponasality?
7. Why is yawn–sigh effective for reducing stridency?

REFERENCES

Abdel-Aziz, M. (2008). Palatopharyngeal sling: A new technique in treatment of velopharyngeal insufficiency. *International Journal of Pediatric Otorhinolaryngology, 72,* 173–177.

Abitbol, J., Abitbol, R., & Abitbol, B. (1999). Sex hormones and the female voice. *Journal of Voice, 13,* 3.

Adler, R. K., Hirsch, S., & Mordaunt, M. (Eds). (2006). *Voice and communication therapy for the transgender/transsexual client.* San Diego, CA: Plural Publishing.

Agency for Healthcare Research and Quality. (2002). Criteria for determining disability in speech-language disorders. *Evidence Report/Technology Assessment, 52.*

Ahlstrom, R. H. (1984). Speech pathology: Views from medicine and dentistry. In S. C. McFarlane (Ed.), *Coping with communicative handicaps.* San Diego, CA: College Hill Press.

Akerlund, L., Gramming, P., & Sundberg, J. (1992). Phonetogram and averages of sound pressure levels and fundamental frequencies of speech: Comparison between female singers and nonsingers. *Journal of Voice, 6,* 55–63.

Alliance for Gender Awareness. (2008). *1st national Transgiving.* Bloomsbury, NJ: Author.

Altman, K. W., Atkinson, C., & Lazarus, C. (2005). Current and emerging concepts in muscle tension dysphonia: A 30-month review. *Journal of Voice, 19,* 261–267.

Altman, K. W., Mirza, N., Ruiz, C., & Sataloff, R. T. (2000). Paradoxical vocal fold motion: Presentation and treatment options. *Journal of Voice, 14,* 99–103.

American Joint Committee for Cancer Staging and End-Results Reporting. (1998). *Manual for stages of cancer* (2nd ed.). Philadelphia: Lippincott.

American Psychiatric Association (APA). (1987). Briquet's syndrome. In *Diagnostic and statistical manual of mental disorders* (3rd ed., pp. 261–264). Washington, DC: Author.

American Speech-Language-Hearing Association. (1991). Amplification as a remediation technique for children with normal peripheral hearing. *ASHA, 33,* 22–24.

American Speech-Language-Hearing Association. (1998a). *The roles of otolaryngologists and speech-language pathologists in the performance and interpretation of strobovideolaryngoscopy* [Paper]. Rockville, MD: Author. Available from www.asha.org/policy.

American Speech-Language-Hearing Association. (1998b). *Training guidelines for laryngeal videoendoscopy/stroboscopy* [Guidelines]. Rockville, MD: Author. Available from www.asha.org/policy.

American Speech-Language-Hearing Association. (2004a). Evaluation and treatment for tracheoesophageal puncture and prosthesis: Technical report. *ASHA (Supplement 24).*

American Speech-Language-Hearing Association. (2004b). Knowledge and skills for speech language pathologists with respect to vocal tract visualization and imaging. *ASHA (Supplement 24).*

American Speech-Language-Hearing Association. (2004c). *Knowledge and skills for speech-language pathologists with respect to vocal tract visualization and imaging* [Knowledge and Skills]. Rockville, MD: Author. Available from www.asha.org/policy.

American Speech-Language-Hearing Association. (2004d). *Preferred practice patterns for the profession of speech-language pathology* [Preferred Practice Patterns]. Rockville, MD: Author. Available from www.asha.org/policy.

American Speech-Language-Hearing Association. (2004e). *Vocal tract visualization and imaging* [Position Statement]. Rockville, MD: Author. Available from www.asha.org/policy.

American Speech-Language-Hearing Association. (2004f). *Vocal tract visualization and imaging* [Technical Report]. Rockville, MD: Author. Available from www.asha.org/policy.

American Speech-Language-Hearing Association. (2007). *Scope of practice in speech-language pathology* [Scope of Practice]. Rockville, MD: Author. Available from www.asha.org/policy.

American Speech-Language-Hearing Association, National Association of Teachers of Singing, & Voice and Speech Trainers Association. (2005). The role of the speech-language pathologist, the teacher of singing, and the speaking voice trainer in voice habilitation. *ASHA/NATS/VASTA Joint Statement.* Rockville, MD: ASHA.

Amir, O., Biron-Shental, T., & Shabtai, E. (2006). Birth control pills and nonprofessional voice: Acoustic analyses. *Journal of Speech, Language, and Hearing Research, 49*(5), 1114–1126.

Anders, L., Hollien, H., Hurme, P., Soninen, A., & Wendler, J. (1988). Perception of hoarseness by several classes of listeners. *Folia Phoniatrica et Logopaedica, 40,* 91–100.

Andreassen, M. L., Leeper, H. A., MacRae, D. L., & Nicholson, I. R. (1994). Aerodynamic, acoustic, and perceptual changes following adenoidectomy. *Cleft Palate-Craniofacial Journal, 31,* 261–270.

Andreassen, M., Smith, B., & Guyette, T. (1992). Pressure-flow 6 measurements for selected oral and nasal sound segments produced by normal adults. *Cleft Palate Journal, 29*(1), 1–9.

Andrews, M. L. (1995). *Manual of voice treatment: Pediatrics through geriatrics.* San Diego, CA: Singular.

Andrews, M. L., with Summers, A. C. (2002). *Voice treatment for children and adolescents.* San Diego, CA: Singular.

Andrus, J., & Shapshay, S. (2006). Contemporary management of laryngeal papilloma in adults and children. *Otolaryngologic Clinics of North America, 39*(1), 135–158.

Anvari, M., & Allen, C. (2003). Surgical outcome in gastroesophageal reflux disease patients with inadequate response to proton pump inhibitors. *Surgical Endoscopy, 17,* 1029–1035.

Armour, A., Fischbach, S., Klaiman, P., & Fisher, D. (2005). Does velopharyngeal closure pattern affect the success of pharyngeal flap pharyngoplasty? *Plastic & Reconstructive Surgery, 115,* 45–52.

Armstrong, S., & Schumann, L. (2003). Myasthenia gravis: Diagnosis and treatment. *Journal of the American Academy of Nurse Practitioners, 15*(2), 72–78.

Arndt, W. B., Shelton, R. L., & Bradford, L. J. (1965). Articulation, voice, and obturation in persons with acquired and congenital palate defects. *Cleft Palate Journal, 2,* 377–383.

Arnold, G. E. (1962). Vocal rehabilitation of paralytic dysphonia. *Archives of Otolaryngology, 76,* 358–368.

Aronson, A. E. (1985). *Clinical voice disorders* (2nd ed.). New York: Thieme-Stratton.

Aronson, A. E. (1990). *Clinical voice disorders: An interdisciplinary approach* (3rd ed.). New York: Thieme-Stratton.

Aronson, A. E., & DeSanto, L. W. (1983). Adductor spastic dysphonia: Three years after recurrent laryngeal nerve resection. *Annals of Otolaryngology, Rhinology, and Laryngology, 93,* 1–8.

Arvedson, J. C. (2002). Gastroesophageal/extra-esophageal reflux and voice disorders in children. *ASHA Division 3, Perspectives on Voice and Voice Disorders, 12*(1), 17–19.

Awan, S. N. (1991). Phonetographic profiles and Fo-SLP characteristics of untrained versus trained vocal groups. *Journal of Voice, 5,* 41–50.

Awan, S. N., (2001). *The voice diagnostic protocol: A practical guide to the diagnosis of voice disorders.* Gaithersburg, MD: Aspen.

Awan, S. N. (2006). The aging female voice: Acoustic and respiratory data. *Clinical Linguistics & Phonetics, 20,* 171–180.

Awan, S. N., & Frenkel, M. L. (1994). Improvements in estimating the harmonics-to-noise ratio of the voice. *Journal of Voice, 8,* 255–262.

Baken, R. J. (1996). *Clinical measurement of speech and voice.* Boston: College Hill Press.

Baken, R. J. (2005). The aged voice: A new hypothesis. *Journal of Voice, 19*(3), 317–325.

Baken, R. J., & Orlikoff, R. F. (1988). Changes in vocal fundamental frequency at the segmental level. *Journal of Speech and Hearing Research, 31,* 207–211.

Baker, J., Ben-Tovim, D. I., Butcher, A., Esterman, A., & McLaughlin, K. (2007). Development of a modified diagnostic classification system for voice disorders with inter-rater reliability study. *Logopedics Phoniatrics Vocology, 32,* 99–112.

Baker, S., Sapienza, C. M., & Collins, S. (2003). Inspiratory pressure threshold training in a case of congenital bilateral abductor vocal fold paralysis. *International Journal of Pediatric Otorhinolaryngology, 67,* 414–416.

Balestrieri, F., & Watson, C. B. (1982). Intubation granuloma. *Otolaryngologic Clinics of North America, 15*(3), 567–579.

Barkmeier, J. M., & Case, J. L. (2000). Differential diagnosis of adductor-type spasmodic dysphonia, vocal tremor, and muscle tension dysphonia. *Current Opinion in Otolaryngology & Head and Neck Surgery, 8,* 174–179.

Barkmeier, J. M., Case, J. L., & Ludlow, C. L. (2001). Identification of symptoms for spasmodic dysphonia and vocal tremor: A comparison of expert and non-expert judges. *Journal of Communication Disorders, 34*(102), 21–37.

Barry, H. C., & Eathorne, S. W. (1994). Exercise and aging: Issues for the practitioner. *Medical Clinics of North America, 78,* 357–376.

Bassich, C. J., & Ludlow, C. L. (1986). The use of perceptual methods by new clinicians for assessing voice quality. *Journal of Speech and Hearing Disorders, 51*, 125–133.

Beaver, M. E., Stasney, C. R., Weitzel, E., Stewert, M. G., Donovan, D. T., Parke, R. B., & Rodriguez, M. (2003). Diagnosis of laryngopharyngeal reflux disease with digital imaging. *Otolaryngology-Head and Neck Surgery, 128*(1), 103–108.

Behrman, A. (2005). Common practices of voice therapists in the evaluation of patients. *Journal of Voice, 19*, 454–469.

Behrman, A. (2006). Facilitating behavioral change in voice therapy: The relevance of motivational interviewing. *American Journal of Speech-Language Pathology, 15*, 215–225.

Behrman, A. (2007). *Speech and voice science.* San Diego, CA: Plural Publishing.

Behrman, A., Agresti, C., Blumstein, E., & Sharma, G. (1996). Meaningful features of voice range profiles from patients with organic vocal fold pathology: A preliminary study. *Journal of Voice, 10*, 269–283.

Behrman, A., Dahl, L. D., Abramson, A. L., & Schutte, H. K. (2003). Anterior-posterior and medial compression of the supraglottis: Signs of nonorganic dysphonia or normal postures? *Journal of Voice, 17*, 403–410.

Belafsky, P. C., Postma, G. N., & Koufman, J. A. (2002a). The association between laryngeal pseudosulcus and laryngopharyngeal reflux. *Otolaryngology-Head and Neck Surgery, 126*(6), 649–652.

Belafsky, P. C., Postma, G. N., & Koufman, J. A. (2002b). Quality and reliability of the reflux symptom index (RSI). *Journal of Voice, 16*, 274–277.

Bele, I. V. (2005). Reliability in perceptual analysis of voice quality. *Journal of Voice, 19*, 555–573.

Benito-Leon, J., Bermejo-Pareja, F., & Louis, E. D. (2005). Incidence of essential tremor in three elderly populations of central Spain. *Neurology, 64*(10), 1721–1725.

Benjamin, B. (1997). Speech production of normally aging adults. *Seminars in Speech and Language, 18*, 135–141.

Bennett, S., & Netsell, R. W. (1999). Possible roles of the insula in speech and language processing: Directions for research. *Journal of Medical Speech-Language Pathology, 7*(4), 255–272.

Benninger, M. S. (2000). Microdissection or microspot CO_2 laser for limited vocal fold benign lesions: A predictive randomized trial. *Laryngoscope, 110*, 1–17.

Benninger, M. S., & Jacobson, B. (1995). Vocal nodules, microwebs, and surgery. *Journal of Voice, 9*(3), 326–331.

Berg, E., Hapner, E., Klein, A., & Johns, M. (2008). Voice therapy improves quality of life in age-related dysphonia: A case-control study. *Journal of Voice, 22*, 70–74.

Berke, G. S., Blackwell, K. E., Gerratt, B. R., Verneil, A., Jackson, K. S., & Sercarz, J. A. (1999). Selective laryngeal adductor denervation-renervation: A new surgical treatment for adductor spasmodic dysphonia. *Annals of Otology, Rhinology, and Laryngology, 108*, 3.

Berkow, R., Beers, M. H., & Fletcher, A. J. (1997). *Merck manual.* West Point, PA: Merck & Co.

Bernsen, R. A., de Jager, A. E., Schmitz, P. I., & van der Meche, F. G. (2002). Long-term impact on work and private life after Guillain-Barré syndrome. *Journal of Neurology Science, 201*(1–2), 13–17.

Berry, W. R. (1983). *Clinical dysarthria.* San Diego, CA: College Hill Press.

Beukelman, D. R., & Mirenda, P. (2005). *Augmentative and alternative communication: Supporting children & adults with complex communication needs* (3rd ed.). Baltimore: Paul H. Brookes.

Bhatia, M. S., & Vaid, L. (2000). Hysterical aphonia—An analysis of 25 cases. *Indian Journal of Medical Sciences, 54*(8), 335–338.

Bhattacharyya, N., Kotz, T., & Shapiro, J. (2002). Dysphagia and aspiration with unilateral vocal cord immobility: Incidence, characterization, and response with surgical treatment. *Annals of Otolaryngology, Rhinology, and Laryngology, 111*(8), 672–679.

Bickley, C. A., & Stevens, K. N. (1987). Effects of vocal tract constriction of the glottal source: Data from voiced consonants. In T. Baer, C. Sasaki, & K. Harris (Eds.), *Laryngeal functioning phonation and respiration.* Boston: Little, Brown.

Birchall, M., & Macchiarini, P. (2008). Airway transplantation: A debate worth having? *Transplantation, 85*(8), 1075–1080.

Blager, F. B. (1995). Treatment of paradoxical vocal cord dysfunction. *Voice and Voice Disorders, 5*, 8–11.

Blager, F. B. (2006). Vocal cord dysfunction. *ASHA Special Interest Division 3, Perspectives on Voice and Voice Disorders, 16*(1), 7–9.

Blakeley, R. W. (1991). Voice assessment without instrumentation. *Seminars in Speech and Language, 12*, 142–153.

Blakiston, J. (1985). *Blakiston's Gould medical dictionary.* New York: McGraw-Hill.

Bless, D., & Baken, R. (1992). International Association of Logopedics and Phoniatrics (IALP) Voice

Committee Discussion of Assessment topics. *Journal of Voice, 6,* 194–210.

Blitzer, A., & Brin, M. F. (1991). Laryngeal dystonia: A series with botulinum toxin therapy. *Annals of Otolaryngology, Rhinology, and Laryngology, 100,* 85–90.

Blitzer, A., Brin, M. F., Fahn, S., & Lovelace, R. E. (1988). Localized injections of botulinum toxin for the treatment of vocal laryngeal dystonia (spastic dysphonia). *Laryngoscope, 98,* 195–197.

Bloch, I., & Behrman, A. (2001). Quantitative analysis of videostroboscopic images in presbylarynges. *Laryngoscope, 111,* 2022–2027.

Blom, E. D. (1995). Tracheoesophageal speech. *Seminars in Speech & Language, 12,* 191–204.

Blom, E. D., & Singer, M. I. (1979). Surgical prosthetic approaches for postlaryngectomy voice restoration. In R. L. Keith & F. L. Darley (Eds.), *Laryngectomee rehabilitation.* Houston, TX: College Hill Press.

Blom, E. D., Singer, M. I., & Hamaker, R. D. (1998). *Tracheoesophageal voice restoration following total laryngectomy.* San Diego, CA: Singular.

Blonigen, J. (1994). *Remediation of vocal hoarseness.* Austin, TX: Pro-Ed.

Blood, G. W., & Hyman, M. (1977). Children's perceptions of nasal resonance. *Journal of Speech and Hearing Disorders, 42,* 446–448.

Blood, G. W., Luther, A. R., & Stemple, J. C. (1992). Coping and adjustment in alaryngeal speakers. *American Journal of Speech-Language Pathology, 1,* 63–69.

Blood, G. W., Mahan, B. W., & Hyman, M. (1979). Judging personality and appearance from voice disorders. *Journal of Communication Disorders, 12,* 63–68.

Bogaardt, H. C., Hakkesteegt, M. M., Grolman, W., & Lindeboom, R. (2007). Validation of the Voice Handicap Index using Rasch analysis. *Journal of Voice, 21,* 337–344.

Bogardus, S. T., Yueh, B., & Shekelle, P. G. (2003). Screening and management of adult hearing loss in primary care: Clinical applications. *Journal of the American Medical Association, 289*(15), 1986–1990.

Bohnenkamp, T. (2008). The effects of a total laryngectomy on speech breathing. *Current Opinion in Otolaryngology & Head and Neck Surgery, 16*(3), 200–204.

Boone, D. R. (1966a). Modification of the voices of deaf children. *Volta Review, 68,* 686–692.

Boone, D. R. (1966b). Treatment of functional aphonia in a child and an adult. *Journal of Speech and Hearing Disorders, 31,* 69–74.

Boone, D. R. (1974). Dismissal criteria in voice therapy. *Journal of Speech and Hearing Disorders, 39,* 133–139.

Boone, D. R. (1982). *The Boone voice program for adults.* Austin, TX: Pro-Ed.

Boone, D. R. (1983). *The voice and voice therapy* (3rd ed.). Englewood Cliffs, NJ: Prentice Hall.

Boone, D. R. (1993). *The Boone voice program for children* (2nd ed.). Austin, TX: Pro-Ed.

Boone, D. R. (1997). *Is your voice telling on you?* (2nd ed.). San Diego, CA: Singular.

Boone, D. R. (1998). *Facilitator application manual.* Lincoln Park, NJ: Kay Elemetrics.

Boone, D. R., & McFarlane, S. C. (1993). A critical study of the yawn-sigh technique. *Journal of Voice, 7,* 75–80.

Boone, D. R., & McFarlane, S. C. (1994). *The voice and voice therapy* (5th ed.). Englewood Cliffs, NJ: Prentice Hall.

Boone, D. R., McFarlane, S. C., & Von Berg, S. L. (2005). *The voice and voice therapy* (7th ed.). Boston: Allyn & Bacon.

Boone, D. R., & Plante, E. (1993). *Human communication and its disorders* (2nd ed.). Englewood Cliffs, NJ: Prentice Hall.

Boone, D. R., & Wiley, K. D. (2000). *The Boone voice program for adults* (2nd ed.). Austin, TX: Pro-Ed.

Boonin, J. (2006). Rate and volume. In R. K. Adler, S. Hirsch, & M. Mordaunt (Eds.), *Voice and communication therapy for the transgender/transsexual client.* San Diego, CA: Plural Publishing.

Borden, G. J., Harris, K. S., & Raphael, L. J. (1994). *Speech science primer: Physiology, acoustics, and perception of speech* (4th ed.). Baltimore: Lippincott.

Boseley, M. E., Cunningham, M. J., Volk, M. S., & Hartnick, C. J. (2006). Validation of the Pediatric Voice-Related Quality-of-Life Survey. *Archives of Otolaryngology-Head and Neck Surgery, 132,* 717–720.

Bosone, Z. T. (1994). Tracheoesophageal fistulization/puncture for voice restoration: Presurgical considerations and troubleshooting procedures. In R. L. Keith & F. L. Darley (Eds.), *Laryngectomee rehabilitation.* Austin, TX: Pro-Ed.

Bouchayer, M., & Cornut, G. (1991). Instrumental microscopy of benign lesions of the vocal folds. In C. N. Ford & D. M. Bless (Eds.), *Phonosurgery: Assessment and surgical management of voice disorders* (pp. 143–165). New York: Raven Press.

Bovo, R., Galceran, M., Petruccelli, J., & Hatzopoulos, S. (2007). Vocal problems among teachers: Evaluation of a preventive voice program. *Journal of Voice, 21,* 705–722.

Bowers, M., Adler, R. K, Hirsch, S., & Mordaunt, M. (2006). Endocrinology: Questions and answers. In R. K. Adler, S. Hirsch, & M. Mordaunt (Eds.), *Voice and communication therapy for the transgender/transsexual client* (pp. 91–100). San Diego, CA: Plural Publishing.

Boyden, K. M. (2000). The pathophysiology of demyelination and the ionic basis of nerve conduction in multiple sclerosis: An overview. *Journal of Neuroscience Nursing, 32,* 49–58.

Boyle, B. (2000). Voice disorders in school children. *Support for Learning, 15,* 71–75.

Bradford, L. I., Brooks, A. R., & Shelton, R. L. (1964). Clinical judgment of hypernasality in cleft palate children. *Cleft Palate Journal, 1,* 329–335.

Bressman, T. (2005). Comparison of nasalance scores obtained with the Nasometer, the NasalView, and the OroNasal System. *Cleft Palate-Craniofacial Journal, 42,* 423–433.

Broaddus-Lawrence, P. L., Treole, K., McCabe, R. B., Allen, R. L., & Toppin, L. (2000). The effects of preventive vocal hygiene education on the vocal hygiene habits and perceptual characteristics of training singers. *Journal of Voice, 14,* 58–71.

Brodnitz, F. S. (1971). *Vocal rehabilitation.* Rochester, MN: Whiting Press.

Brodnitz, F. S., & Froeschels, E. (1954). Treatment of nodules of vocal cords by the chewing method. *Archives of Otolaryngology, 59,* 560–566.

Brookshire, R. H. (2007). *Introduction to neurogenic communication disorders* (7th ed.). St. Louis, MO: Mosby.

Broomfield, J., & Dodd, B. (2004). Children with speech and language disability: Caseload characteristics. *International Journal of Language and Communication Disorders, 39,* 303–325.

Brown, O. L. (1996). *Discover your voice.* San Diego, CA: Singular.

Brown, W., Morris, R., Hollien, H., & Howell, E. (1991). Speaking fundamental frequency characteristics as a function of age and professional singing. *Journal of Voice, 5,* 310–315.

Brown, W. S., Vinson, B. P., & Crary, M. A. (1996). *Organic voice disorders: Assessment and treatment.* San Diego, CA: Singular.

Buller, A. (1942). Nasality: Cause and remedy of our American blight. *Quarterly Journal of Speech, 28,* 83–84.

Butler, C., & Darrah, J. (2001). Effects of a neurodevelopment treatment (NDT) for cerebral palsy: An AACPDM evidence report. *Developmental Medicine and Child Neurology, 43,* 778–790.

Bzoch, K. R. (1989). *Communicative disorders related to cleft lip and palate* (3rd ed.). Austin, TX: Pro-Ed.

Cady, J. (2002). Laryngectomy: Beyond loss of voice—caring for the patient as a whole. *Clinical Journal of Oncology Nursing, 6,* 1–5.

Carding, P., Carlson, E., Epstein, R., Mathieson, L., & Shewell, C. (2000). Formal perceptual evaluation of voice quality in the United Kingdom. *Logopedics Phoniatrics Vocology, 25,* 133–138.

Carding, P. N., Horsley, I. A., & Docherty, G. J. (1999). A study of the effectiveness of voice therapy in the treatment of 45 patients with nonorganic dysphonia. *Journal of Voice, 13,* 72–104.

Carmines, E. G., & Zeller, R. A. (1979). Reliability and validity assessment. In M. S. Lewis-Beck (Ed.), *Quantitative applications in the social science* (pp. 9–27). Thousand Oaks, CA: Sage Publications.

Caruso, A. J., & Mueller, P. B. (1997). Age-related changes in speech, voice and swallowing. In B. B. Shaden & M. A. Toner (Eds.), *Aging and communication: For clinicians, by clinicians* (pp. 117–134). Austin, TX: Pro-Ed.

Case, J. L. (2002). *Clinical management of voice disorders* (4th ed.). Austin, TX: Pro-Ed.

Casper, J. (2000). Confidential voice. In J. C. Stemple (Ed.), *Voice therapy: Clinical studies* (2nd ed.). San Diego, CA: Singular.

Chan, K. M. K., & Yiu, E. M. L. (2002). The effect of anchors and training on the reliability of perceptual voice evaluation. *Journal of Speech, Language, and Hearing Research, 45,* 111–126.

Chan, K. M. K., & Yiu, E. M. L. (2006). A comparison of two perceptual voice evaluation training programs for naive listeners. *Journal of Voice, 20,* 229–241.

Chapey, R. (2001). *Language intervention strategies in aphasia and related neurogenic communication disorders* (4th ed.). Philadelphia: Lippincott.

Chen, Y., Robb, M. P., & Gilbert, H. R. (2002). Electroglottographic evaluation of gender and vowel effects during modal and vocal fry phonation. *Journal of Speech, Language, and Hearing Research, 45,* 821–829.

Cheyne, H. A., Hanson, H. M., Genereaux, R. P., Stevens, K. N., & Hillman, R. E. (2003). *Journal of Speech, Language, and Hearing Research, 46,* 1457–1467.

Chhetri, D. K., Blumin, J. H., Vinters, H. V., & Berke, G. S. (2003). Histology of nerves and muscles in adductor spasmodic dysphonia. *Annals of Otology, Rhinology, and Laryngology, 112*(4), 334–341.

Chodzko-Zajko, W. J. (1997). Normal aging and human physiology. *Seminars in Speech and Language, 18*(2), 95–106.

Clements, K. S., Rassekh, C. H., Seikaly, H., Hokanson, J. A., & Calhoun, K. H. (1997). Communication after laryngectomy: An assessment of patient satisfaction. *Archives of Otolaryngology Head and Neck Surgery, 123*(5), 493–496.

Cleveland, T. F. (1994). A clearer view of singing voice production: 25 years of progress. *Journal of Voice, 8,* 18–23.

Coffin, B. (1981). *Overtones of Bel Canto.* Metuchen, NJ: Scarecrow.

Cohen, S. M., Dupont, W. D., & Courey, M. S. (2006). Quality of life impact of non-neoplastic voice disorders: A meta-analysis. *Annals of Otology, Rhinology, and Laryngology, 115,* 128–134.

Cohen, S. M., & Garrett, C. G. (2007). Utility in voice therapy management of vocal fold polyps and cysts. *Otolarynology Head and Neck Surgery, 136,* 742–746.

Cohen, S. M., Jacobson, B. H., & Garrett, C. G. (2007). Creation and validation of the Singing Voice Handicap Index. *Annals of Otology, Rhinology, & Laryngology, 116,* 402–406.

Cohen, S. M., Jacobson, B. H., Garrett, C. G., Nordzij, J. P., Stewart, M. G., Attia, A., et al. (2007). Creation and validation of the Singing Voice Handicap Index. *Annals of Otology, Rhinology & Laryngology 116,* 402–406.

Coletti, R. B., Christei, D. L., & Orenstein, S. R. (1995). Indications for pediatric esophageal pH monitoring. *Pediatric Gastroenterology Nutrition, 21,* 253–262.

Colton, R. H., & Casper, J. K. (1996). *Understanding voice problems: A physiological perspective for diagnosis and treatment* (2nd ed.). Baltimore: Lippincott.

Colton, R. H., Casper, J. K., & Leonard, R. (2006). *Understanding voice problems: A physiological perspective for diagnosis and treatment* (3rd ed.). Baltimore: Lippincott.

Congdon, N. G., Friedman, D. S., & Lietman, T. (2004). Important causes of visual impairment in the world today. *Journal of the American Medical Association, 290,* 2057–2060.

Connor, N., Cohen, S., Theis, S., Thibeault, S., Heatley, D., & Bless, D. (2008). Attitudes of children with dysphonia. *Journal of Voice, 22,* 197–209.

Consensus Auditory-Perceptual Evaluation of Voice (CAPE-V). Retrieved March 2008 from www .professional.asha.org/resources/divs/div_3.cfm.

Cooper, M. (1990). *Winning with your voice.* Hollywood, FL: Fell.

Costa, H. O., & Matias, C. (2005). Vocal impact on quality of life of elderly female subjects. *Revista Brasileira Otorrinolaringologia, 71,* 172–178.

Cotton, R. T., Gray, S. D., & Miller, R. P. (1989). Update of the Cincinnati experience in pediatric laryngotracheal reconstruction. *Laryngoscope, 99*(11), 1111–1116.

Courey, M. S., Garrett, C. G., & Ossoff, R. H. (1997). Medial microflap for excision of benign vocal fold lesions. *Laryngoscope, 107,* 340–344.

Courey, M. S., Shohet, J. A., Scott, M. A., & Ossoff, R. H. (1996). Immunohistochemical characterization of benign laryngeal lesions. *Annals of Otology, Rhinology, and Laryngology, 105,* 525–531.

Crumley, R. L., & Izdebski, K. (1986). Voice quality following laryngeal reinnervation by ansa hypoglossi transfer. *Laryngoscope, 96,* 611–616.

Culton, G. L., & Gerwin, J. M. (1998). Current trends in laryngectomy rehabilitation: A survey of speech-language pathologists. *Otolaryngology Head and Neck Surgery, 118*(4), 458–463.

Daniloff, R. G. (1985). *Speech science.* San Diego, CA: College Hill Press.

Darley, F. L., Aronson, A. E., & Brown, J. R. (1975). *Motor-speech disorders.* Philadelphia: Saunders.

Davis, A., Stephens, D., Rayment, A., & Thomas, K. (1997). Hearing impairments in middle age: The acceptability, benefit and cost of detection (ABCD). *British Journal of Audiology, 26,* 1–14.

Davis, C. N., & Harris, T. B. (1992). Teachers' ability to accurately identify disordered voices. *Language, Speech, and Hearing Services in Schools, 23,* 136–140.

Davis, P. J., Boone, D. R., Carroll, R. L., Darveniza, F., & Harrison, G. A. (1988). Adductor spastic dysphonia: Heterogeneity of physiological and phonatory characteristics. *Archives of Otolaryngology, 97,* 179–185.

Davis, P. J., Zhang, S. P., Winkworth, A., & Bandler, R. (1996). Neural control of vocalization: Respiratory and emotional influences. *Journal of Voice, 10*(1), 23–38.

Dean, C. M., Ahmarani, C., Bettez, M., & Heuer, R. J. (2001). The adjustable laryngeal implant. *Journal of Voice, 15*(1), 141–150.

Deary, I. J., Wilson, J. A., Carding, P. N., & MacKenzie, K. (2003). VoiSS: A patient-derived voice symptom scale. *Journal of Psychosomatic Research, 54,* 483–489.

De Bodt, M. S., Ketelslagers, K., Peeters, T., Wuyts, F., Mertens, F., Pattyn, J., et al. (2007). Evolution of vocal fold nodules from childhood to adolescence. *Journal of Voice, 21,* 151–156.

De Bodt, M. S., Wuyts, F. L., Van de Heyning, P. H., & Croux, C. (1997). Test-retest study of the GRBAS scale: Influence of experience and professional background on perceptual rating of voice quality. *Journal of Voice, 11,* 74–80.

De Bodt, M. S., Wuyts, F. L., Van de Heyning, P. H., & Lambrechts, L. (1996). The perceptual evaluation of voice disorders. *Acta Oto-Rhino-Laryngologica, 50,* 283–291.

Decoster, W., & Debruyne, F. (1997). The ageing voice: Changes in fundamental frequency, waveform stability and spectrum. *Acta Oto-Rhino-Laryngologica Belgium, 51,* 102–112.

Dedo, H. H. (1976). Recurrent laryngeal nerve section for spastic dysphonia. *Annals of Otology, Rhinology, and Laryngology, 85,* 451–459.

Dedo, H. H. (1997). *Comments at Tenth Annual Pacific Voice Conference,* San Francisco.

Dedo, H. H., & Izdebski, K. (1983). Intermediate results of 306 recurrent laryngeal nerve sections for spastic dysphonia. *Laryngoscope, 93,* 9–16.

Dedo, H. H., & Jackler, R. K. (1982). Laryngeal papilloma: Results of treatment with the CO_2 laser and podophyllum. *Annals of Otolaryngology, Rhinology, and Laryngology, 93,* 425–430.

DeJonckere, P. H., Obbens, C., de Moor, G. M., & Wieneke, G. H. (1993). Perceptual evaluation of dysphonia: Reliability and relevance. *Folia Phoniatrica et Logopaedica, 45,* 76–83.

DeJonckere, P. H., Remacle, M., Fresnel-Elbaz, E., Woisard, V., Crevier, L., & Millet, B. (1996). Differentiated perceptual evaluation of pathological voice quality: Reliability and correlations with acoustic measurements. *Revue Laryngologie Otologie Rhinologie, 117,* 219–224.

DeJonckere, P. H., Remacle, M., Fresnel-Elbaz, E., Woisard, V., Crevier, L., & Millet, B. (1998). Reliability and clinical relevance of perceptual evaluation of pathological voices. *Revue Laryngologie Otologie Rhinologie, 119,* 247–248.

DeJonckere, P. H., van Wijck, I., & Speyer, R. (2003). Efficacy of voice therapy assessed with the Voice Range Profile. *Revue Laryngologie Otologie Rhinologie, 124,* 285–289.

de Krom, G. (1995). Some spectral correlates of pathological breathy and rough voice quality for different types of vowel fragments. *Journal of Speech and Hearing Research, 38,* 794–811.

Denoyelle, F., Mondain, M., Gresillon, N., Roger, G., Chaudre, F., & Garabedian, E. N. (2003). Failures and complications of supraglottoplasty in children. *Archives of Otolaryngology-Head and Neck Surgery, 129*(10), 1077–1080.

Derkay, C. S. (2001). Recurrent respiratory papillomatosis. *Laryngoscope, 11,* 57–69.

de Swart, B. J., Willemse, S. C., Maassen, B. A., & Horstink, M. W. (2003). Improvement in voicing in patients with Parkinson's disease by speech therapy. *Neurology, 60*(3), 498–500.

Dickson, D. R. (1962). Acoustic study of nasality. *Journal of speech and Hearing Research, 5,* 103–111.

Diedrich, W. M., & Youngstrom, K. A. (1966). *Alaryngeal speech.* Springfield, IL: Charles C. Thomas.

Dietrich, M., Verdolini-Abbott, K., Gartner-Schmidt, J., & Rosen, C. A. (2008). The frequency of perceived stress, anxiety, and depression in patients with common pathologies affecting voice. *Journal of Voice 22*(4), 472–488. Retrieved April 7, 2008, from www.jvoice.org/inpress.

Djukanovíc, R., Homeyard, S., Gratziou, C., Madden, J., Walls, A., Montefort, S., et al. (1997). The effect of treatment with oral corticosteroids on asthma symptoms and airway inflammation. *American Journal of Respiratory Critical Care Medicine, 155,* 826–832.

Downie, A., Low, J. M., & Lindsay, D. D. (1981). Speech disorders in Parkinsonism: Usefulness of delayed auditory feedback in selected cases. *British Journal of Disorders of Communication, 16,* 135–139.

Doyle, P. C., Danhauer, J. L., & Reed, C. G. (1988). Listeners' perceptions of consonants produced by esophageal and tracheoesophageal talkers. *Journal of Speech and Hearing Disorders, 53,* 400–407.

Dronkers, N. F. (1996). A new brain region for coordinating speech articulation. *Nature, 384,* 159–161.

Dronkers, N. F., Redfern, B., & Shapiro, J. K. (1993). Neuroanatomic correlates of production deficits in severe Broca's aphasia. *Journal of Clinical Experimental Neuropsychology, 15,* (abstract), 59.

Duff, M. C., Proctor, A., & Yairi, E. (2004). Prevalence of voice disorders in African American and European American preschoolers. *Journal of Voice, 18,* 348–353.

Duffy, J. R. (2005). *Motor speech disorders: Substrates, differential diagnosis and management.* St. Louis, MO: Elsevier Mosby.

Duffy, J. R., & Folger, W. N. (1986). *Dysarthria in unilateral central nervous system lesions*. Paper presented at the annual convention of the American Speech-Language-Hearing Association, Detroit, MI.

Duffy, O. M., & Hazlett, D. E. (2004). The impact of preventive voice care programs for training teachers. *Journal of Voice, 18,* 63–70.

Dursun, G., Boynukalin, S., Bagis Ozgursoy, O., & Coruh, I. (2008). Long-term results of different treatment modalities for glottic insufficiency. *American Journal of Otolaryngology, 29*(1), 7–12.

Dursun, G., Ozgursoy, O. B., Kemal, O., & Coruh, I. (2007). One-year follow-up results of combined use of CO_2 laser and cold instrumentation for Reinke's edema surgery in professional voice users. *European Archives of Otorhinolaryngology, 264,* 1027–1032.

Dursun, G., Sataloff, R. T., Spiegel, J. R., Mandel, S., Heurer, R. J., & Rosen, D. C. (1996). Superior laryngeal nerve paresis and paralysis. *Journal of Voice, 10*(2), 206–211.

Dworkin, J. P. (2008). Laryngitis: Types, causes, and treatments. *Otolaryngologic Clinics of North America, 41,* 419–436.

Dworkin, J. P., & Culatta, R. A. (1996). *Dworkin-Culatta oral mechanism examination and treatment system*. Nicholasville, KY: Edgewood Press, Inc.

Dworkin, J. P., Marunick, M. T., & Krouse, J. H. (2004). Velopharyngeal dysfunction: Speech characteristics, variable etiologies, evaluation techniques and differential treatments. *Language, Speech, and Hearing in Schools, 35,* 333–352.

Dworkin, J. P., Meleca, R. J., & Abkarian, G. G. (2000). Muscle tension dysphonia. *Current Opinion in Otolaryngology & Head and Neck Surgery, 8,* 169–173.

Eadie, T. L. (2003). A proposed framework for comprehensive rehabilitation of individuals who use laryngeal speech. *American Journal of Speech Language Pathology, 12,* 189–197.

Eadie, T. L., & Baylor, C. R. (2006). The effect of perceptual training on inexperienced listeners' judgments of dysphonic voice. *Journal of Voice, 20,* 527–544.

Eckel, F. C., & Boone, D. R. (1981). The s/z ratio as an indicator of laryngeal pathology. *Journal of Speech and Hearing Disorders, 46,* 147–150.

Eisenberg, L. S., & Johnson, K. C. (2008). Audiologic contributions to pediatric cochlear implants. *The ASHA Leader,* March 25, 10–12.

Eisenberg, L. S., Johnson, K. C., Martinez, A. S., DesJardin, J. L., Stika, C. J., & Dzubak, D. (2008). Comprehensive evaluation of a child with an auditory brainstem implant. *Otology and Neurotology, 29,* 251–257.

El Hakim, H., Waddell, A. N., & Crysdale, W. S. (2002). Observations on the early results of treatment of recurrent respiratory papillomatosis using cidfovir. *Journal of Otolaryngology, 31*(6), 333–335.

Eliot, R. S. (1994). *From stress to strength: How to lighten your load*. New York: Chelsea House.

El-Kashian, H. K., Carroll, W. R., Hogikyan, N. D., Chepeha, D. B., Kileny, P. R., & Esclamado, R. M. (2001). Selective cricothyroid muscle reinnervation by muscle-nerve-muscle neurotization. *Archives of Otolaryngology Head and Neck Surgery, 127*(10), 1211–1215.

Ellis, P. D. M., & Bennett, J. (1977). Laryngeal trauma after prolonged endotracheal intubation. *Journal of Laryngology, 91,* 69–76.

Elluru, R. G. (2006). Reconstruction techniques for the treatment of anatomical upper respiratory tract anomalies in children. *Perspectives in Voice and Voice Disorders, 15*(3), 3–11.

Emami, A., Morrison, L., Rammage, L., & Bosch, D. (1999). Treatment of laryngeal contact ulcers and granulomas: A 12-year retrospective analysis. *Journal of Voice, 13*(4), 612–617.

Emerich, K. (2003). Nontraditional tools helpful in the treatment of certain types of voice disturbances. *Current Opinion in Otolaryngology & Head and Neck Surgery, 11*(3), 149–153.

Emerich, K., Titze, I., Svec, J., Popolo, P., & Logan, G. (2005). Vocal range and intensity in actors: A studio versus stage comparison. *Journal of Voice, 19,* 78–83.

Erlmer, D. J. (2003). *Contrasts for auditory and speech training (CAST)*. East Moline, IL: Linguisystems.

Eskenazi, L., Childers, D. G., & Hicks, D. M. (1990). Acoustic correlates of voice quality. *Journal of Speech and Hearing Research, 33,* 298–306.

Evans, M. K., & Deliyski, D. D. (2007). Acoustic voice analysis of prelingually deaf adults before and after cochlear implantation. *Journal of Voice, 21*(6), 669–682.

Fahr, S., Elton, R. I., & UPDRS Development Committee. (1987). Unified Parkinson's disease rating scale. In S. Fahr, C. D. Marsden, D. B. Calne, & M. Goldstein (Eds.), *Recent developments in Parkinson's disease* (pp. 153–304). New York: MacMillan.

Fairbanks, G. (1960). *Voice and articulation drillbook*. New York: Harper Brothers.

Faust, R. A. (2003). Childhood voice disorders: Ambulatory evaluation and operative diagnosis. *Clinical Pediatrics, 42,* 1–9.

Feldman, R. S. (1992). *Understanding stress*. New York: Venture.

Ferrand, C. T. (2000). Harmonics-to-noise ratios in normally speaking prepubescent girls and boys. *Journal of Voice, 14*, 17–21.

Ferrand, C. T. (2002). Harmonics-to-noise ratio: An index of vocal aging. *Journal of Voice, 16*, 480–487.

Ferrand, C. T. (2006). Relationship between masking levels and phonatory stability in normal-speaking women. *Journal of Voice, 20*, 223–228.

Ferrand, C. T. (2007). *Speech science: An integrated approach to theory and clinical practice* (2nd ed.). Boston: Allyn and Bacon.

Fex, S. (1992). Perceptual evaluation. *Journal of Voice, 6*, 155–158.

Filter, M. D., & Urioste, K. (1981). Pitch imitation abilities of college women with normal voices. *Journal of Speech and Hearing Association, 22*, 20–26.

Finitzo, T., & Freeman, F. (1989). Spasmodic dysphonia, whether and where: Results of seven years of research. *Journal of Speech and Hearing Research, 32*, 541–555.

Fisher, H. B. (1975). *Improving voice and articulation* (2nd ed.). New York: Houghton Mifflin.

Fitzsimmons, M., Sheahan, N., & Staunton, H. (2001). Gender and the integration of acoustic dimensions of prosody. *Brain and Language, 78*, 84–108.

Fletcher, S. (1973). *Manual for measurement and modification of nasality with TONAR II.* Birmingham: University of Alabama Press.

Fletcher, S. G. (1972). Contingencies for bioelectronic modification of nasality. *Journal of Speech and Hearing Disorders, 37*, 329–346.

Fletcher, S. G. (1978). *Diagnosing speech disorder for cleft palate.* New York: Grune & Stratton.

Fletcher, S. G., Adams, L. E., & McCutcheon, M. J. (1989). Cleft palate speech assessment through oral-nasal acoustic measures. In K. R. Bzoch (Ed.), *Communicative disorders related to cleft lip and palate* (3rd ed.). Boston: College Hill Press.

Folstein, M. F., Folstein, S. E., & McHugh, P. R. (1975). Mini-mental state: A practical method for grading the cognitive state of patients for the clinician. *Journal of Psychiatric Research, 12*, 189–198.

Ford, C. N., Inagi, K., Bless, D. M., Khidr, A., & Gilchrist, K. W. (1996). Sulcus vocalis: A rational analytical approach to diagnosis and management. *Annals of Otolaryngology, Rhinology and Laryngology, 105*, 189–200.

Ford, C. N., Staskowski, P. A., & Bless, D. M. (1995). Autologous collagen vocal fold injections: A preliminary clinical study. *Laryngoscope, 105*, 944–948.

Franic, D. M., Bramlett, R. E., & Bothe, A. C. (2004). Psychometric evaluation of disease specific quality of life instruments in voice disorders. *Journal of Voice, 19*, 300–315.

Froeschels, E. (1952). Chewing method as therapy. *Archives of Otolaryngology, 56*, 427–434.

Froeschels, E., Kastein, S., & Weiss, D. A. (1955). A method of therapy for paralytic conditions of the mechanisms of phonation, respiration, and glutination. *Journal of Speech and Hearing Disorders, 20*, 365–370.

Fujimoto, F. A., Madison, C. L., & Larrigan, L. B. (1991). The effects of a tracheostoma valve on the intelligibility and quality of tracheoesophageal speech. *Journal of Speech and Hearing Research, 34*, 33–36.

Galli, G., Cammarota, M., Rigante, E., De Corso, C., Parrilla, G. C., Passali, G., et al. (2007). High resolution magnifying endoscopy: A new diagnostic tool also for laryngeal examination? *Acta Otorhinolaryngologica Italica, 27*, 233–236.

Gallivan, G. J., Hoffman, L., & Gallivan, K. H. (1996). Episodic paroxysmal laryngospasm: Voice and pulmonary function assessment and management. *Journal of Voice, 10*(1), 93–105.

Garcia, I., Krishna, P., & Rosen, C. A. (2006). Severe laryngeal hyperkeratosis secondary to laryngopharyngeal reflux. *Ear, Nose and Throat Journal, 85*(7), 417.

Gelfer, M. P., & Schofield, K. J. (2000). Comparison of acoustic and perceptual measures of voice in male-to-female transsexuals. *Journal of Voice, 14*, 22–33.

Gerratt, B. R., Kreiman, J., Antonanzas-Barroso, N., & Berke, G. S. (1993). Comparing internal and external standards in voice quality judgments. *Journal of Speech and Hearing Research, 36*, 14–20.

Gerritsma, E. J. (1991). An investigation into some personality characteristics of patients with psychogenic aphonia and dysphonia. *Folia Phoniatrica et Logopaedica, 42*(1), 13–20.

Gilger, M. A. (2003). Pediatric otolaryngologic manifestations of gastroesophageal reflux disease. *Current Gastroenterology Reports, 5*(3), 247–252.

Gillivan-Murphy, P., Drinnan, M. J., O'Dwyer, T. P., Ridha, H., & Carding, P. (2006). The effectiveness of a voice treatment approach for teachers with self-reported voice problems. *Journal of Voice, 20*, 423–431.

Giovanni, A., Chanteret, C., Lagier, A. (2007). Sulcus Vocalis: A review. *European Archives of Otorhinolaryngology, 264*(4), 337–344.

Glicklich, R. E., Glovsky, R. M., & Montgomery, W. W. (1999). Validation of a voice outcome survey for unilateral vocal cord paralysis. *Otolaryngology-Head & Neck Surgery, 120,* 153–158.

Goffman, L., Ertmer, D., & Erdle, C. (2002). Changes in speech production in a child with cochlear implant: Acoustic and kinematic evidence. *Journal of Speech, Language, and Hearing Research, 45,* 891–901.

Goldman-Eisler, F. (1968). *Psycholinguistics: Experiments in spontaneous speech.* New York: Academic Press.

Golub, J. S., Chen, P., Otto, K. J., Hapner, E., & Johns, M. M. (2006). Prevalence of perceived dysphonia in a geriatric population. *Journal of the American Geriatric Society, 54,* 1736–1739.

Gorham-Rowan, M. M., & Laures-Gore, J. (2006). Acoustic-perceptual correlates of voice quality in elderly men and women. *Journal of Communication Disorders, 39,* 171–184.

Gould, W. J. (1975). Quantitative assessment of voice function in microlaryngology. *Folia Phoniatrica et Logopaedica, 27,* 190–200.

Grace, S. G. (1984). Speech pathology: Views from medicine and dentistry. In S. C. McFarlane (Ed.), *Coping with communicative handicaps.* San Diego, CA: College Hill Press.

Green, G. (1989). Psycho-behavioral characteristics of children with vocal nodules: WPBIC ratings. *Journal of Speech and Hearing Disorders, 54,* 306–312.

Greene, M. C. L. (1980). *The voice and its disorders* (4th ed.). Philadelphia: J. B. Lippincott.

Greene, M. C. L., & Mathieson, L. (1991). *The voice and its disorders* (5th ed.). London: Whurr.

Grillone, G. A., & Chan, T. (2006). Laryngeal dystonia. *Otolaryngologic Clinics of North America, 39,* 87–100.

Guss, J., & Mirza, N. (2006). Methacholine challenge testing in the diagnosis of paradoxical vocal fold motion. *Laryngoscope, 116*(9), 1558–1561.

Guyette, T., Polley, J., Botts, J., Figueroa, A., & Smith, B. (2001). Changes in speech following mandibular distraction osteogenesis. *The Cleft Palate-Craniofacial Journal, 38,* 179–184.

Guyette, T., Polley, J., Figueroa, A., & Smith, B. (2001). Changes in speech following maxillary distraction osteogenesis. *The Cleft Palate-Craniofacial Journal, 38,* 199–205.

Hagen, P., Lyons, G. D., & Nuss, D. W. (1996). Dysphonia in the elderly: Diagnosis and management of age-related voice changes. *Southern Medical Journal, 89,* 204–207.

Hall, S. W., & Merricourt, R. D. (1995). Chemotherapy and radiation therapy for laryngeal cancer. *Seminars in Speech and Language, 12,* 233–239.

Hamaker, R. C., & Hamaker, R. A. (1995). Surgical treatment of laryngeal cancer. *Seminars in Speech and Language, 12,* 221–232.

Hamdan, A. L., Sharara, A. I., Younes, A., & Fuleihan, N. (2001). Effect of aggressive therapy on laryngeal symptoms and voice characteristics in patients with gastroesophageal reflux. *Acta Otolaryngology, 121,* 868–872.

Hamel, W., Fietzek, U., Morsnowski, A, Schrader, B., Herzog, J., Weinert, D., et al. (2003). Deep brain stimulation of the subthalamic nucleus in Parkinson's disease: Evaluation of active electrode contacts. *Journal of Neurology, Neurosurgery and Psychiatry, 74*(8), 1036–1046.

Hammarberg, B., Fritzell, B., Gauffin, J., Sundberg, J., & Wedin, L. (1980). Perceptual and acoustic correlates of abnormal voice qualities. *Acta Otolaryngologica, 90,* 441–451.

Hanson, W., & Metter, E. (1983). DAF speech rate modification in Parkinson's disease: A report of two cases. In W. Berry (Ed.), *Clinical dysarthria.* Austin, TX: Pro-Ed.

Harrison, G. A., Davis, P. J., Troughear, R. H., & Winkworth, A. L. (1992). Inspiratory speech as a management option for spastic dysphonia. *Annals of Otology, Rhinology, and Laryngology, 101,* 375–382.

Hartnick, C. J. (2002). Validation of a pediatric voice quality-of-life instrument: The Pediatric Voice Outcome Survey. *Archives of Otolaryngology-Head and Neck Surgery, 128,* 919–922.

Harvey-Woodnorth, G. (2004). Assessing and managing medically fragile children: Tracheostomy and ventilatory support. *Language, Speech, and Hearing Services in Schools, 35*(4), 363–373.

Hayden, C., & Klimacka, L. (2000). Inter-rater reliability in cleft palate speech assessment. *Journal of Clinical Excellence, 2,* 169–173.

HBIGDA. (2005). *Harry Benjamin International Gender Dysphoria Association's standard of care for gender identity disorders.* Minneapolis: University of Minnesota Press.

Herrington-Hall, B., Lee, L., Stemple, J. C., Niemi, K. R., & McHone, M. M. (1988). Description of laryngeal pathologies by age, sex, and occupation in a treatment-seeking sample. *Journal of Speech and Hearing Disorders, 53,* 57–64.

Heylen, D., Wuyts, F., Mertens, F., De Bodt, M., Pattyn, J., Croux, C., et al. (1998). Evaluation of the vocal performance of children using a voice range profile index. *Journal of Speech, Language, and Hearing Research, 41,* 232–238.

Heylen, L., Wuyts, F. L., Mertens, F., DeBodt, M., & Van De Heyning, P. (2002). Normative voice range profiles of male and female professional voice users. *Journal of Voice, 16,* 1–7.

Higgins, M. B., Carney, A. E., & Schulte, L. (1994). Physiological assessment of speech and voice production of adults with hearing loss. *Journal of Speech and Hearing Research, 37,* 510–521.

Higgins, M. B., McCleary, E. A., Ide-Helvie, D. L., & Carney, A. E. (2005). Speech and voice physiology of children who are hard of hearing. *Ear and Hearing, 26,* 546–558.

Hillman, R. E., & Verdolini, K. (1999). Management of hyperfunctional voice disorders: Unifying concepts and strategies. *ASHA and RTN HealthCare Group, 99S05.*

Hillman, R. E., Walsh, M. J., Wolf, G. T., Fisher, S. G., & Hong, W. K. (1998). Functional outcomes following treatment of advanced laryngeal cancer. *Annals of Otolaryngology, Rhinology, and Laryngology, 172,* 1–27.

Hirano, M. (1981). *Clinical examination of the voice.* New York: Springer-Verlag.

Hirano, M. (1989). Objective evaluation of the human voice: Clinical aspects. *Folia Phoniatrica et Logopaedica, 41,* 89–144.

Hirano, M., & Bless, D. M. (1993). *Videostroboscopic examination of the larynx.* San Diego, CA: Singular.

Hirano, M., Kurita, S., & Nakashima, T. (1983). Growth, development and aging of human vocal folds. In D. Bless (Ed.), *Vocal fold physiology: Contemporary research and clinical issues* (pp. 22–43). San Diego, CA: College Hill Press.

Hirano, M., Yoshida, T., Tanaka, S., & Hibi, S. (1990). Sulcus vocalis: Functional aspects. *Annals of Otology, Rhinology, and Laryngology, 99,* 679–683.

Hirano, S., Kojima, H., Tateya, I., & Ito, J. (2002). Fiberoptic laryngeal surgery for vocal process granuloma. *Annals of Otology, Rhinology, and Laryngology, 111*(9), 789–793.

Hirano, S., Yamashita, M., Ohno, T., Kitamura, M., Kanemaru, S., & Ito, J. (2008). Phonomicrosurgery for posterior glottic lesions using triangular laryngoscope. *European Archives of Otorhinolaryngology, 265,* 435–440.

Hirsch, S., & Van Dorsel, J. (2006). Nonverbal communication: A multicultural view. In R. K. Adler, S. Hirsch, & M. Mordaunt (Eds.), *Voice and communication therapy for the transgender/transsexual client.* San Diego, CA: Plural Publishing.

Hixon, T. J., & Abbs, J. H. (1980). Normal speech production. In T. J. Hixon, L. D. Shriberg, & J. H. Saxman (Eds.), *Introduction to Communication Disorders.* Upper Saddle River, NJ: Prentice Hall.

Hixon, T. J., Hawley, J. L., & Wilson, K. J. (1982). An around the house device for the clinical determination of respiratory driving pressure: A note on making the simple even simpler. *Journal of Speech and Hearing Disorders, 47,* 413.

Hixon, T. J., & Hoit, J. D. (1998). Physical examination of the diaphragm by the speech-language pathologist. *American Journal of Speech-Language Pathology, 7,* 37–45.

Hixon, T. J., & Hoit, J. D. (1999). Physical examination of the abdominal wall by the speech-language pathologist. *American Journal of Speech-Language Pathology, 8,* 35–46.

Hixon, T. J., & Hoit, J. D. (2000). Physical examination of the rib cage by the speech-language pathologist. *American Journal of Speech-Language Pathology, 9,* 179–196.

Hixon, T. J., & Hoit, J. D. (2005). *Evaluation and management of speech breathing disorders: Principles and methods.* Tucson, AZ: Reddington Brown.

Hixon, T. J., Mead, J., & Goldman, M. D. (1976). Dynamics of the chest wall during speech production: Function of the thorax, rib cage, diaphragm, and abdomen. *Journal of Speech and Hearing Research, 19*(2), 297–356.

Hobbs, F., & Stoops, N. (2002). *Demographic trends in the 20th century.* U. S. Census Bureau, Census 2000 Special Reports, Series CENSR-4. Washington, DC: U.S. Government Printing Office.

Hocevar-Boltezar, I., Jarc, A., & Kozelj, D. D. (2006). Ear, nose and voice problems in children with orofacial clefts. *The Journal of Laryngology & Otology, 120,* 276–281.

Hochman, I. I., & Zeitels, S. M. (2000). Phonomicrosurgical management of vocal fold polyps: The subepithelial microflap resection technique. *Journal of Voice, 14,* 112–118.

Hoffman, L., Bolton, J., & Ferry, S. (2008). Passy-Muir speaking valve use in a children's hospital: An interdisciplinary approach. *ASHA Special Interest Division 3, Perspectives, Voice and Voice Disorders, 18,* 2.

Hoffman Ruddy, B., & Sapienza, C. M. (2004). Treating voice disorders in the school-based setting: Working within the framework of IDEA. *Language,*

Speech, and Hearing Services in Schools, 35(4), 327–332.

Hogikyan, N. D., & Sethuraman, G. (1999). Validation of an instrument to measure voice-related quality of life (V-RQOL). *Journal of Voice, 13,* 557–569.

Hoit, J. D. (1995). Influence of body position on breathing and its implications for the evaluation and treatment of speech and voice disorders. *Journal of Voice, 9,* 341–347.

Hoit, J. D., & Hixon, T. J. (1987). Age and speech breathing. *Journal of Speech and Hearing Research, 30,* 351–366.

Hoit, J. D., Hixon, T. J., Altman, M. E., & Morgan, W. J. (1989). Speech breathing in women. *Journal of Speech and Hearing Research, 32,* 353–365.

Hoit, J. D., Hixon, T. J., Watson, P. J., & Morgan, W. J. (1990). Speech breathing in children and adolescents. *Journal of Speech and Hearing Research, 33,* 51–69.

Holden, P. K., Vokes, D. E., Taylor, M. B., Till, J. A., & Crumley, R. L. (2007). Long-term botulinum toxin dose consistency for treatment of adductor spasmodic dysphonia. *Annals of Otology, Rhinology and Laryngology, 116*(12), 891–896.

Hollien, H. (1974). On vocal registers. *Journal of Phonetics, 2,* 125–143.

Hollien, H. (1987). Old voices: What do we really know about them? *Journal of Voice, 1,* 2–17.

Hollien, H., Dew, D., & Philips, P. (1971). Data on adult phonational ranges. *Journal of Speech and Hearing Research, 14,* 755–760.

Holmberg, E. B., Hillman, R. E., Hammarberg, B., Södersten, M., & Doyle, P. (2001). Efficacy of a behavioral based voice therapy protocol for vocal nodules. *Journal of Voice, 15,* 395–412.

Holmberg, E. B., Ihre, E., & Södersten, M. (2007). Phonetograms as a tool in the voice clinic: Changes across voice therapy for patients with vocal fatigue. *Logopedics Phoniatrics Vocology, 32*(3), 113–127.

Hooper, C. R. (2006). Language: Syntax and semantics. In R. K. Adler, S. Hirsch, & M. Mordaunt (Eds.), *Voice and communication therapy for the transgender/transsexual client.* San Diego, CA: Plural Publishing.

Horga, D., & Liker, M. (2006). Voice and pronunciation of cochlear implant speakers. *Clinical Linguistics and Phonetics, 20,* 211–217.

Horii, Y., & Fuller, B. (1990). Selected acoustic characteristics of voices before intubation and after extubation. *Journal of Speech and Hearing Research, 33,* 505–510.

Hsiung, M. W., Woo, P., Minasian, A., Schaefer Mojica, J. (2000). Fat augmentation for glottic insufficiency. *Laryngoscope, 110*(6), 1026–1033.

Hughes, C. A., Troost, S., Miller, S., & Troost, T. (2000). Unilateral true vocal fold paralysis: Cause of right-sided lesions. *Otolaryngology Head and Neck Surgery, 122*(5), 678–680.

Hull, R. H. (2001). *Aural rehabilitation: Serving children and adults.* San Diego, CA: Singular Publishing Group.

Hummert, M. L., Mazloff, D., & Henry, C. (1999). Vocal characteristics of older adults and stereotyping. *Journal of Nonverbal Behavior, 23,* 111–132.

Hunter, E., Svec, J., & Titze, I. (2006). Comparison of the produced and perceived voice range profile in untrained and trained classical singers. *Journal of Voice, 20,* 513–526.

Huntley, R., Hollien, H., & Shipp, T. (1980). Influences of listener characteristics on perceived age estimations. *Journal of Voice, 1,* 49–52.

Hutchinson, J., Robinson, K., & Nerbonne, M. (1978). Patterns of nasalance in a sample of normal gerontologic subjects. *Journal of Communication Disorders, 11,* 469–481.

Inagi, K., Ford, C. N., Bless, D. M., & Heisey, D. (1996). Analysis of factors affecting botulinum toxin results in spasmodic dysphonia. *Journal of Voice, 10,* 306–313.

Isenberg, J. S., Crozier, D. L., & Dailey, S. H. (2008). Institutional and comprehensive review of laryngeal leukoplakia. *Annals of Otology, Rhinology and Laryngology, 117*(1), 74–79.

Ishi, C., Ishiguro, H., & Hagita, N.(2006). Acoustic analysis of pressed voice. *The Journal of the Acoustical Society of America, 120,* 3374.

Iskowitz, M. (1998, April 20). In pursuit of natural sound. *Advance,* 7–9.

Isshiki, N., Shoji, K., Kojima, H., & Hirano, S. (1996). Vocal fold atrophy and its surgical treatment. *Annals of Otology, Rhinology and Laryngology, 105,* 182–188.

Issing, W. J. (2003). Gastroesophageal reflux—A common illness? *Laryngorhinootologie, 82*(2), 118–122.

Izdebski, J. (1986). Current views on the pathomechanism of bronchial hyperactivity. *Polskie Archiwun Medycyny Wewnetrzej, 76*(5–6), 278–284.

Izdebski, K., Dedo, H. H., & Boles, L. (1984). Spastic dysphonia: A patient profile of 200 cases. *American Journal of Otolaryngology, 5,* 7–14.

Jacobson, B. H., Johnson, A., Grywalski, C., Silbergleit, A., Jacobson, G. & Benninger, M. S. (1997). The voice handicap index (VHI): Development and validation. *American Journal of Speech-Language Pathology, 6,* 66–70.

Jamison, W. (1996). Some practical considerations when evaluating the exceptional adolescent singing voice. *Language, Speech, and Hearing Services in Schools, 27,* 292–300.

Jankovic, J. (1986). Cranial-cervical dyskinesias. In S. H. Appel (Ed.), *Current neurology* (p. 6). Chicago: Mosby-Year Book.

Johns, D. F., Rohrich, R. J., & Awada, M. (2003). Velopharyngeal incompetence: A guide for clinical evaluation. *Plastic & Reconstructive Surgery, 112,* 1890–1898.

Kahane, J. (1981). Anatomic and physiologic changes in the aging peripheral speech mechanism. In D. S. Beasley & G. A. Davis (Eds.), A*ging communication processes and disorders* (pp. 21–45). New York: Grunne and Stratton.

Kahane, J., & Beckford, N. (1991). The aging larynx and voice. In D. Ripich (Ed.), *Handbook of geriatric communication disorders* (pp. 165–186). Austin, TX: Pro-Ed.

Kahane, J., & Mayo, R. (1989). The need for aggressive pursuit of healthy childhood voices. *Language, Speech, and Hearing Services in Schools, 20,* 102–107.

Kandogan, T., Olgun, L., & Gultekin, G. (2003). Causes of dysphonia in patients above 60 years of age. *Kulak Burun Bogaz Ihtis Derg, 11,* 139–143.

Kantner, C. E. (1947). The rationale of blowing exercises for patients with repaired cleft palates. *Journal of Speech Disorders, 12,* 281–286.

Karnell, M., Melton, S., Childes, J., Coleman, T., Dailey, S., & Hoffman, H. (2007). Reliability of clinician-based (GRBAS and CAPE-V) and patient-based (V-RQOL and IPVI) documentation of voice disorders. *Journal of Voice, 21,* 576–590.

Kawaida, M., Fukuda, H., & Kohno, N. (2002). Digital image processing of laryngeal lesions by electronic videoendoscopy. *Laryngoscope, 112,* 559–564.

Kazandijian, M., & Dikeman, K. (2008). Communication options for tracheostomy and ventilator-dependent patients. In E. N. Myers & J. T. Jonas (Eds.), *Tracheostomy: Airway management, communication and swallowing* (pp. 187–214). San Diego, CA: Plural Publishing.

Keith, R. L., & Darley, F. L. (1994). *Laryngectomee rehabilitation* (3rd ed.). Austin, TX: Pro-Ed.

Kempster, G. B., Gerratt, B. R., Verdolini Abbott, K., Barkmeier-Kraemer, J., Hillman, R. E. (2008). Consensus auditory-perceptual evaluation of voice: Development of a standardized clinical protocol. *American Journal of Speech-Language Pathology,* in press.

Kendall, K. (2007). Presbyphonia: A review. *Current Opinion in Otolaryngology & Head and Neck Surgery, 15,* 137–140.

Kendall, K. A., Browning, M. M., & Skovlund, S. M. (2005). Introduction to high-speed imaging of the larynx. *Current Opinion in Otolaryngology & Head and Neck Surgery, 13,* 135–137.

Kent, R. D. (1994). *Reference manual for communicative sciences and disorders: Speech and language.* Austin, TX: Pro-Ed.

Kent, R. D. (1996). Hearing and believing: Some limits to the auditory-perceptual assessment of speech and voice. *American Journal of Speech-Language Pathology, 5,* 7–23.

Kent, R. D., Kent, J. F., & Rosenbek, J. C. (1987). Maximum performance tests of speech production. *Journal of Speech and Hearing Disorders, 52,* 367–387.

Kent, R., Vorperian, H., Kent, J., Duffy, J. (2003). Voice dysfunction in dysarthria: Application of the Multi-Dimensional Voice Program. *Journal of Communication Disorders, 36*(4), 281–306.

Kent, R. D., Kim, H., Weismer, G., & Kent, J. (1994). Laryngeal dysfunction in neurological disease: Amyotrophic lateral sclerosis, Parkinson disease, and stroke. *Journal of Medical Speech-Language Pathology, 2*(3), 157–175.

Kent, R. D., & Read, C. (2002). *The acoustic analysis of speech.* Albany, NY: Thomson Learning.

Kingdom, T. T., & Lee, K. C. (1996). Invasive aspergillosis of the larynx in AIDS. *Otolaryngology-Head and Neck Surgery, 115,* 135–137.

Kirchner, J. A., & Wyke, B. D. (1965). Articular reflex mechanisms in the larynx. *Annals of Otology, Rhinology, and Laryngology, 74,* 749–768.

Klein, S., Piccirillo, J. F., & Painter, C. (2000). Comparative contrast of voice measurements. *Otolaryngology-Head and Neck Surgery, 123,* 164–169.

Kleinsasser, O. (1979). *Microlaryngoscopy and endolaryngeal microsurgery: Technique and typical findings.* Baltimore: University Park.

Kleinsasser, O. (1982). Pathogenesis of vocal cord polyps. *Annals of Otology, Rhinology and Laryngology, 91,* 378–381.

Koike, M., Kobayashi, N., Hirose, H., & Hara, Y. (2002). Speech rehabilitation after total laryngectomy. *Acta Otolaryngology Supplement 122*(547), 107–112.

Konst, E. M., Rietveld, T., Peters, H. F., & Prahl-Andersen, B. (2003). Phonological development of toddlers with unilateral cleft lip and palate who were treated with and without infant orthopedics: A randomized clinical trial. *Cleft Palate-Craniofacial Journal, 40*(1), 32–39.

Kooijman, P. G., de Jong, F. I., Oudes, M. J., Huinck, W., van Acht, H., & Graamans, K. (2005). Muscular tension and body posture in relation to voice handicap and voice quality in teachers with persistent voice complaints. *Folia Phoniatrica et Logopaedica, 57*(3), 134–147.

Koschkee, D. L., & Rammage, L. (1997). *Voice care in the medical setting.* San Diego, CA: Singular.

Kotby, M. N. (1995). *The accent method of voice therapy.* San Diego, CA: Singular.

Kotby, M., El-Sady, S., Baslouny, S., Abou-Rass, Y., & Hegazi, M. (1991). Efficacy of the accent method of voice therapy. *Journal of Voice, 5*, 316–320.

Koufman, J. A. (1991). The otolaryngologic manifestations of gastroesophageal reflux disease (GERD). *Laryngoscope, 101*, 1–78.

Koufman, J. A. (2003). Evaluation of laryngeal biomechanics by fiberoptic laryngoscopy. In J. S. Rubin, R. T. Sataloff, & G. S. Korovin (Eds.), *Diagnosis and treatment of voice disorders* (2nd ed.). New York: Delmar Learning.

Koufman, J. A., & Belafsky, P. C. (2001). Unilateral or localized Reinke's edema (pseudocyst) as a manifestation of vocal fold paresis: The paresis podule. *Laryngoscope, 111*(4), 576–580.

Koufman, J. A., & Blalock, P. D. (1991). Functional voice disorders. In J. A. Kougman & G. Isaacson (Eds.), *Voice disorders: Otolaryngologic clinics in North America.* Philadelphia: W. B. Saunders.

Koufman, J. A., Radomski, T. A., Joharji, G. M., Russell, G. B., & Pillsbury, D. C. (1996). Laryngeal biomechanics of the singing voice.*Otolaryngology-Head and Neck Surgery, 115*, 527–537.

Krauss, J., & Jankovic, A. (1996). Surgical treatment of Parkinson's disease. *American Family Physician, 54*, 1621–1629.

Krauss, R. M., Freyberg, R., & Morsella, E. (2002). Inferring speakers' physical attributes from their voices. *Journal of Experimental Social Psychology, 38*, 618–625.

Kreiman, J., & Gerratt, B. R. (2000). Sources of listener disagreement in voice quality assessment. *Journal of the Acoustical Society of America, 108*, 1867–1879.

Kreiman, J., & Gerratt, B. R. (2005). Perception of aperiodicity in pathological voice. *Journal of the Acoustical Society of America, 117*, 2201–2211.

Kreiman, J., Gerratt, B. R., Kempster, G. B., Erman, A., & Berke, G. S. (1993). Perceptual evaluation of voice quality: Review, tutorial, and a framework for future research. *Journal of Speech and Hearing Research, 36*, 21–40.

Kuehn, D. P. (1997). The development of a new technique for treating hypernasality: CPAP. *American Journal of Speech-Language Pathology, 6*, 5–8.

Kuehn, D. P., & Moller, K. T. (2000). Speech and language issues in the cleft palate population: The state of the art. *Cleft Palate-Craniofacial Journal, 37*, 348–354.

Kummer, A. W., & Lee, L. (1996). Evaluation and treatment of resonance disorders. *Language, Speech, and Hearing Services in Schools, 27*, 271–281.

La, F. M., Ledger, W. L., Davidson, J. W., Howard, D. M., & Jones, G. L. (2007). The effects of a third-generation combined oral contraceptive pill on the classical singing voice. *Journal of Voice, 21*(6), 754–761.

Lallh, A. K., & Rochet, A. P. (2000). The effect of information on listeners' attitudes toward speakers with voice or resonance disorders. *Journal of Speech, Language, and Hearing Research, 43*, 782–795.

Lam, D. J., Starr, J. R., Perkins, J. A., Lewis, C. W., Eblen, L. E., Dunlap, J., & Sie, K. C. (2006). A comparison of nasendoscopy and multiview videofluoroscopy in assessing velopharyngeal insufficiency. *Otolaryngology-Head and Neck Surgery, 134*, 394–402.

LaRossa, D. (2000). The state of the art in cleft palate surgery. *Cleft Palate-Craniofacial Journal, 37*, 225–228.

LaRossa, D., Jackson, O. H., Kirschner, R. E., Low, D. W., Solot, C. B., Cohen, M. A., Mayro, R., Wang, P., Minugh-Purvis, N., & Randall, P. (2004). The Children's Hospital of Philadelphia modification of the Furlow double-opposing z-palatoplasty: Long-term speech and growth results. *Clinics in Plastic Surgery, 31*, 243–249.

Lauder, E. (2000). *Self-help for the laryngectomee.* Carpinteria, CA: Author.

Laver, J. (1980). *The phonetic description of voice quality.* Cambridge, UK: Cambridge University Press.

Laver, J. (1994). *Principles of phonetics.* Oxford, UK: Oxford University Press.

Laver, J., Wirz, S., MacKenzie, J., & Hiller, S. M. (1981). A perceptual protocol for the analysis of vocal profiles. *Edinburgh University Department of Linguistics Work in Progress, 14*, 139–155.

Lavorato, A. S., & McFarlane, S. C. (1983). Treatment of the professional voice. In W. H. Perkins (Ed.), *Current therapy of communication disorders: Voice disorders*. New York: Thieme-Stratton.

LeBorgne, W. (2007). Clinical applications and use of the Voice Range Profile. *Perspectives on Voice and Voice Disorders, 17,* 18–24.

LeBorgne, W., & Weinrich, B. (2002). Phonetogram changes for trained singers over a nine-month period of vocal training. *Journal of Voice, 16,* 37–43.

Lecoq, M., & Drape, F. (1996). Epidemiological survey of dysphonia in children at primary school. *Revue de Laryngologie Otologie Rhinologie, 117*(4), 323–325.

Leder, S. B., Ross, D. A., Briskin, K. B., & Sasaki, C. T. (1997). A prospective, double-blind, randomized study on the use of a topical anesthetic, vasoconstrictor, and placebo during transnasal flexible fiberoptic endoscopy. *Journal of Speech and Hearing Research, 40,* 1352–1357.

Lee, E. K., & Son, Y. I. (2005). Muscle tension dysphonia in children: Voice characteristics and outcome of voice therapy. *International Journal of Pediatric Otorhinolaryngology, 69,* 911–917.

Lee, G. S., Hsiao, T. Y., Yang, C. C. H., & Kuo, T. B. J. (2007). Effects of speech noise on vocal fundamental frequency using power spectral analysis. *Ear and Hearing, 28,* 343–350.

Lee, L., Stemple, J. C., & Glaze, L. (2005). *Quick screen for voice*. San Diego, CA: Plural Publishing.

Lee, L., Stemple, J. C., Glaze, L., Kelchner, L. N. (2004). Quick screen for voice and supplementary documents for identifying pediatric voice disorders. *Language, Speech, and Hearing Services in Schools, 35*(4), 308–320.

Lee, M., Drinnan, M., & Carding, P. (2005). The reliability and validity of patient self-rating of their own voice quality. *Clinical Otolaryngology, 30,* 357–361.

Lee, S. W., Son, Y. I., Kim, C. H., Lee, J. Y., Kim, S. C., & Koh, Y. W. (2007). Voice outcomes of polyacrylamide hydrogel injection laryngoplasty. *Laryngoscope, 117*(10), 1871–1875.

Leeper, H. A., Tissington, M. L., & Munhall, K. G. (1998). Temporal characteristics of velopharyngeal function in children. *Cleft Palate Journal, 35,* 215–221.

Lehmann, Q. H. (1965). Reverse phonation: A new maneuver for eliminating the larynx. *Radiology, 84,* 215–222.

Leonard, R., & Kendall, K. (1997). *Dysphagia assessment and treatment planning: A team approach*. San Diego, CA: Singular.

Leonard, R., & Kendall, K. (1999). Differentiation of spasmodic and psychogenic dysphonias with phonoscopic evaluation. *Laryngoscope, 109,* 295–300.

Leonard, R., & Kendall, K. (2001). Phonoscopy—A valuable tool for otolaryngologists and speech-language pathologists in the management of dysphonic patients. *Laryngoscope, 111*(10), 1760–1766.

Leonard, R., & Kendall, K. (2005). Effects of voice therapy on vocal process granuloma: A phonoscopic approach. *American Journal of Otolaryngology, 26*(2), 101–107.

Lewin, J. S., Lemon, J., Bishop-Leone, J. K., Leyk, S., Martin, J. W., & Gillenwater, A. M. (2000). Experience with Barton button and peristomal breathing valve attachments for hands-free tracheoesophageal speech. *Head and Neck, 22*(2), 142–148.

Lewis, K., & Watterson, T. (2003). Comparison of nasalance scores obtained from the Nasometer and the NasalView. *Cleft Palate-Craniofacial Journal, 40*(1), 40–45.

Lewis, K. E., Watterson, T. L., & Houghton, S. M. (2003). The influence of listener experience and academic training on ratings of nasality. *Journal of Communication Disorders, 36,* 49–58.

Lindestadt, P., Hertegard, S., & Bjorck, G. (2004). Laryngeal adduction asymmetries in normal speaking. *Logopedics, Phoniatrics, and Vocology, 29,* 128–134.

Lindestadt, P. A., Sodersten, M., Merker, B., & Granqvist, S. (2001). Voice source characteristics in Mongolian "throat singing" studied with high speed imaging technique, acoustic spectra, and inverse filtering. *Journal of Voice, 15,* 1.

Linebaugh, C. W. (1983). Treatment of flaccid dysarthria. In W. H. Perkins (Ed.), *Current therapy in communication disorders: Dysarthria and apraxia* (pp. 78–85). New York: Thieme-Stratton.

Linville, S. E. (1996). The sound of senescence. *Journal of Voice, 10,* 190–200.

Linville, S. E. (2001). *Vocal aging*. San Diego, CA: Singular.

Linville, S. E. (2002). Source characteristics of aged voice assessed from long-term average spectra. *Journal of Voice, 16,* 472–479.

Linville, S. E., & Fisher, H. B. (1985). Acoustic characteristics of women's voices with advancing age. *Journal of Gerontology, 40,* 324–330.

Linville, S. E., & Korabic, E. W. (1987). Fundamental frequency stability characteristics of elderly women's voices. *Journal of the Acoustical Society of America, 81,* 1196–1199.

Linville, S. E., & Rens, J. (2001). Vocal tract resonance analysis of aging voice using long-term average spectra. *Journal of Voice, 15,* 323–330.

Linville, S. E., Skarin, B. D., & Fornatto, E. (1989). The interrelationship of measures related to vocal function, speech rate, and laryngeal appearance in elderly women. *Journal of Speech & Hearing Research, 32,* 323–330.

Liotti, M., Ramig, L. O., Vogel, D., New, P., Cook, C. I., Ingham, R. J., Ingham, J. C., & Fox, P. T. (2003). Hypophonia in Parkinson's disease: Neural correlates of voice treatment revealed by PET. *Neurology, 1160*(3), 432–440.

Liss, J. M., Weismer, G., & Rosenbek, J. C. (1990). Selected acoustic characteristics of speech production in very old males. *Journal of Gerontology, 45,* 35–45.

Liu, H., & Ng, M. L. (2007). Electrolarynx in voice rehabilitation. *Auris Nasus Larynx, 34*(3), 327–332.

Liu, X. Z., & Yan, D. (2007). Ageing and hearing loss. *Journal of Pathology, 211,* 188–197.

Llabrés, M., Molina-Martinez, F. J., & Miralles, F. (2005). Dysphagia as the sole manifestation of myasthenia gravis. *Journal of Neurology, Neurosurgery and Psychiatry, 76*(9), 1297–1300.

Loder, E., & Biondi, D. (2002). Use of botulinum toxin for chronic headaches: A focused review. *Clinical Journal of Pain, 18*(6 Suppl), S169–S176.

Logemann, J. A. (1998). *Evaluation and treatment of swallowing disorders* (2nd ed.). Austin, TX: Pro-Ed.

Lohmander, A., & Olsson, M. (2004). Methodology for perceptual assessment of speech in patients with cleft palate: A critical review of the literature. *Cleft Palate-Craniofacial Journal, 41,* 64–70.

Lorenz, R. R., Esclamado, R. M., Teker, A. M., Strome, M., Scharpf, J., Hicks, D., Milstein, C., & Lee, W. T. (2008). Ansa cervicalis-to-recurrent laryngeal nerve anastomosis for unilateral vocal fold paralysis: Experience of a single institution. *Annals of Otology, Rhinology and Laryngology, 117*(1), 40–45.

Loughran, S., Alves, C., & MacGregor, F. B. (2002). Current aetiology of unilateral vocal fold paralysis in a teaching hospital in the West of Scotland. *Journal of Laryngology and Otology, 116*(11), 907–910.

Luchsinger, R., & Arnold, G. E. (1965). *Voice-speech-language clinical communicology: Its physiology and pathology.* Belmont, CA: Wadsworth.

Ludlow, C. L. (2005). Central nervous system control of the laryngeal muscles in humans. *Respiratory Physiology and Neurobiology, 147,* 205–222.

Lundquist, P. G., Haglund, S., Carlson, B., Strander, H., & Lundgren, E. (1984). Interferon therapy in juvenile laryngeal papillomatosis. *Otolaryngology-Head and Neck Surgery, 92,* 386–391.

Ma, E., Robertson, J., Radford, C., Vagne, S., El-Halabi, R., & Yiu, E. (2007). Reliability of speaking and maximum voice range measures in screening for dysphonia. *Journal of Voice, 21,* 397–406.

Ma, E., & Yiu, E. (2001). Voice activity and participation profile: Assessing the impact of voice disorders on daily activities. *Journal of Speech, Language, and Hearing Research, 44,* 511–524.

Maier, W., Lohle, E., & Welte, V. (1994). Pathogenic and therapeutic aspects of contact granuloma. *Laryngorhinootologie, 73*(9), 488–491.

Makowska, W., Bogacka-Zatorska, E., & Rogozinski, T. (2001). Human papillomavirus in laryngeal leukoplakia. *Otolaryngology Polska, 55*(4), 395–398.

Malik, T., Bruce, I., & Cherry, J. (2007). Surgical complications of tracheooesophageal puncture and speech valves. *Current Opinion in Otolaryngology & Head and Neck Surgery, 15*(2), 117–122.

Marchant, H., Supiot, F., Choufani, G., & Hassid, S. (2003). Bilateral vocal fold palsy caused by chronic axonal neuropathy. *Journal of Laryngology and Otology, 117*(5), 414–416.

Marcotullio, D., Magliulo, G., & Pezone, T. (2002). Reinke's edema and risk factors: Clinical and histopathologic aspects. *American Journal of Otolaryngology, 23*(2), 81–84.

Marsh, J. (2004). The evaluation and management of velopharyngeal dysfunction. *Clinics in Plastic Surgery, 31,* 261–269.

Martin, D. P., & Wolfe, V. I. (1996). Effects of perceptual training based upon synthesized voice signals. *Perceptual Motor Skills, 83,* 1291–1298.

Maryn, Y., De Bodt, M. S., & Van Cauwenberge, P. (2003). Ventricular dysphonia: Clinical aspects and therapeutic options. *Laryngoscope, 113,* 859–866.

Mason, M. F. (1993). *Speech pathology for tracheostomized and ventilator dependent patients.* Newport Beach, CA: Voicing.

Mason, R. M., & Warren, D. W. (1980). Adenoid involution and developing hypernasality in cleft palate. *Journal of Speech and Hearing Disorders, 45,* 469–480.

Mathers-Schmidt, B. A. (2001). Paradoxical vocal fold motion: A tutorial on a complex disorder and the speech language pathologist's role. *American Journal of Speech-Language Pathology, 10,* 111–125.

Max, L., DeBruyn, W., & Steurs, W. (1997). Intelligibility of oesophageal and tracheooesophageal speech: Preliminary observations. *European Journal of Disorders of Communication, 32,* 429–440.

Mazaheri, M. (1979). Prosthodontic care. In H. K. Cooper, R. L. Harding, M. M. Krogman, M. Mazaheri, & R. T. Millard (Eds.), *Cleft palate and cleft lip: A team approach.* Philadelphia: Saunders.

McColl, D., Hooper, A., Von Berg, S. (2006, Spring). Counseling in laryngectomy. *Contemporary Issues in Communication Sciences and Disorders, 33.*

McFarlane, S. C. (1990). Videolaryngoendoscopy and voice disorders. *Seminars in Speech and Language, 11,* 162–171.

McFarlane, S. C., Fujiki, M., & Brinton, B. (1984). *Coping with communicative handicaps: Resources for the practicing clinician.* San Diego, CA: College Hill Press.

McFarlane, S. C., Holt-Romeo, T. L., Lavorato, A. S., & Warner, L. (1991). Unilateral vocal fold paralysis: Perceived vocal quality following three methods of treatment. *American Journal of Speech-Language Pathology, 1,* 45–48.

McFarlane, S. C., & Lavorato, A. S. (1984). The use of videoendoscopy in the evaluation and treatment of dysphonia. *Communicative Disorders, 9,* 117–126.

McFarlane, S. C., Nelson, W., & Watterson, T. L. (1998). Acoustic, physiologic and aerodynamic effects of tongue protrusion /i/ in dysphonia. *ASHA Leader, 18,* 72.

McFarlane, S. C., & Shipley, K. G. (1979). Spastic dysphonia: Laryngeal stuttering? *ASHA Leader, 21,* 710.

McFarlane, S. C., & Von Berg, S. (1998). Facilitative techniques in intervention for dysphonia. *Current Opinion in Otolaryngology & Head and Neck Surgery, 6,* 161–165.

McFarlane, S. C., & Watterson, T. L. (1990). Vocal nodules: Endoscopic study of their variations and treatment. *Seminars in Speech and Language, 11,* 47–59.

McFarlane, S. C., & Watterson, T. L. (1995a). General principles of working to develop alaryngeal speech. *Seminars in Speech and Language, 12,* 175–180.

McFarlane, S. C., & Watterson, T. L. (1995b). Laryngectomee rehabilitation. *Seminars in Speech and Language, 12,* 175–239.

McFarlane, S. C., Watterson, T. L., & Brophy, J. (1990). Transnasal videoendoscopy of the laryngeal mechanisms. *Seminars in Speech and Language, 11,* 8–16.

McFarlane, S. C., Watterson, T. L., Lewis, K., & Boone, D. R. (1998). Effect of voice therapy facilitation techniques on airflow in unilateral paralysis patients. *Phonoscope, 1,* 187–191.

McFerran, D. J., Abdullah, V., Gallimore, A. P., Pringle, M. B., & Croft, C. B. (1994). Vocal process granulomata. *Journal of Laryngology and Otology, 108,* 216–220.

McKinney, J. C. (1994). *The diagnosis and correction of vocal faults.* San Diego, CA: Singular.

McKinnon, S. L., Hess, C. W., & Landry, R. G. (1986). Reactions of college students to speech disorders. *Journal of Communication Disorders, 19,* 75–82.

McMurray, J. S. (2003). Disorders of phonation in children. *Pediatric Clinics of North America, 50,* 363–380.

McWilliams, B. J., Morris, H. L., & Shelton, R. L. (1990). *Cleft palate speech* (2nd ed.). Philadelphia: B. C. Decker.

Merati, A. L., Keppel, K., Braun, N. M., Blumin, J. H., & Kerschner, J. E. (2008). Pediatric voice-related quality of life: Findings in healthy children and in common laryngeal disorders. *Annals of Otology, Rhinology and Laryngology 117*(4), 259–262.

Merchant, H., Supiot, F., Choufani, G., & Hassid, S. (2003). Bilateral vocal palsy caused by chronic motor axonal neuropathy. *Journal of Laryngology and Otology, 117*(5), 414–416.

Metter, E. J. (1985). *Speech disorders: Clinical evaluation and diagnosis.* Jamaica: Spectrum Publications.

Milisen, R. (1957). Methods of evaluation and diagnosis of speech disorders. In L. E. Travis (Ed.), *Handbook of speech pathology.* New York: Appleton-Century-Crofts.

Miller, S. (2004). Voice therapy for vocal fold paralysis. *Otolaryngologic Clinics of North America, 3,* 105–119.

Millet, B., & Dejonckere, P. H. (1998). What determines the differences in perceptual rating of dysphonia between experienced raters? *Folia Phoniatrica et Logopaedica, 50,* 305–310.

Minckler, J. (1972). Functional organization and maintenance. *Introduction to neuroscience.* St. Louis, MO: Mosby.

Minifie, F. D. (1994). *Introduction to communication sciences and disorders.* San Diego, CA: Singular.

Miyamoto, R. C., Cotton, R. T., Rope, A. F., Hopkin, R. J., Cohen, A. P., Shott, S. R., et al. (2004). Association of anterior glottic webs with velocardiofacial syndrome (chromosome 22q11.2 deletion). *Otolaryngology-Head and Neck Surgery, 130*(4), 415–417.

Mokhemar, M. A. (2002). *The central auditory processing kit.* East Moline, IL: Linguisystems.

Moll, K. L. (1968). Speech characteristics of individuals with cleft lip and palate. In D. C. Spriestersbach & D. Sherman (Eds.), *Cleft palate and communication*. New York: Harper & Row.

Monsen, R. B. (1976). Second formant transitions in speech of deaf and normal-hearing children. *Journal of Speech and Hearing Research, 19,* 279–289.

Moore, G. P., & von Leden, H. (1958). Dynamic variations of the vibratory pattern in the normal larynx. *Folia Phoniatrica et Logopaedica, 10,* 205–238.

Morgan, J. E., Zraik, R. I., Griffin, A. W., Bowen, T. L., & Johnson, F. L. (2007). Injection versus medialization laryngoplasty for the treatment of unilateral vocal fold paralysis. *Laryngoscope, 117*(11), 2068–2074.

Morris, R., & Brown, W. (1994). Age-related differences in speech intensity among adult females. *Folia Phoniatrica et Logopaedica, 46,* 64–69.

Morris, H. L., & Smith, J. K. (1962). A multiple approach evaluating velopharyngeal competency. *Journal of Speech and Hearing Disorders, 27,* 218–226.

Morrison, M., & Rammage, L. (1994). *The management of voice disorders*. San Diego, CA: Singular.

Morrison, M. D., Rammage, L. A., Belisle, G. M., Pullan, C. B., & Nichol, H. (1983). Muscular tension dysphonia. *Journal of Otolaryngology, 12,* 302–306.

Mulrow, C. D., & Lichtenstein, M. J. (1991). Screening for hearing impairment in the elderly: Rationale and strategy. *Journal of General Internal Medicine, 6,* 249–258.

Munier, C., & Kinsella, R. (2008). The prevalence and impact of voice problems in primary school teachers. *Occupational Medicine, 58,* 74–76.

Munoz, J., Mendoza, E., Fresneda, M. D., Carballo, G., & Ramirez, I. (2002). Perceptual analysis in different voice samples: Agreement and reliability. *Perceptual Motor Skills, 94,* 1187–1195.

Murdoch, B. E., Thompson, E. C., & Stokes, P. D. (1994). Phonatory and laryngeal dysfunction following upper motor neuron vascular lesions. *Journal of Medical Speech-Language Pathology, 2,* 177–190.

Murphy, P. J., & Akande, O. O. (2007). Noise estimation in voice signals using short-term cepstral analysis. *Journal of the Acoustical Society of America, 121,* 1679–1690.

Murray, J. F., & Nadel, J. A. (1994). *Textbook of respiratory medicine*. Philadelphia: Saunders.

Murry, T., Tabaee, A., & Aviv, J. E. (2004). Respiratory retraining of refractory cough and laryngopharyngeal reflux in patients with paradoxical vocal fold movement disorder. *Laryngoscope, 114*(8), 1341–1345.

Murry, T., Tabaee, A., Owczarzak, V., & Aviv, J. E. (2006). Respiratory retraining therapy and management of laryngopharyngeal reflux in the treatment of patients with cough and paradoxical vocal fold movement disorder. *Annals of Otology, Rhinology and Laryngology, 115*(10), 754–758.

Murry, T., & Woodson, G. E. (1995). Combined-modality treatment of adductor spasmodic dysphonia with botulinum toxin and voice therapy. *Journal of Voice, 9,* 460–465.

Nagata, K., Kurita, S., Yasumoto, S., Maeda, T., Kawaski, H., & Hirano, M. (1983). Vocal fold polyps and nodules: A 10-year review of 1,156 patients. *Auris Nasus Larynx, 10*(Suppl), S27–S35.

Nash, E. A., & Ludlow, C. L. (1996). Laryngeal muscle activity during speech breaks in adductor spasmodic dysphonia. *Laryngoscope, 106,* 484–489.

Nasseri, S. S., & Maragos, N. E. (2000). Combination thyroplasty and the "twisted larynx" combined type IV and type I thyroplasty for superior laryngeal nerve weakness. *Journal of Voice, 14*(1), 104–111.

National Academy on an Aging Society (1999). *Hearing loss: A growing problem that affects quality of life*. Washington, DC: Author. Retrieved from www .agingsociety.org.

National Emphysema Foundation (NEF). (2007). Archives.

National Institute for Deafness and Other Communication Disorders (NIDCD). (2007). *Strategic plan*. Bethesda, MD: Author.

Negus, V. E. (1957). The mechanism of the larynx. *Laryngoscope, 67,* 961–986.

Nemetz, M. A., Pontes, P. A., & Vieira, V. P. (2005). Vestibular fold configuration during phonation in adults with and without dysphonia. *Revista Brasileira Otorrinolaringologia, 71,* 6–12.

Newby, H. A. (1972). *Audiology*. New York: Appleton-Century-Crofts.

Nishiyama, K., Hirose, H., Iguchi, Y., Yamamoto, K., Suzuki, T., Yamanaka, J., Hirayama, M., & Okamoto, M. (2001). A new surgical technique combining autologous intracordal transplantation of fat and fascia for sulcus vocalis. *Nippon Jibiinkoka Gakkai Kaiho, 104*(12), 1151–1155.

Noyes, B. E., &. Kemp, J. S. (2007). Vocal cord dysfunction in children. *Paediatric Respiratory Reviews, 8,* 155–163.

Oates, J. (2004). The evidence base for the management of individuals with voice disorders. In S. Reilly,

J. Douglas, & J. Oates (Eds.), *Evidence based practice in speech pathology* (pp. 140–184). London: Whurr.

Oates, J. (2006). Evidence based practice. In R. K. Adler, S. Hirsch, & M. Mordaunt (Eds.), *Voice and communication therapy for the transgender/transsexual client* (pp. 23–44). San Diego, CA: Plural Publishing.

Oates, J. M., & Dacakis, G. (1983). Speech pathology considerations in the management of transsexualism. *British Journal of Disorders of Communication, 18*, 139–151.

O'Brien, C. F. (2002). Treatment of spasticity with botulinum toxin. *Clinical Journal of Pain, 18* (6 Suppl), S182–S190.

O'Connor, R. (2004). *Measuring quality of life in health.* New York: Elsevier.

Offer, D. (1980). Normal adolescent development. In H. I. Kaplan, A. M. Freedman, & B. J. Sadock (Eds.), *Comprehensive textbook of psychiatry* (3rd ed.). Baltimore: Lippincott.

O'Hollaren, M. T. (1995). Dysphea and the larynx. *Annals of Allergy, Asthma, and Immunology, 75,* 1–4.

O'Hollaren, M. T., & Everts, E. C. (1991). Evaluating the patient with stridor. *Annals of Allergy, Asthma, and Immunology, 67,* 301–306.

Orlikoff, R. (1990). The relationship of age and cardiovascular health to certain acoustic characteristics of male voices. *Journal of Speech and Hearing Research, 33,* 450–457.

O'Sullivan, B. P., Finger, L., & Zwerdling, R. G. (2004). Use of nasopharyngoscopy in the evaluation of children with noisy breathing. *Chest, 125*(4), 1265–1269.

Park, J. B., Simpson, L. L., Anderson, T. D., & Sataloff, T. (2003). Immunologic characterization of spasmodic dysphonia patients who develop resistance to botulinum toxin. *Journal of Voice, 17*(2), 255–264.

Park, W., Hicks, D. M., Khandwala, F., Richter, J. E., Abelson, T. I., Milstein, C., & Vaezi, M. F. (2005). Laryngopharyneal reflux: Prospective cohort study evaluating optimal dose of proton-pump inhibitor therapy and pretherapy predictors of response. *Laryngoscope, 115*(7), 1230–1238.

Patel, R., Dailey, S., & Bless, D. M. (2008). Comparison of high-speed digital imaging with stroboscopy for laryngeal imaging of glottal disorders. *Annals of Otology, Rhinology and Laryngology, 117*(6), 413–424.

Paul, R. (2002). *Introduction to clinical methods in communication disorders.* Baltimore: Brookes Publishing Co.

Pauloski, B. R., Fisher, H. B., Kempster, G. B., & Blom, E. D. (1989). Statistical differentiation of tracheoesophageal speech produced under four prosthetic/occlusion speaking conditions. *Journal of Speech and Hearing Research, 32,* 591–599.

Pawar, S., Lim, H. J., Gill, M., Smith, T. L., Merati, A., Toohill, R. J., Loehri, T. A. (2007). Treatment of postnasal drip with proton pump inhibitors: A prospective, randomized, placebo-controlled study. *American Journal of Rhinology, 21*(6), 695–701.

Pearl, N. B., & McCall, G. N. (1986). *Laryngeal function during two types of whisper: A fiberoptic study.* Paper presented at ASHA convention, Detroit.

Pedersen, M., Beranova, A., & Moller, S. (2004). Dysphonia: Medical treatment and a medical voice hygiene advice approach. A prospective randomised pilot study. *European Archives of Otorhinolaryngology, 261,* 312–315.

Pedersen, M., & McGlashan, J. (2001). Surgical versus non-surgical interventions for vocal cord nodules. *Cochrane Database of Systematic Reviews, 2.* Art. No.: CD001934. DOI: 10.1002/14651858 .CD001934.

Perkins, W. H. (1983). Optimal use of voice: Prevention of chronic vocal abuse. *Seminars in Speech and Language, 4,* 273–286.

Pershall, K. E., & Boone, D. R. (1986). A videoendoscopic and computerized tomographic study of hypopharyngeal and supraglottic activity during assorted vocal tasks. In V. Lawrence (Ed.), *Transcripts of the Fourteenth Symposium: Care of the professional voice.* New York: Voice Foundation.

Peterson, G. E., & Barney, H. L. (1952). Control methods used in a study of the vowels. *Journal of the Acoustical Society, 24,* 175–184.

Peterson-Falzone, S. J., Hardin-Jones, M. A., & Karnell, M. P. (2001). *Cleft palate speech* (3rd ed.). St. Louis, MO: Mosby.

Phillips, M. A. (2002). *On developing a female voice* (Video). Burbank, CA: Heart Corps.

Pillsbury, H. C., & Sasaki, C. T. (1982). Granulomatous diseases of the larynx. *Otolaryngologic Clinics of America, 15*(3), 539–551.

Pinto, J., da Silva Freitas, M., Carpes, A., Zimath, P., Marquis, V., & Godoy, L. (2007). Autologous grafts for treatment of vocal sulcus and atrophy. *Head and Neck Surgery, 137*(5), 785–791.

Plassman, B. L., & Lansing, R. W. (1990). Perceptual cues used to reproduce an inspired lung volume. *Journal of Applied Physiology, 69,* 1123–1130.

Pontes, P., & Behlau, M. (1993). Treatment of sulcus vocalis: Auditory perceptual and acoustic analysis of the slicing mucosa surgical technique. *Journal of Voice, 7,* 365–376.

Pontes, P., Brasolotto, A., & Behlau, M. (2005). Glottic characteristics and voice complaints in the elderly. *Journal of Voice, 19,* 84–94.

Pontes, P., Yamasaki, R., & Behlau, M. (2006). Morphological and functional aspects of the senile larynx. *Folia Phoniatrica et Logopaedica, 58,* 151–158.

Popolo, P. S., Švec, J. G., & Titze, R. I. (2005). Adaptation of a pocket PC for use as a wearable voice dosimeter. *Journal of Speech, Language, and Hearing Research, 48*(4), 780–791.

Portone, C. R., Hapner, E. R., McGregor, L., Otto, K., & Johns, M. M., III. (2007). Correlation of the Voice Handicap Index (VHI) and the Voice-Related Quality of Life Measure (V-RQOL). *Journal of Voice, 21,* 723–734.

Prater, R. J., Swift, R. W., Miller, L., & Deem, J. L. (1999). *Manual of voice therapy* (2nd ed.). Austin, TX: Pro-Ed.

Ptacek, P. H., & Sander, E. K. (1966). Age recognition from voice. *Journal of Speech and Hearing Research, 9,* 273–277.

Ramig, L. O., Bonitati, C. M., Lemke, J. H., & Horii, Y. (1994). Voice treatment for patients with Parkinson disease: Development of an approach and preliminary efficacy data. *Journal of Medical Speech-Language Pathology, 2*(3), 191–209.

Ramig, L. O., & Ringel, R. (1983). Effects on physiologic aging on selected acoustic characteristics of voice. *Journal of Speech and Hearing Research, 26,* 22–30.

Ramig, L. O., Sapir, S., Fox, S., & Countryman, S. (2001). Changes in vocal loudness following intensive voice treatment (LSVT) in individuals with Parkinson's disease: A comparison with untreated patients and normal age-matched controls. *Movement Disorders, 16,* 79–83.

Ramig, L. O., & Verdolini, K. (1998).Treatment efficacy: Voice disorders. *Journal of Speech, Language, and Hearing Research, 41,* 101–116.

Rastatter, M. P., & Hyman, M. (1982). Maximum phoneme duration of /s/ and /z/ by children with vocal nodules. *Language, Speech, and Hearing Services in Schools, 13,* 197–199.

Rastatter, M., & Jacques, R. (1990). Formant frequency structure of the aging male and female vocal tract. *Folia Phoniatrica et Logopaedica, 42,* 312–319.

Raza, S. A., Mahendran, S., Rahman, N., & Williams, R. G. (2002). Familial vocal fold paralysis. *Journal of Laryngology and Otology, 116*(12), 1047–1049.

Ringel, R. L., & Chodzko-Zajko, W. J. (1987). Vocal indices of biological age. *Journal of Voice, 1,* 31–37.

Robb, P. J. (2007). Adenoidectomy: Does it work? *Journal of Laryngology and Otology, 121,* 209–214.

Rochet, A. (1991). Aging and the respiratory system. In D. Ripich (Ed.), *Handbook of geriatric communication disorders* (pp. 145–163). Austin, TX: Pro-Ed.

Rosen, C., Lee, A. S., Osborne, J., Zullo, T., & Murry, T. (2004). Development and validation of the Voice Handicap Index-10. *Laryngoscope, 114,* 1549–1556.

Rosen, C. A., & Murry, T. (2000a). Nomenclature of voice disorders and vocal pathology. *Otolaryngologyic Clinics of North America, 33,* 1035–1045.

Rosen, C. A., & Murry, T. (2000b). Voice Handicap Index in singers. *Journal of Voice, 14,* 370–377.

Rosen, C. A., Woodson, G. E., Thompson, J. W., Hengesteg, A. P., & Bradlow, H. L. (1998). Preliminary results of the use of indole-3-carginol for recurrent respiratory papillomatosis. *Current Opinion in Otolaryngology & Head and Neck Surgery, 118*(6), 810–815.

Rothberg, M. B., Haessler, S. D., & Brown, R. B. (2008). Complications of viral influenza. *American Journal of Medicine, 121*(4), 258–264.

Roy, N., Bless, D. M., Heisey, D., & Ford, C. N. (1997). Manual circumlaryngeal therapy for functional dysphonia: An evaluation of short- and long-term treatment outcomes. *Journal of Voice, 11*(3), 321–331.

Roy, N., Ford, C. N., & Bless, D. M. (1996). Muscle tension dysphonia and spasmodic dysphonia: The role of manual laryngeal tension reduction in diagnosis and management. *Annals of Otology, Rhinology and Laryngology, 105,* 851–856.

Roy, N., Gouse, M., Mauszycki, S. C., Merrill, R. M., & Smith, M. (2005). Task specificity in adductor spasmodic dysphonia versus muscle tension dysphonia. *Laryngoscope, 115,* 311–316.

Roy, N., Gray, S., Simon, M., Dove, H., Corbin-Lewis, K., & Stemple, J. (2001). An evaluation of the effects of two treatment approaches for teachers with voice disorders: A prospective randomized clinical trial. *Journal of Speech, Language, and Hearing Research, 44,* 286–296.

Roy, N., Holt, K. I., Redmond, S., & Muntz, H. (2007). Behavioral characteristics of children with vocal fold nodules. *Journal of Voice, 21,* 157–168.

Roy, N., & Leeper, H. A. (1993). Effects of the manual laryngeal musculoskeletal tension reduction technique as a treatment for functional voice disorders: Perceptual and acoustic measures. *Journal of Voice, 7,* 242–249.

Roy, N., Mauszycki, S. C., Merrill, R. M., Gouse, M., & Smith, M. (2007). Toward improved differential diagnosis of adductor spasmodic dysphonia and muscle tension dysphonia. *Folia Phoniatrica et Logopaedica, 59,* 83–90.

Roy, N., Merrill, R. M., Gray, S. D., & Smith, E. M. (2005). Voice disorders in the general population: Prevalence, risk factors, and occupational impact. *Laryngoscope, 115,* 1988–1995.

Roy, N., Merrill, R. M., Thibeault, S., Gray, S. D., & Smith, E. M. (2004). Voice disorders in teachers and the general population: Effects on work performance, attendance, and future career choices. *Journal of Speech, Language, and Hearing Research, 47,* 542–551.

Roy, N., Smith, M. E., Allen, B., & Merrill, R. M. (2007). Adductor spasmodic dysphonia versus muscle tension dysphonia: Examining the diagnostic value of recurrent laryngeal nerve lidocaine block. *Annals of Otology, Rhinology and Laryngology, 116,* 161–168.

Roy, N., Stemple, J. C., Merrill, R. M., & Thomas, L. (2007). Epidemiology of voice disorders in the elderly: Preliminary findings. *Laryngoscope, 117,* 628–633.

Roy, N., Weinrich, B., Gray, S. D., Tanner, K., Stemple, J. C., & A Sapienza, C. M. (2003). Three treatments for teachers with voice disorders: A randomized clinical trial. *Journal of Speech-Language Hearing Research, 46*(3), 670–688.

Roy, N., Weinrich, B., Gray, S. D., Tanner, K., Toledo, S. W., Dove, H., Corbin-Lewis, K., & Stemple, J. C. (2002). Voice amplification versus vocal hygiene instruction for teachers with voice disorders: A treatment outcomes study. *Journal of Speech, Language, and Hearing Research, 45*(4), 625–638.

Roy, S., & Vivero, R. J. (2008). Recurrent respiratory papillomatosis. *Ear, Nose & Throat Journal, 87*(1), 18–19.

Rubin, A., & Sataloff, R. (2007). Vocal fold paresis and paralysis. *Otolaryngologic Clinics of North America, 40*(5), viii–ix, 1109–1131.

Rubin, J. S., & Yanagisawa, E. (2003). Benign vocal fold pathology through the eyes of the laryngologist. In J. S. Rubin, R. T. Sataloff, & G. S. Korovin (Eds.), *Diagnosis and treatment of voice disorders* (2nd ed.). New York: Delmar Learning.

Rundell, K. W., & Spiering, B. A. (2003). Inspiratory stridor in elite athletes. *Chest, 123*(2), 468–474.

Ruotsalainen, J. H., Sellman, J., Lehto, L., Jauhiainen, M., & Verbeek, J. H. (2007). Interventions for treating functional dysphonia in adults. *Cochrane Database of Systematic Reviews, 3.* Art. No.: CD006373. DOI: 10.1002/14651858.CD006373.pub2.

Ruscello, D. M., Lass, N. J., & Podbesek, J. (1988). Listeners' perceptions of normal and voice-disordered children. *Folia Phoniatrica et Logopaedica, 40*(6), 290–296.

Ryan, E. B., & Capadano, H. L. (1978). Age perceptions and evaluative reactions toward adult speakers. *Journal of Gerontology, 33,* 98–102.

Ryan, W., & Burk, K. (1974). Perceptual and acoustic correlates in the speech of males. *Journal of Communication Disorders, 7,* 181–192.

Sander, E. K. (1989). Arguments against the aggressive pursuit of voice therapy for children. *Language, Speech, and Hearing Services in the Schools, 20,* 94–101.

Sanli, A., Celebi, O., Eken, M., Oktay, A., Aydin, S., & Ayduran, E. (2008). Role of the 30° telescope in evaluation of laryngeal masses during direct laryngoscopy. *Journal of Voice, 2,* 238–244.

Sapienza, C. M., Cannito, M. P., Murray, T., Branski, R., & Woodson, G. (2002). Acoustic variations in reading produced by speakers with spasmodic dysphonia pre-botox injections and within early stages of post-botox injection. *Journal of Speech, Language, and Hearing Research, 45*(5), 830–843.

Sapienza, C. M., Ruddy, B. H., Baker, S. (2004). Laryngeal structure and function in the pediatric larynx. *Language, Speech, and Hearing Services in Schools, 35,* 299–307.

Sapir, S., Ramig, L. O., Hoyt, P., Countryman, S., O'Brien, C., & Hoehn, M. (2002). Speech loudness and quality 12 months after intensive voice treatment (LSVT) for Parkinson's disease: A comparison with an alternative speech treatment. *Folia Phoniatrica et Logopaedica, 54*(6), 296–303.

Sasaki, C. T., & Toolhill, R. J. (2000). Ambulatory pH monitoring for extraesophageal reflux—Introduction. *Annals of Otology, Rhinology and Laryngology, 109*(Suppl), 2–3.

Sataloff, R. T. (1981). Professional singers: The science and art of clinical care. *American Journal of Otolaryngology, 2,* 251–266.

Sataloff, R. T. (1997a). Common infections and inflammations and other conditions. In R. T. Sataloff (Ed.), *Professional voice: The science and art of clinical care* (2nd ed., pp. 429–436). San Diego, CA: Singular.

Sataloff, R. T. (Ed.). (1997b). *Professional voice: The science and art of clinical care* (2nd ed.). San Diego, CA: Singular.

Sataloff, R. T. (1997c). Voice surgery. In R. T. Sataloff (Ed.), *Professional voice: The science and art of clinical care* (2nd ed.). San Diego, CA: Singular.

Sataloff, R. T., Spiegel, J. R., & Hawkshaw, M. J. (2003). History and physical examination of patients with voice disorders. In J. S. Rubin, R. T. Sataloff, & G. S. Korovin (Eds.), *Diagnosis and treatment of voice disorders* (2nd ed.). New York: Delmar Learning.

Sataloff, R. T., Spiegel, J. R., Hawkshaw, M., & Caputo Rosen, D. (1996). Severe hyperkeratosis mimicking carcinoma. *Ear, Nose & Throat Journal, 75*(10), 647.

Scarsellone, J. M., Rochet, A. P., & Wolfaardt, J. F. (1999). The influence of dentures on nasalance values in speech. *Cleft Palate-Craniofacial Journal, 36,* 51–56.

Schindler, A., Bottero, A., Capaccio, P., Ginocchio, D., Adorni, F., & Ottaviani, F. (2008). Vocal improvement after voice therapy in unilateral vocal fold paralysis. *Journal of Voice, 22*(1), 113–118.

Schulz, G. M. (2002). The effects of speech therapy and pharmacological treatment on voice and speech in Parkinson's disease: A review of the literature. *Current Medicinal Chemistry, 9,* 1359–1366.

Schulz, G. M., Greer, M., & Friedman, W. (2000). Changes in vocal intensity in Parkinson's disease following pallidotomy surgery. *Journal of Voice, 14*(4), 589–606.

Schuster, M., Lohscheller, J., Kummer, P., Hoppe, U., Eysholdt, U., & Rosanowski, F. (2003). Quality of life in laryngectomees after prosthetic voice restoration. *Folia Phoniatrica et Logopaedica, 55*(5), 211–219.

Schweinfurth, J. M., Billante, M., & Courey, M. S. (2002). Risk factors and demographics in patients with spasmodic dysphonia. *Laryngoscope, 112*(2), 220–223.

Scukanec, G., Petrosino, L., & Squibb, K. (1991). Formant frequency characteristics of children, young adult and aged female speakers. *Perceptual and Motor Skills, 73,* 203–208.

Sedory, S. E., Hamlet, S. L., & Conner, N. P. (1989). Comparisons of perceptual and acoustic characteristics of tracheoesophageal and excellent esophageal speech. *Journal of Speech and Hearing Disorders, 49,* 202–210.

Seifert, E., & Kollbrunner, J. (2005). Stress and distress in non-organic voice disorders. *Swiss Medical Weekly, 135,* 387–397.

Seifert, E., Oswald, M., Bruns, U., Vischer, M., Kompis, M., & Haeusler, R. (2002). Changes of voice and articulation in children with cochlear implants. *International Journal of Pediatric Otorhinolaryngology, 66,* 115–123.

Sell, D., Mars, M., & Worrell, E. (2006). Process and outcome study of multidisciplinary prosthetic treatment for velopharyngeal dysfunction. *International Journal of Language and Communication Disorders, 41,* 495–511.

Shadden, B. B., & Toner, M. A. (1997). Introduction: The continuum of life functions. In B. B. Shaden & M. A. Toner (Eds.), *Aging and communication: For clinicians, by clinicians* (pp. 3–17). Austin, TX: Pro-Ed.

Shah, R. K., Feldman, H. A., & Nuss, R. C. (2007). A grading scale for pediatric vocal fold nodules. *Otolaryngology-Head and Neck Surgery, 136,* 193–197.

Shah, R. K., Woodnorth, G. H., Glynn, A., & Nuss, R. C. (2005). Pediatric vocal nodules: Correlation with perceptual voice analysis. *International Journal of Pediatric Otorhinolaryngology, 69,* 903–909.

Shama, K., Krishna, A., & Cholayya, N. U. (2007). Study of harmonics-to-noise ratio and critical-band energy spectrum of speech as acoustic indicators of laryngeal and voice pathology. *Journal on Applied Signal Processing, 1,* 50.

Shelton, R. L., Hahn, E., & Morris, H. L. (1968). Diagnosis and therapy. In D. C. Spriestersbach & D. Sherman (Eds.), *Cleft palate and communication.* New York: Academic Press.

Shelton, R. L., & Trier, W. C. (1976). Issues involved in the evaluation of velopharyngeal closure. *Cleft Palate Journal, 13,* 127–137.

Shipp, T., & Hollien, H. (1969). Perception of the aging male voice. *Journal of Speech and Hearing Research, 12,* 703–712.

Shrivastav, R., Sapienza, C., & Nandur, V. (2005). Application of psychometric theory to the measurement of voice quality using rating scales. *Journal of Speech, Language, and Hearing Research, 48,* 323–335.

Sieron, A., Namysloski, G., Misiolek, M., Adamek, M., & Kawczyk-Krupka, A. (2001). Photodynamic therapy of premalignant lesions and local recurrence of laryngeal and hypopharyngeal cancers. *European Archives of Otorhinolaryngology, 258*(7), 349–352.

Skolnick, M. L., Glaser, E. R., & McWilliams, B. J. (1980). The use and limitations of the barium pharyngogram in detection of velopharyngeal insufficiency. *Radiology, 135,* 301–304.

Slater, S. C. (1992). Omnibus survey: Portrait of the professions. *ASHA Leader, 3,* 61–65.

Smith, B. E., & Guyette, T. (1996). Observation: Pressure-flow differences in performance during production of the CV syllables /pi/ and /pa/. *The Cleft Palate-Craniofacial Journal, 33,* 74–76.

Smith, B. E., Guyette, T., Patil, Y., & Brannan, T. (2003). Pressure-flow measurements for selected nasal sound segments produced by normal children and adolescents: A preliminary study. *The Cleft Palate-Craniofacial Journal, 40,* 158–164.

Smith, B. E., & Kuehn, D. P. (2007). Speech evaluation of velopharyngeal dysfunction. *Journal of Craniofacial Surgery, 18,* 251–261.

Smith, B. E., Patil, Y., Guyette, T., Brannan, T., & Cohen, M. (2004). Pressure-flow measurements for selected oral sound segments produced by normal children and adolescents: A basis for clinical testing. *The Journal of Craniofacial Surgery, 15,* 247–254.

Smitheran, J., & Hixon, T. (1981). A clinical method for estimating laryngeal airway resistance during vowel production. *Journal of Speech and Hearing Disorders, 46,* 138–146.

Sneeuw, K. C. A., Sprangers, M. A. G., & Aaronson, N. K. (2002). The role of healthcare providers and significant others in evaluating the quality of life of patients with chronic disease. *Journal of Clinical Epidemiology, 55,* 1130–1143.

Solomon, N. P., & Charron, S. (1998). Speech breathing in able-bodied children and children with cerebral palsy: A review of the literature and implications for clinical intervention. *American Journal of Speech-Language Pathology, 7,* 61–78.

Solomon, N. P., & Hixon, T. J. (1993). Speech breathing in Parkinson's disease. *Journal of Speech and Hearing Research, 36,* 294–310.

Spielman, J., Ramig, L. O., Mahler, L., Halpern, A., & Gavin, W. (2007). Effects of an extended version of the Lee Silverman Voice Treatment on voice and speech in Parkinson's disease. *American Journal of Speech-Language Pathology, 16,* 95–107.

Spielman, J., Starr, A. C., Popolo, P. S., & Hunter, E. J. (2007). Recommendations for the creation of a voice acoustics laboratory. *The National Center for Voice and Speech Online Technical Memo, 7, Version 1.4.* Available at: www.ncvs.org.

Speyer, R., Speyer, I., & Heijnen, M. A. M. (2008). Prevalence and relative risk of dysphonia in rheumatoid arthritis. *Journal of Voice, 22,* 232–237.

Spieth, L. E., & Harris, C. V. (1996). Assessment of health-related quality of life in children and adolescents: An integrative review. *Journal of Pediatric Psychology, 21,* 175–193.

Stacy, M., & Jankovic, J. (1992). Differential diagnosis of Parkinson's disease and the Parkinsonism plus syndromes. *Neurologic Clinics, 10,* 341–359.

Starcevic, V., & Lipsitt, D. R. (2001). *Hypochondriasis: Modern perspectives on an ancient malady.* New York: Oxford University Press.

Stathopoulos, E. T., & Sapienza, C. M. (1993). Respiratory and laryngeal function of women and men during vocal intensity variation. *Journal of Speech-Language and Hearing Research, 36,* 64–75.

Stathopoulos, E. T., & Sapienza, C. M. (1997). Developmental changes in laryngeal and respiratory function with variations in sound pressure level. *Journal of Speech, Language, and Hearing Researchet Logopaedica, 40,* 595–614.

Stathopoulos, E. T., & Weismer, G. (1985). Oral airflow and air pressure during speech production: A comparative study of children, youths and adults. *Folia Phoniatrica et Logopaedica, 37,* 152–159.

Stemple, J. C. (2000). *Voice therapy: Clinical studies* (2nd ed.). San Diego, CA: Singular.

Stemple, J. C. (2005). A holistic approach to voice therapy. *Seminars in Speech and Language, 26,* 131–137.

Stemple, J. C. (2007). *Principles of physiologic voice therapy.* Short Course. Tempe, AZ: Arizona State University.

Stemple, J. C., Gerdeman, B. K., & Glaze, L. E. (1994). *Clinical voice management.* San Diego, CA: Singular.

Stemple, J. C., Glaze, L. E., & Klaben, B. G. (2000). *Clinical voice pathology: Theory and management* (3rd ed.). San Diego, CA: Thomson Learning.

Stemple, J. C., & Holcomb, B. (1988). *Effective voice and articulation.* Columbus, OH: Merrill.

Stewart, C. F., Allen, E. L., Tureen, P., Diamond, B. E., Blitzer, A., & Brin, M. F. (1997). Adductor spasmodic dysphonia: Standard evaluation of symptoms and severity. *Journal of Voice, 11,* 95–103.

Stoll, C., Hochmuth, M., Meister, P., & Soost, F. (2001). Refinement of velopharyngoplasty in patients with cleft palate by covering the pharyngeal flap with nasal mucosa of the velum. *Journal of Craniomaxillofacial Surgery, 29*(3), 185–186.

Strauss, L., Hejal, R., Galan, G., Dixon, L., & McFadden, E. R., Jr. (1997). Observations on the effects of aerosolized albuterol in acute asthma. *American Journal of Respiratory Critical Care Medicine, 155,* 826–832.

Stroebel, C. (1983). *Quieting reflex training for adults.* York, UK: BMA Audio Cassettes.

Stroh, B. C., Faust, R. A., & Rimell, F. L. (1998). Results of esophageal biopsies performed during triple endoscopy in the pediatric patient. *Archives of Otolaryngology-Head and Neck Surgery, 124,* 545–549.

Strome, M. (1982). Common laryngeal disorders in children. In M. D. Filter (Ed.), *Phonatory voice disorders in children.* Springfield, IL: Charles C. Thomas.

Strome, M., Stein, J., Esclamado, R., Hicks, D., Lorenz, R. R., Braun, W., Yetman, R., Eliachar, I., & Mayes, J. (2001). Laryngeal transplantation and 40-month follow-up. *New England Journal of Medicine, 344*(22), 1676–1679.

Strouse, A., Ashmead, D. H., Ohde, R. N., & Grantham, D. W. (1998). Temporal processing in the aging auditory system. *Journal of Acoustical Society of America, 104*(4), 2385–2399.

Su, C. Y., Tsai, S. S., Chiu, J. F., & Cheng, C. A. (2004). Medialization laryngoplasty with strap muscle transposition for vocal fold atrophy with or without sulcus vocalis. *Laryngoscope, 114,* 1106–1112.

Su, C. Y., Tsai, S. S., Chuang, H. C., & Chiu, J. F. (2005). Functional significance of arytenoid adduction with the suture attaching to cricoid cartilage versus to thyroid cartilage for unilateral paralytic dysphonia. *Laryngoscope, 115*(10), 1752–1759.

Subtelny, J., Whitehead, R., & Klueck, E. (1989). Therapy to improve pitch in young adults with profound hearing loss. *Volta Review, 91,* 261–268.

Sullivan, M. D., Heywood, B. M., & Beukelman, D. R. (2001). A treatment for vocal cord dysfunction in female athletes: An outcome study. *Laryngoscope, 111,* 1751–1755.

Svirsky, M. A., Lane, H., Perkell, J. S., & Wozniak, J. (1992). Effects of short-term auditory deprivation on speech production in adult cochlear implant users. *Journal of the Acoustical Society of America, 92,* 1284–1300.

Tachimura, T., Nohara, K., & Wada, T. (2000). Effect of placement of speech appliance on levator veli palatini muscle activity during speech. *Cleft Palate-Craniofacial Journal, 37*(5), 478–482.

Tait, N. A., Michel, J. F., & Carpenter, M. A. (1980). Maximum duration of sustained /s/ and /z/ in children. *Journal of Speech and Hearing Disorders, 45,* 239–246.

Tanaka, S., Hirano, M., & Umeno, H. (1994). Laryngeal behavior in unilateral superior laryngeal nerve paralysis. *Annals of Otolaryngology, Rhinology and Laryngology, 103,* 93–97.

Tarlov, A. R., Ware, J. E., Greenfield, S., Nelson, E. C., Perrin, E., & Zubkoff, M. (1989). The medical outcomes study. *Journal of the American Medical Association, 262,* 925–930.

Teles-Magalhães, L. C., Pegoraro-Krook, M. I., & Pegoraro, R. (2000). Study of the elderly females' voice by phonetography. *Journal of Voice, 14,* 310–321.

Templin, M. C., & Darley, F. L. (1980). *The Templin-Darley Tests of Articulation.* Iowa City, IA: Bureau of Education Research and Service.

Thibeault, S. (2007). What are the roles of the laryngologist and speech language pathologist in management of patients with dysphonia? *ASHA Special Interest Division 3, Voice and Voice Disorders, 17*(3), 4–8.

Thibeault, S. L. (2005). Advances in our understanding of the Reinke space. *Current Opinion in Otolaryngology & Head and Neck Surgery, 13,* 148–151.

Thomas, L. B., Harrison, A. L., & Stemple, J. C. (2007). Aging thyroarytenoid and limb skeletal muscle: Lessons in contrast. *Journal of Voice* (in press).

Thomas, L. B., & Stemple, J. C. (2007). Voice therapy: Does science support the art? *Communication Disorders Review, 1,* 49–77.

Titze, I. R. (1994). *Principles of voice production.* New York: Prentice Hall.

Tomonaga, T., Awad, Z. T., Filipi, C. J., Hinder, R. A., Selima, M., Tercero, F., Marsh, R. E., Shiino, Y., & Welch, R. (2002). Symptom predictability of reflux induced respiratory disease. *Digestive Diseases and Sciences, 47*(1), 9–14.

Toohill, R. J. (1975). The psychosomatic aspects of children with vocal nodules. *Archives of Otolaryngology, 101,* 591–595.

Trost-Cardamone, J. E. (1990). The development of speech: Cleft palate misarticulations. In D. E. Kernahan & S. W. Rosenstein (Eds.), *Cleft lip and palate: A system of management.* Baltimore: Lippincott.

Trudeau, M. D. (1998). Paradoxical vocal cord dysfunction among juveniles. *Voice and Voice Disorders, 8,* 11–13.

Trudeau, M. D., & Forrest, L. A. (1997). The contributions of phonatory volume and transglottal airflow to the s/z ratio. *American Journal of Speech-Language Pathology, 6,* 65–69.

Tsukahara, K., Tokashiki, R., Hiramatsu, H., & Suzuki, M. (2005). A case of high-pitched diplophonia that resolved after a direct pull of the lateral cricoarytenoid muscle. *Acta Otolaryngologica, 125,* 331–333.

Tucker, H. M., & Lavertu, P. (1992). Paralysis and paresis of the vocal folds. In A. Blitzer, M. F. Brin, C. T. Sasaki, & K. S. Harris (Eds.), *Neurologic disorders of the larynx.* New York: Thieme Medical.

United States Administration on Aging (2004). Retrieved May 16, 2008, from www.aoa.gov.

United States Bureau of the Census (2000). Retrieved May 16, 2008, from www.census.gov.

van den Berg, J. (1958). Myoelastic-aerodynamic theory of voice production. *Journal of Speech and Hearing Research, 1,* 227–243.

van den Berg, J. W. (1968). Register problems. In M. Krauss (Ed.), *Sound production in man.* New York: New York Academy of Sciences.

Van Riper, C., & Irwin, J. V. (1958). *Voice and articulation.* Englewood Cliffs, NJ: Prentice Hall.

Varvares, M. A., Montgomery, W. W., & Hillman, R. E. (1995). Teflon granuloma of the larynx: Etiology, pathophysiology, and management. *Annals of Otology, Rhinology and Laryngology, 104*(7), 511–515.

Verdolini, K. (2000). Resonant voice therapy. In J. C. Stemple (Ed.), *Voice therapy: Clinical studies* (2nd ed.). San Diego, CA: Singular.

Verdolini, K., & Ramig, L. (2001). Review: Occupational risks for voice problems. *Logopedics, Phoniatrics, and Vocology, 26,* 37–46.

Verdolini, K., Rosen, C. A., & Branski, R. C. (2006). *Classification manual for voice disorders-I.* Mahwah, NJ: Lawrence Erlbaum Associates.

Verdolini-Marston, K., Burke, M. K., Lessac, A., Glaze, L., & Caldwell, E. (1995). Preliminary study of two methods of treatment for laryngeal nodules. *Journal of Voice, 9*(1), 74–85.

Verdonck-de Leeuw, I. M., & Mahieu, H. F. (2004). Vocal aging and the impact on daily life: A longitudinal study. *Journal of Voice, 18,* 193–202.

Vertigan, A. E., Theodoros, D. G., Winkworth, A. L., & Gibson, P. G. (2007). Perceptual voice characteristics in chronic cough and paradoxical vocal fold movement. *Folia Phoniatrica et Logopaedica, 59,* 256–267.

Vogel, D., Carter, J. E., & Carter, P. B. (2000). *The effects of drugs on communication disorders* (2nd ed.). San Diego, CA: Singular.

Von Berg, S., & McFarlane, S. C. (2002a). A collaborative approach to the diagnosis and treatment of child voice disorders. *ASHA Special Interest Division 3,*

Perspectives on Voice and Voice Disorders, 12(1), 19–22.

Von Berg, S., & McFarlane, S. C. (2002b). *Differential diagnosis of dysphonia in an adolescent with complex medical history.* Paper presented at the annual convention of the American Speech-Language-Hearing Association, Atlanta, GA.

Von Berg, S., Watterson, T. L., & Fudge, L. A. (1999). Behavioral management of paradoxical vocal fold movement. *Phonoscope, 2*(3), 145–149.

Walner, D. L., & Cotton, R. T. (1999). Acquired anomalies of the larynx and trachea. In R. T. Cotton & C. M. Meyer (Eds.), *Practical pediatric otolaryngology* (3rd ed., pp. 515–538). Philadelphia: Lippincott-Raven.

Ward, E. C., Koh, S. K., Frisby, J., & Hodge, R. (2003). Differential modes of alaryngeal communication and long-term voice outcomes following pharyngolaryngectomy and laryngectomy. *Folia Phoniatrica et Logopaedica, 55*(1), 39–49.

Ware, J. E., & Sherbourne, C. D. (1992). The MOS 36-item short-form health survey (SF-36). *Medical Care, 30,* 473–481.

Warren, D. W. (1979). PERCI: A method for rating palatal efficiency. *Cleft Palate Journal, 16,* 279–285.

Watterson, T. L., Hansen-Magorian, H., & McFarlane, S. C. (1990). A demographic description of laryngeal contact ulcer patients. *Journal of Voice, 4,* 71–75.

Watterson, T. L., Hinton, J., & McFarlane, S. C. (1996). Novel stimuli for obtaining nasalance measures from young children. *Cleft Palate- Craniofacial Journal, 33,* 67–73.

Watterson, T. L., Lewis, K. E., & Deutsch, C. (1998). Nasalance and nasality in low pressure and high pressure speech. *Cleft Palate-Craniofacial Journal, 35,* 293–298.

Watterson, T. L., & McFarlane, S. C. (1990). Transnasal videoendoscopy of the velopharyngeal port mechanism. *Seminars in Speech and Language, 11,* 27–37.

Watterson, T. L., & McFarlane, S. C. (1991). Transoral and transnasal laryngeal endoscopy. *Seminars in Speech and Language, 12,* 77–87.

Watterson, T. L., & McFarlane, S. C. (1992). Adductor and abductor spasmodic dysphonia: Different disorders. *American Journal of Speech- Language Pathology, 1,* 19–20.

Watterson, T. L., & McFarlane, S. C. (1995). The artificial larynx. *Seminars in Speech and Language, 12,* 205–215.

Watterson, T., McFarlane, S. C., & Diamond, K. L. (1993). Phoneme effects on vocal effort and vocal quality. *American Journal of Speech and Language Pathology, 2,* 74–78.

Watterson, T., McFarlane, S. C., & Menicucci, A. (1990). Vibratory characteristics of Teflon-injected and noninjected paralyzed vocal folds. *Journal of Speech and Hearing Disorders, 55,* 61–66.

Watterson, T. L., York, S. L., & McFarlane, S. C. (1994). Effect of vocal loudness on nasalance measures. *Journal of Communication Disorders, 27,* 257–262.

Watts, C., Murphy, J., & Barnes-Burroughs, K. (2003). Pitch matching accuracy of trained singers, untrained subjects with talented singing voices, and untrained subjects with nontalented singing voices in conditions of varying feedback. *Journal of Voice, 17*(2), 185–194.

Webb, A. L., Carding, P. N., Deary, I. J., MacKenzie, K., Steen, N., & Wilson, J. A. (2004). The reliability of three perceptual evaluation scales for dysphonia. *European Archives of Otorhinolaryngology, 261,* 429–434.

Weed, D. T., Jewett, B. S., Rainey, C., Zealear, D. L., Stone, R. E., Ossoff, R. H., & Netterville, J. L. (1996). Long-term follow-up of recurrent laryngeal nerve avulsion for the treatment of spastic dysphonia. *Annals of Otology, Rhinology and Laryngology, 105,* 592–601.

Weinrich, B. (2002). Common voice disorders in children. *ASHA Special Interest Division 3, Perspectives on Voice and Voice Disorders, 12*(1), 13–16.

Weiss, L., & McFarlane, S. C. (1998). Responses to clinical stimulation as prognostic indicators of vocal recovery. *Phonoscope, 1,* 165–177.

Wetmore, S. I., Key, J. M., & Suen, J. Y. (1985). Complications of laser surgery for laryngeal papillomatosis. *Laryngoscope, 95,* 798–803.

Whited, R. E. (1979). Laryngeal dysfunction following prolonged intubation. *Annals of Otolaryngology, Rhinology and Laryngology, 88,* 474–478.

Williamson, A. B. (1945). Diagnosis and treatment of seventy-two cases of hoarse voice. *Quarterly Journal of Speech, 31,* 189–202.

Wilson, D. K. (1987). *Voice problems of children* (3rd ed.). Baltimore: Lippincott.

Wilson, F. B., Oldring, D. J., & Mueller, J. (1980). Recurrent laryngeal nerve dissection: A case report involving return of spastic dysphonia after initial surgery. *Journal of Speech and Hearing Disorders, 45,* 112–118.

Wingate, J., Brown, W., Shrivastav, R., Davenport, P., & Sapienza, C. (2007). Treatment outcomes for professional voice users. *Journal of Voice, 21,* 433–449.

Wingate, J., & Collins, S. (2005, November). *Consistency of voice range profiles in normal speakers.* Paper presented at the annual ASHA Convention, San Diego, CA.

Wingfield, W. L., Pollock, D., Gunert, R. R. (1969). Therapeutic efficacy of amantadine-HCL and rumantidine-HCL in naturally occurring influence A2 respiratory illness in many. *New England Journal of Medicine, 281,* 579–584.

Winkler, R., & Sendlmeier, W. (2006). EGG open quotient in aging voices—Changes with increasing chronological age and its perception. *Logopedics Phoniatrics Vocology, 31,* 51–56.

Wirz, S. (1986). The voice of the deaf. In M. Fawcus (Ed.), *Voice disorders and their management.* London: Croom Helm.

Witt, P., Cohen, D., Grames, L. M., & Marsh, J. (1999). Sphincter pharyngoplasty for the surgical management of speech dysfunction associated with velocardiofacial syndrome. *British Journal of Plastic Surgery, 52*(8), 613–618.

Wolfe, V. I., Martin, D. P., & Palmer, C. I. (2000). Perception of dysphonic voice quality by naive listeners. *Journal of Speech, Language, and Hearing Research, 43,* 697–705.

Wolpe, J. (1987). *Essential principles and practices of behavior therapy.* Phoenix, AZ: Milton H. Erickson Foundation.

Woo, P. (2006). Office-based laryngeal procedures. *Otolaryngologic Clinics of North America, 39,* 111–133.

Woo, P., Casper, J., Colton, R., & Brewer, D. (1992). Dysphonia in the aging: Physiology versus disease. *Laryngoscope, 102,* 139–144.

Wuyts, F. L., De Bodt, M. S., & Van de Heyning, P. H. (1999). Is the reliability of a visual analog scale higher than an ordinal scale? An experiment with the GRBAS scale for the perceptual evaluation of dysphonia. *Journal of Voice, 13,* 508–517.

Xu, Z., Xia, Z., Wang, Z., & Jiang, F. (2007). Pediatric sulcus vocalis. *Lin Chung Er Bi Yan Hou Tou Jing Wai Ke Za Zh, 21*(12), 550–551.

Xue, S. A., & Deliyski, D. (2001). Effects of aging on selected voice parameters: Preliminary normative data and educational implications. *Educational Gerontology, 27,* 159–168.

Yamaguchi, H., Shrivastav, R., Andrews, M. L., & Niimi, S. A. (2003). Comparison of voice quality ratings made by Japanese and American listeners using the GRBAS scale. *Folia Phoniatrica et Logopaedica, 55,* 147–157.

Yiu, E. M. L., Chan, K. M. K., & Mok, R. S. M. (2007). Reliability and confidence in using a paired comparison paradigm in perceptual voice quality evaluation. *Clinical Linguistics and Phonetics, 21,* 129–145.

Yorkston, K. M., Beukelman, D. R., Strand, E. A., & Bell, K. R. (1999). *Management of motor speech disorders in children and adults.* Austin, TX: Pro-Ed.

Yorkston, K. M., Miller, R. M., & Strand, E. A. (2004). *Management of speech and swallowing in degenerative diseases.* Tuscon, AZ: Communication Skill Builders.

Yumoto, E., Gould, W. J., & Baer, T. (1982). Harmonics-to-noise ratio as an index to the degree of hoarseness. *Journal of the Acoustical Society of America, 71,* 1544–1550.

Zealer, D. L., Billante, C. R., Courey, M. S., Netterville, J. L., Paniello, R. C., Sanders, I., et al. (2003). Reanimation of the paralyzed human larynx with an implantable electrical stimulation device. *Laryngoscope, 113*(7), 1149–1156.

Zeine, L., & Walter, K. L. (2002). The voice and its care: Survey findings from actors' perspectives. *Journal of Voice, 16,* 229–243.

Zeitels, S. M., Hillman, R. E., Desloge, R., Mauri, M., & Doyle, P. B. (2002). Phonomicrosurgery in singers and performing artists: Treatment outcomes, management theories, and future directions. *Annals of Otology, Rhinology and Laryngology, Supplement 190,* 21–40.

Zemlin, W. R. (1988). *Speech and Hearing Science: Anatomy and Physiology* (3rd ed.). Englewood Cliffs, NJ: Prentice Hall.

Zemlin, W. R. (1998). *Speech and hearing science: Anatomy and physiology* (4th ed.). Englewood Cliffs, NJ: Prentice Hall.

Zraick, R. I., Birdwell, K. Y., & Smith-Olinde, L. K. (2005). The effect of speaking sample duration on determination of habitual pitch. *Journal of Voice, 19,* 197–201.

Zraick, R. I., Davenport, D. J., Tabbal, S. D., Hicks, G. S., Hutton, T. J., & Patterson, J. (2004). Reliability of speech intelligibility ratings using the Unified Huntington's Disease Rating Scale. *Journal of Medical Speech-Language Pathology, 12,* 31–40.

Zraick, R. I., Dennie, T. M., Tabbal, S. D., Hutton, T. J., Hicks, G. S., & O'Sullivan, P. (2003). Reliability of speech intelligibility ratings using the Unified Parkinson's Disease Rating Scale. *Journal of Medical Speech-Language Pathology, 11,* 227–240.

Zraick, R. I., Gentry, M. A., Smith-Olinde, L., & Gregg, B. A. (2006). The effect of speaking context on determination of habitual pitch. *Journal of Voice, 20,* 545–554.

Zraick, R. I., Gregg, B. A., & Whitehouse, E. L. (2006). Speech and voice characteristics of geriatric speakers: A review of the literature and a call for research and training. *Journal of Medical Speech-Language Pathology, 14,* 133–142.

Zraick, R. I., Keyes, M., Montague, J., & Keiser, J. (2002). Mid-basal-to-ceiling versus mid-ceiling-to-basal elicitation of maximum phonational frequency range. *Journal of Voice, 16,* 317–322.

Zraick, R. I., Klaben, B., Connor, N., Thiebault, S., Kempster, G., Glaze, L., et al. (2007 November). *Results of the CAPE-V validation study.* Seminar at the Annual Convention of the American Speech-Language-Hearing Association, Boston.

Zraick, R. I. & Liss, J. M. (2000). A comparison of equal-appearing interval scaling and direct magnitude estimation of nasal voice quality. *Journal of Speech and Hearing Research, 43*(4), 979–988.

Zraick, R. I., Liss, J. M., Dorman, M. F., Case, J. L., LaPointe, L. L., & Beals, S. P. (2000). Multidimensional scaling of nasal voice quality. *Journal of Speech and Hearing Research, 43*(4), 989–996.

Zraick, R. I., Marshall, W. C., Smith-Olinde, L., & Montague, J. C. (2004).The effect of speaking task on determination of habitual loudness. *Journal of Voice, 18,* 176–182.

Zraick, R. I., Nelson, J. C., Montague, J. C., & Monoson, P. K. (2000). The effect of task on determination of maximum phonational frequency range. *Journal of Voice, 14,* 154–160.

Zraick, R. I., & Risner, B. Y. (2008). Assessment of quality of life in persons with voice disorders. *Current Opinion in Otolaryngology & Head and Neck Surgery, 16,* 188–193.

Zraick, R. I., Risner, B. Y., Smith-Olinde, L., Gregg, B. A., Johnson, F. L., & McWeeny, E. K. (2006). Patient versus partner perception of voice handicap. *Journal of Voice, 21,* 485–494.

Zraick, R. I., & Skaggs, S. D., & Montague, J. C. (2000). The effect of task on determination of habitual pitch. *Journal of Voice, 14,* 484–489.

Zraick, R. I., Wendel, K. W., & Smith-Olinde, L. (2005). The effect of speaking task on perceptual judgment of the severity of dysphonic voice. *Journal of Voice, 19,* 574–581.

Zur, K., Cotton, S., Kelchner, L., Baker, S., Weinrich, B., & Lee, L. (2007). Pediatric Voice Handicap Index (pVHI): A new tool for evaluating pediatric dysphonia.

International Journal of Pediatric Otorhinolaryngology, 71, 77–82.

Zwitman, D. H. (1990). Utilization of transoral endoscopy to assess velopharyngeal closure. *Seminars in Speech and Language, 11,* 38–46.

Zwitman, D. H., & Calcaterra, T. C. (1973). The "silent cough" method for vocal hyperfunction. *Journal of Speech and Hearing Disorders, 38,* 119–125.

Zwitman, D. H., Gyepes, M. T., & Ward, P. H. (1976). Assessment of velar and lateral wall movement by oral telescope and radiographic examination in patients with velopharyngeal inadequacy and in normal subjects. *Journal of Speech and Hearing Disorders, 41,* 381–389.

Products and Organizations

American Cancer Society, The National Cancer Information Center.

B & K Real-Time Frequency Analyzer. Naerum, Denmark: Bruel & Kjaer.

Blue Tree Tri Pack, Vocal Pathology. Lynnwood, WA: Blue Tree Publishing.

Computerized Speech Lab. Lincoln Park, NJ: KayPENTAX.

Dr. Speech. Neu-Anspach, Germany: Tiger DRS, Inc.

Facilitator. Lincoln Park, NJ: KayPENTAX.

FonoView. Sound card-CD Windows. Milwaukee, WI: Speech Bin.

Hearit. Tucson, AZ:

International Association of Laryngectomees, P.O. Box 691060, Stockton, CA 95269.

Language Master. Chicago: Bell and Howell.

Nasometer. Lincoln Park, NJ: KayPENTAX.

National Association of Teachers of Singing (NATS). www.NATS.org.

Phonatory Function Analyzer, FS-77. Nagashima Medical Instruments. Richmond, VA: Kelleher Medical Instruments.

Phonic Ear Vois. Mill Valley, CA: H. C. Electronics.

PM 100 Pitch Analyzer. Lincoln Park, NJ: KayPENTAX.

Self-Help for the Laryngectomee (Lauder).

Tonar II. This instrument, developed by S. G. Fletcher in 1970, is no longer commercially available.

Tunemaster III. Ridgewood, NJ: Berkshire Instruments.

VASTA. Voice and Speech Trainers Association, www.VASTA.org

Visi-Pitch. Lincoln Park, NJ: KayPENTAX.

Vocaid. Tucson, AZ: Texas Instruments, Communication Builders.

Vocal Loudness Indicator. Moline, IL: LinguiSystems.

Voice Instrumentation. Minneapolis, MN: Artic Arion Products.

Voice Monitor. Hollins, VA: Communication Research Unit.

VoxMetria. Software analysis of voice and voice quality. Milwaukee, WI: Speech Bin.

CONTENTS TO THE DVD

Case Studies

CS.1 Differential Diagnosis of a Complex Voice Disorder

CS.2 Ventricular Dysphonia with Laryngocele

CS.3 Unilateral Vocal Fold Paralysis

CS.4 Child Voice Dyad

CS.5 Functional Aphonia

CS.6 Functional Dysphonia Associated with Reflux

CS.7 Open-Mouth Approach

CS.8 Parkinson's Disease

CS.9 Spastic Dysarthria

CS.10 Vocal Nodules

CS.11 Vocal Overuse

Facilitating Approaches (See Table 7.1 in text)

FA.1 Auditory Feedback

FA.2 Change of Loudness

FA.3 Chant Talk

FA.4 Chewing

FA.5 Confidential Voice

FA.6 Counseling

FA.7 Digital Manipulation

FA.8 Elimination of Abuses

FA.9 Establishing a New Pitch

FA.10 Focus

FA.11 Glottal Fry

FA.12 Head Positioning

FA.13 Hierarchy Analysis

FA.14 Inhalation Phonation

FA.15 Laryngeal Massage

FA.16 Masking

FA.17 Nasal/Glide Stimulation

FA.18 Open-Mouth Approach

FA.19 Pitch Inflections

FA.20 Redirected Phonation

FA.21 Relaxation

FA.22 Respiration Training

FA.23 Tongue-Protrusion /i/

FA.24 Visual Feedback

FA.25 Yawn–Sigh

Laryngeal Images Photo Gallery

Normal Vocal Folds

Polypoid Degeneration

Presbylaryngis

Recurrent Respiratory Papilloma

Reflux Laryngitis

Vocal Fold Atrophy (Right Vocal Fold Paralysis)

Vocal Fold Cyst

Vocal Fold Ectasia-Varice

Vocal Fold Hemorrhage

Vocal Fold Nodules

Vocal Fold Polyp

Vocal Process Granuloma

Acknowledgements

Words cannot praise the London Library highly enough. It is a private institution where a member has access not only to an extensive library but can carry off great numbers of books, even reference books, for loans that can extend crucially into years. My only dread was the call of another member in need of one of "my" volumes. Heartfelt thanks go to this great, individualistic institution and its unfailingly helpful staff. There are many individuals who have helped me write this book.

Thanks first to Sheila Murphy, who fifteen years ago or so first suggested the queens as a marvellous subject for a book. The idea lurked in my subconscious during my next two writing marathons. Only then was I able to begin. Sheila has been the first critical eye to read every one of my books, and her suggestions and generous editorial comments on *Elizabeth and Mary* were invaluable. Others I should like to thank include Lola Bubbosh, the late Sheila Dickinson, Sue Greenhill, Beryl Hislop, Rosalind Oxenford, Dr. Peter Shephard, the late David Thesen, and Elizabeth Walston. Particular thanks to Robin Bell for permission to quote from his elegant translations of Mary Queen of Scots' poems, previously published as *Bittersweet Within My Heart*.

On a professional front, I could not have a better agent than Derek Johns and his great team at A. P. Watt. Derek has transformed my working life. Warm thanks to him and his assistant, Anjali Pratap. Derek's greatest gifts to me as his author are my editors, Carol Janeway at Knopf in the United States and Arabella Pike at HarperCollins. Arabella has brought an incisive intelligence to everything, applied with such warmth and humour that it has been a delight to work with her. Around her are a team whose extraordinary quality was epitomized by a magical candle-lit banquet and firework display at Hampton Court Palace. Tilly Ware organised it, and nobody lucky enough to be there will ever forget it.

The last year of writing this book was inextricably linked for me with the final illness of my father. A great family enterprise brought our whole band of brothers and sisters together to care for him: so Karen, Mark, Isabel, Brigid, Tricia, Andy and Sue, with their own generous families, have all become a part of it, and none more than our mother, Ellinor, with her zest for life and instinctive understanding of death.

The writer's life is inevitably isolated and hard for those closest to her. My own family, Lily, Ben, Jess and Nick's daughter Sophia, have brought patience, insight and support to me during difficult times. And Ellie and Theo have arrived to gladden our hearts. Closest of all to the rock face is Nick, my partner in most things, my linguist, lightning conductor and love.

Moray and his counter charges against the Queen of Scots would be heard. The commissioners representing both antagonists gathered at the beginning of October 1568. Moray came himself and although Mary was not present she had Lord Herries and the Bishop of Ross amongst others to make her case. The Duke of Norfolk, Earl of Sussex and Sir Ralph Sadler were there to represent Elizabeth in her role of arbitrator, given express instructions by her that Mary's responsibility for murdering her husband had to be established beyond doubt otherwise she would be instrumental in returning her cousin to her rightful throne, "having regard to the princely state wherein she was born."[30]

Moray was not slow to produce what he considered to be his *coup de grâce*, the letters purportedly written in Mary's hand, found in the silver-gilt casket in the keeping of a servant of Bothwell after his defeat at Carberry Hill. He revealed privately to Norfolk and his fellow commissioners these eight letters and a series of sonnets, astonishingly torrid with sexual feeling and suggestively conspiratorial in the murder of Darnley.

If these "casket letters" were in fact genuine, they were unambiguously incriminating both of Mary's complicity in, if not incitement of, the murder of her husband, the King, and in her illicit and overwhelming sexual passion for the man who was the chief suspect in his death. There was much circumstantial detail which was reinforced by other sources, and the central strand of emotion in them had a certain sincerity and truth. However, the originals disappeared soon after their exposure, some said destroyed by James VI in the 1580s to protect his mother's reputation. Relying only on copies in the absence of the originals, debate has raged for nearly four and a half centuries, and the truth cannot now be known. Mary was never allowed to examine them and consistently denied their authenticity. Buchanan, knowing the Queen personally, having been her Latin tutor and therefore also in close contact with her handwriting and phraseology, declared the letters and poems were genuine. By this time, however, he had become a hostile witness, basing much of his subsequent notorious attack* on Mary on the revelations of these letters. The likelihood is that they were partly, or even wholly, forgeries; genuine letters from Mary interpolated with incriminating words and phrases, genuine letters from another of Bothwell's lovers that had been made to appear to be from Mary, possibly amalgamations of more than one source, or out and out fabrications.

Norfolk was horrified by what he read. In his letter to Elizabeth on

* *Detectio Mariae Reginae Scotorum (A Detection of Mary Queen of Scots)*, George Buchanan, 1571.

11 October 1568, he could not disguise his shock: "they shewed unto us one horrible and longe lettre of her owne hand, as they saye, contayninge foule matteir and abhominable, to be either thowght of, or to be written by a prince . . . The said lettres and ballades do discover suche inordinate 'and filthie' [scored out] love betwene her and Bothaill, her loothesomnes and abhorringe of her husband that was murdered. . ." He concluded that the writings contained so much circumstantial evidence "unknowen to anie other then to herselfe and Bothaill [Bothwell]"[31] that it would have been hard to counterfeit them: yet if they were genuine then a judgement as to Mary's guilt as an accomplice to the murder of her husband could not be avoided. He awaited Elizabeth's response as to how they should proceed.

Elizabeth seemed not overtly alarmed, and certainly not concerned to press to establish Mary's guilt. Even when she eventually saw the letters for herself a couple of months later, after the inquiry had reconvened in London, she told Knollys matter-of-factly that they "conteyned manny matters very unmete *to come from a 'quene'* [scored out] to be repeated before honest eares, and easely drawn to be apparent proves ageynst the Quene."[32] She did demand, however, that the inquiry move to Westminster better to assess the evidence, and it was convened on 25 November. To assuage Mary's suspicions, Norfolk was ordered to explain that this move was in order to save time, bypassing some of the delay in sending communications to and fro. Elizabeth was anxious that Mary and her commissioners should continue to think that there was little doubt that her cause would be successful, and that the inquiry was concerned primarily in the detail of her restoration and the safeguarding of her son's interests.

Norfolk's personal ambitions, however, appeared to overcome his disapproval of Mary's unqueenly behaviour as suggested by the casket letters. Soon he was confiding a contrary view to her commissioner, Maitland of Lethington. In his opinion Elizabeth's real purpose was to prolong Mary's confinement, thus allowing Moray to blacken her reputation as much as possible and so damage her popular following in England. In this way, he suggested, Elizabeth meant to undermine the powerful Catholic support that was building around the charismatic image of the unjustly imprisoned Mary.

The Duke of Norfolk was Elizabeth's premier nobleman. A vain, vacillating man, he had grown resentful that his princely status and vast wealth did not translate into greater influence at court. He aspired to something even grander. To be the consort of the Queen of Scotland, with the chance of becoming even, through her, the King of England, suited the amour-propre of this thrice-widowed, thirty-two-year-old

magnate. Knollys had been postulating an English marriage for Mary as the only way, in the event of releasing her, to neutralise the threat she posed of inviting French or Spanish interference into the land. He thought the safest way to rein her in was to marry her to a kinsman of Elizabeth's, specifically his own nephew George Carey, who was a cousin of the Queen's on her Boleyn side. But Norfolk, in need of a wife himself, could think of no better way to advance his own status. He began making moves to canvass support for his plan almost immediately. By the end of the year the gossip around court was full of his aspirations, but for a while Elizabeth was kept in the dark. This was a perilous act. It meant Norfolk was less than impartial in a murder enquiry where the suspect was the focus of his own high ambitions. The secrecy meant too that his negotiations looked suspiciously like a conspiracy in the making.

Inevitably the rumours reached the Queen. When Elizabeth asked Norfolk frankly if his marriage plans involved the Queen of Scots he theatrically denied everything: "What! . . . Should I seek to marry her, being so wicked a woman, such a notorious adulteress and murderer? I love to sleep upon a safe pillow."[33] Elizabeth was not to forget this and Norfolk's words would return to haunt him.

The inquiry continued at Westminster to the end of the year. With a flourish, Moray produced the pretty casket, engraved with the imperial monogram of François II and unmistakably once belonging to Mary. From it he extracted the treacherous letters, now for everyone to see. Copies were duly made: everyone was pruriently riveted and aghast in equal measure. But Mary refused to answer her accusers except in person, and Elizabeth was not about to allow her sweet eloquence and personal charm any formal airing before the most notable councillors and nobility of her land. With consummate skill she side-stepped her request by pointing out that she could not allow Mary to demean herself by giving credence, through her presence, to charges based on this tawdry evidence.

Although Mary had not been shown the letters, she consistently and forcefully maintained that any such writings were undoubted forgeries.

Moray swore to their authenticity. The truth was probably somewhere between the two. The author of any deception, however, was another area for surmise and debate. The longest letter, known as the second letter, probably caused the most trouble. If true, it revealed a murderous duplicity and contempt by a queen and wife towards her ill and pathetic husband. Doubly damning was the fact that this callousness was united with a venal passion for the masterful lover, and her hus-

band's would-be murderer. Purportedly written from Glasgow, where Mary had gone to bring back the sick Darnley to Edinburgh, having promised to resume conjugal relations with him as an inducement, the writer addressed Bothwell:

> *God forgive me, and God knytt us togither for ever, for the most faythfull couple that ever he did knytt together. This is my fayth, I will dye in it. Excuse it, yf I write yll, you must gesse the one halfe, I can not doo with all, for I am yll at ease, and glad to write unto you when other folkes be asleepe, seeing that I cannot doo as they doo, according to my desyre, that is betwene your armes, my deere lyfe, whom I besech God to preserve from all yll . . . Cursed be this pocky fellow that troublith me thus muche, for I had a pleasanter matter to discourse with you, but for him. He is not muche the worse, but he is yll arayde. I thought I shuld have bene kylled with his breth, for it is worse than your uncles breth, and yet I was sett no neerer to him than in a chayre by his bolster, and he lyeth at the furder syd of the bed.*

The letter continued with a great deal more conversational, rambling detail, and then ended "Burne this lettre, for it is too dangerous . . . Now if to please you my deere lyfe, I spare nether honour, conscience, nor hazard, nor greatnes, take it in good parte . . . I pray you give no credit, against the most faythfull lover that ever you had or shall have. See not also her [his wife Jean?] whose faynid teares you ought not more to regarde than the true travails which I endure to deserve her place, for obtayning of which against my own nature, I doo betraye those that could lett me. God forgive me, and give you my only friend and good luck and prosperitie that your humble and faythfull lover doth wisshe unto you; who hopith shortly to be an other thing unto you, for the reward of my paynes."[34]

The female character that emerged from this letter was obdurately set against her young, frightened and ill husband who was begging for forgiveness and a restoration of his conjugal life with her. She was prepared to sacrifice his life together with her conscience and honour in order to satisfy her own and her lover's desire to be united. The Scottish and English commissioners and nobility who read these apparently most intimate confessions of the Queen of Scots were likely to have found them initially as repellant and frightening as did the Duke of Norfolk. There was however less evidence of contemporary public denunciation of Mary's character as a result, or declaration as to the authenticity of the documents, than followed in the centuries of debate that followed. This

was possibly due to Elizabeth's coolness on the matter and strong disapproval of their public dissemination.

Elizabeth possibly understood better than anyone how the attitudes and emotions unmasked in the "casket letters" were not just a devastating destruction of Mary's reputation but were also an attack on every "unnatural" woman in a position of authority. Her attempts at protecting Mary from public vilification went on throughout her reign with various proclamations against a variety of books and pamphlets. The soldier-poet and playwright George Whetstone,* looking back on this time, commented that Elizabeth "forbad the bookes of [Mary's] faultes, to be conversant among her English subjects which almost in every other nation were made vulgar."[35] Norfolk's view that this was Elizabeth's double-dealing in action, being seen publicly to do well by Mary while allowing the slander of murder and adultery to hang over her head indefinitely, might have been part of the reason for her carefulness of Mary's fame. It was just as likely, however, that highly sensitised as she was to her own reputation, Elizabeth wished to protect them both personally and as female monarchs from defamation. All the worst qualities of emotionalism, weak-mindedness and treachery were still believed to belong to the female and to gain frightening proportions with the promotion of women to power.

Mary's commissioners repudiated the inquiry and withdrew when permission for Mary to appear in front of Elizabeth was refused. Judgement was deferred and the inquiry dismantled with no movement in any direction. As Norfolk had predicted, through sleight of hand Elizabeth had managed to maintain her favourite diplomatic stance, self-righteous and Janus-faced as the guardian of her throne without actually having to take any decisive action at all.

Mary was left bereft of hope. Suddenly the tide was comprehensively against her, and without her being aware of the turn. Peremptorily, she was moved in early February 1569 from Bolton to the medieval castle of Tutbury, a windy, exposed and semi-derelict fortress in Staffordshire. Of all the places Mary was kept during her long English imprisonment, Tutbury was the one she loathed most. Ill-furnished and uncomfortable, freezing cold and plagued with damp, it was one of the properties belonging to the Earl of Shrewsbury, an austere but sympathetic and just man, who had been chosen to replace the overly susceptible Knollys as Mary's keeper.

---

* George Whetstone (1550–87) is principally remembered for his play *Promos and Cassandra*, written in 1578 in rhymed verse, which provided the plot for Shakespeare's *Measure for Measure*.

In an impassioned letter to Elizabeth written later that year from the fastness of Tutbury, Mary's description of the rough treatment of herself and her servants, and the "bodily fear" it occasioned in her, had uneasy echoes of the fear Elizabeth endured at the hands of her own sister while imprisoned during the investigation of the Wyatt rebellion. Mary's pleas not to be left "to waste away in tears and complaints . . . at least let me not be placed in the hands of any one suspicious to my friends and relations, for fear of false reports . . ." reflected the exact anxiety which had haunted Elizabeth. Her valediction was also affecting: "I shall pray God to give you a happy and long life, and me a better share of your favour than to my sorrow I perceive that I have, whereto I shall commend myself affectionately to the end . . . Your very affectionate distressed sister and cousin."[36]

Elizabeth was not happy with the role in which she was cast by Mary in her unhappy imprisonment. She did not see herself as an unjust oppressor, and certainly not as the persecutor of a fellow queen. She was bombarded by Mary with pathetic letters full of complaints and half-suppressed rage. Much of the time she did not answer them, for the answers could only be the same. But the weight of them and the guilt, frustration and self-righteousness they roused in Elizabeth were hard to bear. Running through the letters was the threnody of Mary's close kinship with Elizabeth (daughter, sister, cousin) and her longing to meet her. This she was continually denied, and the anguished impotence of her enforced isolation from the Queen had Mary resorting to the language of unrequited love: if allowed into Elizabeth's presence at last, "I shall discover to you the secrets of my heart . . . I shall devote myself more and more to love, honour, and obey you . . . and if you please so to favour me, I would beg of you first of all to command me when you please, where you please, in what company, to remain as secretly, as long or as short, without seeing or being seen but by you, with whom alone I have to do."[37]

While equivocating and parrying her cousin's pleas for an audience, for fairer treatment, for restoration of her crown, for her place in the succession, Elizabeth still tried to console Mary with warm promises which by now had grown increasingly threadbare. She vowed that she would protect her reputation and keep private the false accusations against her, "praying her to take patience in [Elizabeth's] gentle ward, where she was nearer at hand to get the crown of England set upon her head," and assuring her that she herself, "who was but the eldest sister,"[38] was likely to die before her.

Mary was not consoled. Her expectation of freedom at last was replaced with the depressed realisation that Elizabeth might profess

determination to restore her to her throne but the hard prescriptions of politics and the prerogatives of power made it very difficult for her to do so. On one occasion in April 1569, when she had hoped to keep the French sympathetic in her stand-off with the Spanish over their captured payships, Elizabeth thought the political benefits of releasing Mary might be worth the risks. After procrastinating for months, however, Moray flatly refused to have her back, much to Elizabeth's fury. The problem of what to do with Mary was left explosively in her hands.

By the end of the summer of 1569, the possible restoration of Mary had become bound up in many of the English councillors' minds with the advantage of containing her appetite for trouble by marrying her off to Norfolk. What had begun as Norfolk's singular ambition now involved a motley band of men with mixed, even contradictory, interests in a controversial enterprise initially cooked up behind Elizabeth's back. The most unlikely alliance was between the long-sworn enemies Norfolk and Leicester. Leicester's disingenuous explanation of his careerist involvement was that despite his high regard for the Duke and his low regard for Mary, he was prepared to countenance such a match if it was best for the Queen and her kingdom: "there could be no better Remedie to provide for so dangerous a Woman . . . considering the present state of the World."[39]

Mary's own attempts at release had been focussed more on inveigling support, even armed intervention, from one or other of the Catholic powers. To Philip II of Spain she had sent the rash and over-optimistic message that if he "help me, I shall be Queen of England in three months, and Mass shall be said all over the country."[40] This inflated boast was intended to lure Philip from his usual passivity into some sign of solidarity. It revealed more tellingly, however, the unreality of an indulged woman who had relied always on her charm to effect everything. It led her to believe that now, in a neighbouring kingdom, she could translate her personal charisma into a national fervour powerful enough, with the help of Spanish gold, to dethrone Elizabeth herself.

Her English cousin, after a decade of rule, had established herself beyond doubt as a competent and popular monarch who inspired in her phalanx of advisors a fundamental loyalty. Despite the storms of temper she unleashed periodically at their heads, Elizabeth could be relied on to offer Cecil and her council a reciprocal loyalty and an openness to reason and compromise, an utterly serious acceptance of her obligations as queen. Compromise and obligation were alien concepts to a princess raised in the French court of Henri II, and they were unwelcome

restraints on the character of a queen who had ruled through personal passions, impulse and defiance.

The Norfolk marriage plan had been put to Mary in May 1569 and she had jumped at the chance.* Rather crucially, however, it needed Elizabeth's blessing, and no one was keen to be the one to tell her. Norfolk himself had already denied to her face that her suspicions were well-founded. His subsequent evasions only suggested something sinister was afoot. In fact when Leicester eventually told Elizabeth of the plan in September 1569 she was incensed and unsettled. That Leicester, her greatest intimate, should have supported such a match through his own opportunism, ingratiating himself, it seemed, with someone he thought might be a future sovereign, hurt her feelings. But what threatened her life, Elizabeth felt, was the alliance of her premier nobleman with the greatest rival for her throne. The Catholicism of one and the near Catholicism of the other only added to the danger. She told a chastened Leicester that she believed she would have ended up once more in the dreaded Tower if those two had been allowed to marry. Although this was an outburst sprung in the heat of emotion, the very fact that she could think her position so precarious indicated the extent of Elizabeth's insecurity in the face of Mary's legitimate claim to her throne.

Mary posed much more than a political threat to Elizabeth. For a solitary, unmarried queen, a woman bereft of immediate family, the loyalty of her closest associates was of paramount importance. Leicester was her lifelong intimate: the fever of passion may have passed but a possessive and close affection remained. For him to dilute his loyalty to Elizabeth with his favour of Mary's interests was an emotional betrayal of a particularly poignant kind. Elizabeth was jealous of the effect her Scottish cousin seemed to have on all who encountered her. It was becoming tediously predictable that every male bent a little at the knees and went weak in the head with even short-term exposure to Mary's personal charm. Sir Nicholas Throckmorton, seasoned ambassador, gave some compelling reasons why the Scottish Queen, "a Woman so ill thowght of heretofore," should suddenly be surrounded by English friends: "the first, hir misery; whereof all Men naturallie take Compassion: The second, hir Entertaynment of such as came to hir: And the third, Th'opinion that some had of hir Title in Succession."[41]

One of Elizabeth's officials had spent a night at Tutbury in the foul

---

* Mary was still married to Bothwell and would remain so until his death on 14 April 1578. From 1570 onwards there were various requests from Mary and her envoys to the Pope for nullification of the marriage by reason of it being bigamous, or Bothwell having taken Mary by force. If Mary had a serious suitor there is little doubt that she would have received dispensation from the Pope to marry a fourth husband.

winter of early 1569. One hour in Mary's company had so impressed him that he wrote to Cecil and his queen warning them, "there shulde veray few Subjects in this Land have Accesse to, or Conferens with this Lady. For besyd, that she is a goodly personadge, (and yet in trouthe not comparable to our Souverain) she hathe withall an alluring Grace, a prety *Scottishe* speche, and a serching Witt, clowded with Myldnes [and a searching intelligence softened with sweetness of manner]."[42] The highly infectious and indiscriminate nature of Mary's "alluring Grace" made her the most formidable rival, all the more so given that Elizabeth would never meet her and had to rely only on such reports from her half-smitten nobles and executives. In a time when the supernatural was a companion to daily life, this physical alienation from Mary's human reality meant her power inflated in imagination into something almost like sorcery.

Knollys, Lord Scrope, her own cousin George Carey, Norfolk, Throckmorton, the northern earls and eventually even solid Shrewsbury himself, who could she trust not to be entranced? For a while it seemed only Cecil, Elizabeth's cast-iron Secretary of State, was immune to the Queen of Scots, a fact of which Mary herself was acutely aware. Like all beautiful women who were used to getting what they wanted, she was galled by the rare individual who did not succumb to her charm. When she was not in one of her passions, vilifying him as "hir Enemy," she credited Cecil with intelligence and a respect for the law, for being "a faithefull Servaunt to his Mistress," while wanly wishing "it might be hir Luck to gett the Friendshipp of so wise a Man."[43]

While Mary hankered after an advisor of Cecil's calibre, Elizabeth had to deal with her manoeuvres for a fourth husband in the form of the less intellectually impressive, but more princely, Norfolk. The perfidious duke was immediately summoned to Elizabeth's presence. In fright he feigned illness. His sudden departure from court to return to his estates had caused all kinds of alarmist talk; his disobedience and continued absence set tongues wagging that Norfolk was mustering his forces in a show of treasonous rebellion. Even Elizabeth was worried and moved to the more defensible Windsor Castle. The ports were temporarily closed and extra guard put on the Queen of Scots. Elizabeth recognised that it was essential for her to maintain authority, particularly against the highest nobleman in the land. She could not leave unpunished his defiance of her peremptory order to attend her at court, even if it meant coming in an invalid's litter. Elizabeth knew that strong leadership meant the pack mentality of her nobles worked in her favour but that if she showed any weakness the rogue males could as easily turn on her and establish their own hierarchy of power. With Mary as a legitimate candidate for queen, they could gloss any treason with legality.

Norfolk might have had the desire for power but he lacked the nerve. He had been in urgent communication with the disaffected northern earls, his brother-in-law Westmoreland and Northumberland being the most bellicose. Having sworn he would not answer the Queen's summons, he did set out finally from his estates in Norfolk in the company of forty of his men on the last day of September. Within three days he was under house arrest, and by 10 October imprisoned in the Tower of London ("to[o] great a Terror for a trew Man"[44] as he had exclaimed to Elizabeth just two weeks before). He was to remain there for ten months, unhappy, uncomfortable but with his ambitions towards the Queen of Scots undimmed.

Mary's captivity and the close constraint of her days meant her hopes were artificially inflated and liable to extreme collapse. She was naturally a woman of action not reflection, and to be prevented from riding or hunting, which happened periodically as the political situation in England deteriorated, was a great hardship to her. Her energies were channelled into writing pleading affectionate letters to Elizabeth, angry and inflammatory ones to her family in France and other supporters, and devising plots for escape. Mary delighted in codes and ciphers and hidden messages and this fascination translated into the embroidery work she had enjoyed ever since she was a girl in France. When asked by an English visitor the previous January how she passed the time when the weather kept her indoors, Mary explained "that all that Day she wrought with hir Nydill, and that the Diversitie of the Colors made the Worke seme lesse tedious, and contynued so long at it till veray Payn made hir to give over."[45] The long hours waiting for deliverance were spent in devising motifs to embroider, choosing the colours and investing the images with layers of meaning. Often she worked alongside her jailer's wife.

The Countess of Shrewsbury, better known to posterity as Bess of Hardwick, was a redoubtable woman of exceptional will and ambition. A squire's daughter from Derbyshire, she married four successively wealthier husbands and, remarkably for the age, managed to hang on to all her accumulated wealth. The Earl of Shrewsbury was her last husband and their notoriously quarrelsome marriage took a far greater toll on him than on her. She was a dynamic builder of magnificent houses (Chatsworth and Hardwick Hall being just two of them), property speculator, money lender, dynastic engineer and gale-force personality. She outlived every husband by decades and even outlived her queen, though she was six years her senior, dying at last in 1608 at the defiant age of eighty-one. Perhaps she was more a woman to admire from a distance than to live with in close intimacy. Although Bess and Mary used differ-

ent powers to get what they wanted from the world, neither was capable of neutral relationships. Mary loved and hated with passion, often the same person and within the same week; Bess was more calculating and disciplined but unused to being denied or gainsaid. Their relationship was an interesting one. The Earl of Shrewsbury's custody of Mary lasted fifteen years, an imprisonment as much for him and his family as it was for his ward. It added enormous financial and emotional strains to his life, which no doubt affected his health (he was plagued with gout) and hastened his death.

To begin with, Bess and Mary were friends, although they would end as enemies, with Bess accusing her husband of committing adultery with their royal prisoner. Fifteen years the elder, the Countess of Shrewsbury was cast more as a mother figure to Mary, who was still only twenty-five when they first met. Their main activity together in those early years of captivity was embroidery, during which time they mapped out their images, selected their silks and wools, and practised their needlework. Shrewsbury wrote to Cecil that every day Mary would seek out Bess and they would work on their projects together, only talking of trifling matters he was quick to reassure. In fact the women's talk was full of court gossip, some of it highly malicious, about Elizabeth and her love affairs, her vanity, speculations about her recoil from marriage, all of which Mary later was to recount in a rash defamatory letter to Elizabeth, when she had fallen out with Bess and wanted revenge on the two iron-willed women who had her in their power.

Not only was the gossip anti-Elizabeth, some of the devices that Mary embroidered expressed her simmering anger, resentment against the Queen, and hope for renewed life and glory. The women would leaf through emblem books, popular in France and England during the sixteenth century, or Gesner's book, *Icones Animalium*, a catalogue of fine woodcuts of animals, birds and fishes published in 1560. These gave ideas for their work, some with added detail or Latin mottoes satisfyingly suggestive of hidden meaning. Mary embroidered one small panel of a tabby cat worked in orange wool with a crown on its head (Elizabeth was famously red-headed) and a little mouse, not in the original pattern, was added to the picture to emphasise the threatening nature of the ginger predator.

The most telling piece of embroidery was worked by Mary in about 1570 while Norfolk was still imprisoned but keeping their marriage hopes alive. It was a panel with a large vine at the centre, one half fruitful and laden with grapes, the other half almost leafless and barren of fruit. A large hand with a billhook was shown in the process of pruning

the barren branch under the motto *Virescit Vulnere Virtus*, "virtue flour-
ishes by wounding." This was sent as a cushion to Norfolk. Under the
guise of a pious homily about accepting the necessity of suffering, its
message from his impatient future bride was something much more
aggressive. It was recognised by the protagonists and their supporters as
a veiled encouragement to get rid of Elizabeth, the barren Tudor scion,
possibly even by killing her, so that the fertile, fruitful branch representing Mary could flourish.

Although Elizabeth did not know yet of this lethal embroidered
message, she feared that she was at risk from her disaffected northern
earls attempting precisely this excision. She ordered Mary to be moved
from the more salubrious Shrewsbury house at Wingfield, where she
had spent some of the summer, back to dreaded Tutbury Castle. Mary's
household also was reduced to around thirty, the better to maintain
security. Prior to this she had been much more leniently treated and servants, friends and hangers-on frequently swelled her retinue to twice
that number, all to be supported by Shrewsbury's estate, inadequately
reimbursed by Elizabeth.

Immediately on return to Tutbury, Mary's coffers were searched for
any incriminating correspondence, and her visitors and letters, usually
closely vetted, now were forbidden. Nothing suspicious was found
although Shrewsbury wrote to Elizabeth that before they left Wingfield,
the Queen "consumed with Fier very many Writings."[46] Mary hated
returning to Tutbury and resented deeply the harsh constraints placed
on her activities while the crisis lasted. She was particularly incensed by
the rude way in which she and her servants were treated. In a letter to
Elizabeth on the first day of October 1569, her outrage burnt through
her usual tone of sweet woebegone reason: "they have forbid me to go
out, and have rifled my trunks, entering my chamber with pistols and
arms, not without putting me in bodily fear, and accusing my people,
rifle them, and place them under arrest."[47]

Elizabeth's sharp treatment of Norfolk had certainly reasserted her
authority but it also panicked Northumberland and Westmoreland who
had been in communication not only with Norfolk but with Mary and
her agents too. These northern earls had always been more a law unto
themselves with their own council of the north, distant geographically
and philosophically from the monarch and court centred in the south.
They, like the majority of their people, remained reactionary and wed-
ded to the old religion. They were solely concerned with restoring
Catholicism and their association with Norfolk and his plans to marry
Mary was with this intent, with Mary sprung from jail as their Catholic
queen. Nor were they squeamish at the idea of inviting foreign aid to

help effect this. Norfolk's capitulation without a struggle, however, left them exposed and alarmed.

At the end of October, Elizabeth demanded that Sussex, Lord President of the North, summon the earls to London. Fearful that this meant their freedom, if not their lives, were already forfeit, the reluctant rebels accompanied by a body of armed retainers rode to Durham to raise their standard of rebellion. On 14 November they took possession of the cathedral, threw the book of Common Prayer on the ground, overturned the communion table and demanded that Mass be said. Their aims, however, were confused and their force divided and lacking in conviction or focus. Some wanted to ride south and release the Queen of Scots, but that bold scheme was abandoned when they heard of the prompt action which had confined her more straitly. Others wanted the succession clarified with the Duke of Norfolk's name among the leading contenders; still others thought the main aim was to re-establish the Catholic religion.

Elizabeth's forces were mobilised on all sides. There was general alarm and confusion, some of the nobility hesitantly joining the breakaway earls, more joined the government, patriotic allegiances crossing religious lines. With Durham occupied, Berwick, Newcastle and Carlisle remained loyal. Poorly organised, too hastily initiated, the rebellion was soon over without a shot being fired in anger. By Christmas 1569 the two renegade earls had fled over the border into Scotland. "The earls are old in blood but poor in force,"[48] Elizabeth is reputed to have said to her court as they galloped towards the border, leaving their supporters in disarray.

In retrospect it was easy to dismiss the whole thing as a damp squib, but at the time Elizabeth and her council had real fears that the whole of the north might rise in rebellion, the inflammable borderlands catch fire too and in the ensuing chaos France or Spain gain a foothold. Elizabeth's long letter at the end of November to the Earl of Sussex expressed both anger and fear:

> *these Rebells have nothing so much to Hart, nor seeke any other Thing so gredely in this theyr trayterous Enterprise, as the subduing of this Realme under the Yoke of foraine Princis, to make it the Spoile of Strangers . . . and so brede the Distruction of our faythfull and loving Subjects; and under Colour of Religion, to bring this and other theyr sedicious and lewde Intentions to passe, to the manifest Contempt of Almighty God, to the Troble and Danger of our Estate, and utter Desolation, Spoyle and Ruyne of our whole Realme.*[49]

Every county was ordered to ready itself with men, weapons and ammunition, some of it to be stored in the Tower where the armaments were old and worn out, having been cleaned for too long with sand and "become to a great extent honeycombed from one end to the other." Londoners under obligation to provide horses for military service were ordered to furnish them in readiness, as were "armourers to provide corselets; harquebus makers to provide harquebuses, and the merchants to provide arms, each one according to his ability."⁵⁰ "Confidential estimates" of the numbers of men ready to be called up, according to the French ambassador La Mothe Fenelon, came to six thousand harquebusiers, six thousand men in armour and a further twelve thousand, but with some doubt as to whether there was enough weaponry for all of them. Elizabeth was not taking this threat lightly.

It did not bode well for Mary either. She was moved south from Tutbury to the greater security of Coventry, travelling at night as far as possible to avoid "fond gazing, and confluence of the people,"⁵¹ as Shrewsbury wrote carefully to Cecil. There was real concern from Cecil, Elizabeth and those who guarded Mary that there should be no opportunity for the Scottish Queen to be seen except by authorised persons, for fear that her affecting presence would become a focus for popular sympathy. Once the rebellion had faded, she was moved back, again discreetly through an unwitting populace, to inhospitable Tutbury. Here, in the bitter January of 1570 shortage of wood for fuel made the ancient castle even more evilly favoured.

As she had done in the case of Norfolk's disloyalty, Elizabeth needed to reassert her authority with the northern rebels too. To the Earl of Sussex, her Lord President of the Council of the North, she wrote: "We do marvel that we have heard of no execution by martial law, as was appointed, of the meaner sort of rebels in the North. If the same be not already done, you are to proceed thereunto, for the terror of others, with expedition and to certify us of your doing therein. We understand that some in those parts, in this hour of service, have remained at home, or shown great slackness in our service, having brethren or children with the rebels; have an earnest regard to such, and spare no offenders in that case."⁵² Although only Northumberland forfeited his life, some six months later when he was returned from imprisonment in Lochleven Castle, it was the ordinary foot soldiers, poor country men on the whole who had joined the ill-starred earls in some confusion, who bore the brunt of her salutary revenge for treason. In the first few months of 1570, hundreds of them were summarily hanged, lands and livelihoods were forfeit. In the grim aftermath of rebellion, mercy was hard to come by.

Elizabeth had written a prayer in Greek, published in a 1569 collec-

tion of her prayers, which explained something of her belief that a monarch's duty was to employ just punishment as a cauterising process and thus safeguard the health of the nation: "Grant me to use mildness towards the virtuous, to encourage them still more to their duty and to chastise the wicked and lawless, so that I may turn them from evil and, truly in the manner of a physician, may bring this body of the realm from sickness to health and safety."[53]

This concept of necessary justice was extended to her treatment of Mary too. When the French ambassador had the temerity to tell Elizabeth, soon after the northern earls' rebellion, that his monarch disapproved of the continued imprisonment of the Queen of Scots, she claimed that such treatment was nothing less than her duty as a monarch: "[Mary's] friends have given shelter to the English rebels, and with her aid and connivance they levied war on me with fire and sword. No sovereign in Europe will sit down under such provocation, and I would count myself unworthy of realm, crown and name of queen if I endured it."[54]

Although the imprisonment of Norfolk and the disabling of the northern earls were all significant setbacks to Mary's plans, she was in one of her buoyant periods and was not cast down for long. Scheming and plotting her escape brought meaning and purpose to a monotony of uneventful days. If Mary could envisage a triumphant denouement that involved the utter disarray of her enemies and the award of the greatest prize of all, the scheming gained added piquancy. Marriage to Norfolk still offered her the clearest path to freedom and glory and by the end of January 1570 she was writing to him, still imprisoned in the Tower, with affectionate words and a bold, even foolhardy, plan for a double escape:

> *Mine own lord, I wrote to you before, to know your pleasure if I should seek to make any enterprize; if it please you, I care not for my danger; but I would wish you would seek to do the like; for if you and I could escape both, we should find friends enough . . . If you think the danger great, do as you think best, and let me know what you please that I do; for I will ever be, for your sake, perpetual prisoner, or put my life in peril for your weal [welfare] and myne.*

Although asking for his desires in the matter and promising blind obedience to his commands, Mary was the more adventurous and courageous of the two. She urged action where he seemed hesitant and was full of daring when he was of two minds. Although this alliance with Norfolk certainly suited her ambitions, Mary was also emotionally engaged by

the idea. To a young woman in the prime of life, her imprisonment, inactivity, loneliness and long hours of wishful thinking added an inevitable aura of romance to a man she had not met, did not know, but hoped to marry and eventually love: she addressed herself to "My Norfolk" and signed off "Your own faithful to death, Queen of Scots."[55]

With every year that passed, with each new scare, Mary's presence in England was becoming more clearly an incitement to plotters, religious fanatics, lovelorn noblemen, interventionist foreign powers, ambitious courtiers, to play the hero and rescue her from her pathetic state. There were some who were beginning to call for the death of the Queen of Scots as the only way to safeguard Elizabeth, the reformed religion and the peace of the nation. Knox, never one to pull his punches or choose a discreet word when a dozen rabble-rousing ones would do, wrote to Cecil in the new year of 1570 using the same horticultural analogy, but with different meaning, that Mary was busy embroidering on Norfolk's cushion. Mary's needlework depicting the need for excising a sterile vine threatened Elizabeth's life. Knox's gardening lore on the force of regeneration thundered out the threat to Mary's: "Yf ye strik not att the roote, the branches that appear to be brocken will budd againe (and that mor quicklye then men can beleve)."[56]

In Cecil he had someone not altogether hostile to the idea, but Elizabeth was never to accept wholeheartedly the necessity of Mary's death. She was, however, often exasperated, rattled, intimidated even, by what was fast becoming a double bind, where she was as much imprisoned emotionally and politically by her relationship with Mary as Mary was physically constrained by her. She was reputed to have exclaimed to the French ambassador, "I am just as anxious to see Mary Stuart out of England as she can be to go!"[57] For Mary the way out was continually blocked by decisions and events largely beyond her will, but the dream was kept alive in the letters and messages, the codes and confidences, which streamed from her various prisons. Increasingly, for Elizabeth, there seemed no way of ridding herself of her uninvited guest whose presence attracted such treachery.

The insecurity of life was once again brought home to everyone with news of the assassination of the Earl of Moray, natural brother to Mary and regent to her son. A Hamilton, kinsman of the Duke of Châtelherault, had ambushed Moray as he left Edinburgh on 21 January 1570. Despite the regent being in the company of one hundred and fifty armed horsemen his assassin managed to wound him fatally with a shot from a harquebus. Elizabeth was shocked by Moray's death. They were of similar age and had been mutually helpful colleagues during inchoate

times when the new religion and new reigns were in the process of being established. On hearing of his death, she cried out, "saying this would be the beginning of her ruin."[58]

For Mary, hope rose again. It seemed that without being asked Hamilton had done her job for her. She had little impulse to pity or forgive the brother she had once professed to love and in fact by the summer of the following year she was promising a pension to be paid to his assassin. The Queen's party gained enormous confidence and more noble recruits while the King's men (those supporting James VI and the regency) declined in support, reaching possibly their lowest point. Again the ancient feudal rivalry of Hamilton and Lennox remained the underlying scaffold for this deadly opposition. For six months Scotland was without a regent while the possibility that Mary might be restored seemed as close as it would ever come to reality. Elizabeth then gave her approval to the choice of Lennox, Darnley's father and the child-king's grandfather and a man inveterately opposed to Mary, as the next regent.

Leicester, possibly seeing the greatest threat coming from Spain not France, argued that France should be placated and made an ally. To best achieve that end, Mary needed to be returned to Scotland, albeit with drastically curbed powers. Elizabeth too seemed to be sensitive to the fact she could no longer justify holding her in custody. Writing to Sussex, her loyal lieutenant of the North, she explained her thinking: "if the Queen of Scots shall not refuse reasonable conditions—we do not see how with honour and reason we can continue her in restraint."[59] Reluctantly, but willing to do anything to escape her debilitating situation, Mary did indeed agree to swingeing conditions. Her son would go to England to be brought up there; prominent members of the King's party, her enemies, would occupy the major administrative posts; and Scottish foreign policy would be bent to English will. In exchange Mary would be named as Elizabeth's successor. Desperate for freedom at any cost, and not one to plan ahead or put much value on foresight as a defensive tool, Mary chose to grab the opportunity while she could, and charm or storm her way through the consequences later.

A series of events however were to jeopardise Mary's chances of freedom and push Elizabeth further from the sympathetic solidarity she had felt when first her cousin had fled south. In the last days of February 1570, the aged Pius V acted finally to excommunicate Elizabeth, "that servant of all iniquity . . . pretended Queen of England." The papal bull only reached England in mid-May when a foolhardy Catholic gentleman nailed it to the garden gate of the Bishop of London's palace. This pronouncement, purportedly from God, not only absolved all the faith-

ful from any loyalty or obedience to Elizabeth or her laws, it threatened that anyone who remained loyal to the "pretended queen" "shall incur the same sentence of malediction."[60]

This was a distinct threat to Elizabeth. In a time when the authority of the spiritual prince far outweighed the temporal, the Pope in theory was commanding English Catholics to rebel on pain of similar anathema. In effect, most were happy to continue with the ideologically unsound practice of offering spiritual allegiance to Pius and his successors, and political allegiance to Elizabeth and hers. Elizabeth's policy of equivocation and tolerance towards the private matters of faith of her subjects, however, was forced increasingly during the new decade to become more wary and prescriptive.

Undoubtedly, Mary's presence and the Catholic ambitions that fomented around her, speeded this process of suspicion and division. There seemed to be numerous plots against Elizabeth's throne, even her life. With the benefit of hindsight most were amateurish, but all prior to discovery had the potential for harm. Norfolk's release from the Tower in the summer of 1570 provided a focus once more for the bolder schemes. He remained under a kind of house arrest at Howard House, his residence in London, and appeared to have gone cold temporarily on the plan to marry Mary. Possibly the ordeal of the Tower was still too fresh in memory: possibly he did intend to keep the promise he had given Elizabeth which had persuaded her to release him at last: "from the Bottome of my Harte [I] crave of your Majestie Forgivenes for that which is past . . . with a full Intencion never to deale if that Cause of Mariage of the Quene of *Scottes*, nor in any other Cause belonginge to her, but as your Majestie shall commaund me."

Begging that the omnipotent queen "drawe me owt of the Dongeon of your Displeasure,"[61] he was soon to show he had neither the wisdom nor the self-control to keep from a dungeon of far greater peril. Elizabeth had made a similar promise to Cecil that she would never marry Lord Robert, and had managed to keep it despite her passions being deeply engaged. Norfolk soon failed where ambition was the motive force, and Mary Queen of Scots its seductive charioteer. Too late he was to realise his mistake, and in an affectionate letter of concern and advice to his children written as he awaited execution for treason he warned: "Beware of high degrees! To a vainglorious proud stomacke it seemeth at the first sweet . . . in the end it brings heapes of cares, toyles [snares] in the state, and most commonly in the end utter overthrowe."[62]

The utter overthrow of the Duke of Norfolk caused Elizabeth great anguish, and brought Mary into deepest suspicion and closer to the risk of execution herself. This time, she had accepted Elizabeth's humiliating

conditions for her release whereby she relinquished everything but her title as Queen of Scots and her claim to be a successor to the English throne. The procrastination of the Scottish King's party, concerned for their own power and security should she return, finally exhausted the negotiations. They would not countenance any reversal of the abdication document signed by Mary at Lochleven, nor would they allow the King to be removed into England. By March 1571, Mary's expectation of a legal restitution to her throne was over. In fact, that winter Mary was ill for a month or more, whether of her old complaints or of the strain of frustrated ambition, no one could say. The deadly inertia while she waited, her hopes artificially elevated or plunged into despair, would have driven an impatient nature such as hers into chronic depression or mania. Instead she kept her hopes alive through elaborate schemes of escape and fantasies of derring-do, in the only serious activity left to her.

Roberto Ridolphi had already played a minor role in the conspiracies surrounding the earlier plan to marry Mary to the Duke of Norfolk, and the consequent rebellion of the northern earls in 1569. A Florentine banker and papal agent then living in London, he concocted a grandiose plan which became notorious as the Ridolphi plot. Potentially dangerous to Elizabeth and the security of the realm, its effects in reality were to prove fatal to Norfolk and deeply damaging to Mary. Ridolphi had been busy distributing the papal bull excommunicating Elizabeth and denying her legitimacy on the English throne.

Spurred by this papal authority he aimed to enlist a Spanish army of invasion to support a rising of the English Catholics, under the leadership of Norfolk, and inspired by the prospect of placing a Catholic Queen Mary on the "pretender's" throne. It was inevitable that Mary would put her name to this scheme. She was desperate to be free, and she thrived on the excitement and sense of hope that smuggled letters, encoded messages and clandestine meetings brought to her sorely constrained life. Even the intrigues of court life, the pleasures of dance and music, and the pursuit of love, were much diminished by captivity. All that was left to her was to plot her escape, however madcap and dangerous, and dream of revenge on her enemies by grasping Elizabeth's crown.

At the beginning of February 1571, Mary wrote to Norfolk using the Bishop of Ross as her envoy. She pointed out that Ridolphi intended telling Philip II that there were numbers of the English nobility together with thousands of their men ready to rise in support of her. All they needed was a sign of support from Spain. Norfolk was not immediately enthusiastic. He knew already the force of Elizabeth's displeasure;

he had promised not to promote Mary's interests in any way and must have realised that to be exposed again as a central figure in such a conspiracy would be to forfeit his life. However, his pride and ambition to be elevated to the role of princely consort got the better of his caution. Reluctantly he agreed to join the enterprise.

The inception of this plot coincided exactly with Elizabeth's agreement that her ambassadors could open marriage negotiations with the Duc d'Anjou, Charles IX's younger brother. As Henri III, he was destined to inherit the French throne after Charles's death in 1574. He was not yet twenty years old and Elizabeth was in her thirty-eighth year, but by now she knew, and her closest advisors must have been wearily aware, that this was another proposal that would not develop beyond the fruitless discussion stage. This would prove, however, protracted and artificially sustained, and would secure for England the advantages of being in provisional alliance with a powerful European neighbour, saved for a time from the loneliness and vulnerability of being a renegade Protestant state in a continent of Catholic powers. It also cooled French concern for the fate of Mary, their erstwhile queen.

So far and deep had court gossip spread about Elizabeth's immoderate behaviour with Leicester that Anjou, renowned himself for his promiscuity and later for flamboyant transvestitism and homosexuality, complained to his mother Catherine de Medici about Elizabeth's reputed immorality. He had to be assured she was the model of propriety before he would proceed. Such reservations as to her reputation only served to outrage Elizabeth when she was unfavourably compared to Mary. Upbraided by the French ambassador for not allowing Mary greater liberty, she was determined, she said, to point out to all European princes that her treatment of her cousin was of "such rectitude" that she had no cause for shame or regret, unlike Mary herself. "Would to God that the Queen of Scots had no more occasion to blush at that which can be known of her,"[63] was her sharp riposte.

Sir Francis Walsingham was propelled by this familiar charade into the political foreground, sent as ambassador to France to deal with the marriage negotiations. His talent for intelligence gathering was already well marked. He had been suspicious of Mary's potential as a focus, or even instigator, of rebellion from the moment she had set foot on English soil. From that point on he remained alert to her activities and watchful of those drawn to her flame. He joined the front rank of Elizabeth's ministers with her other great statesman, William Cecil, whom she created Baron Burghley at the end of February 1571: "My stile is, Lord of Burghley, if you meane to know it," he wrote proudly to a colleague, adding the plaint, "the poorest Lord in England."[64] Leicester too

had grown in political stature and experience. From Elizabeth's favourite, willing to assume any stance that would promote his own position, he was showing himself to be a reliable and intelligent councillor and, despite Cecil's personal antipathy to him, took his place with Cecil and Walsingham as the third pillar of the powerful triumvirate that formed the solid base of Elizabeth's rule.

While Elizabeth and her ministers put a preliminary hand of friendship out to the French, Ridolphi set out for Europe in March determined on raising Spanish military aid in his scheme for Elizabeth's overthrow. Spurred with the explicit support of Mary and the covert agreement of Norfolk, his first stop was the Duke of Alva, Philip II's military commander in the Low Countries. Alva was engaged in ferociously suppressing the Protestants who were supported covertly by the English. Where Ridolphi was breezy and over-optimistic, Alva was tough-minded and not susceptible to dreams. He did not like the idea of forcibly deposing Elizabeth and thought Spain could only invade once the Queen was dead or at least captive. Ridolphi passed on to Rome where the Pope gave moral support for his schemes, but not much else. In Madrid, Ridolphi's enthusiastic view of the numbers of English Catholics on the verge of insurrection inflamed the chronically dour and cautious Philip. The Spanish King got carried away with the plan to order an armed incursion into England to get rid of Elizabeth, place Mary on the throne and re-establish Catholicism in that heretic isle.

In fact, nothing came of it. Messengers were apprehended, letters discovered, ciphers broken, confessions wrung out under torture.* Mary was immediately and incontrovertibly implicated. Her ambassador, the Bishop of Ross, threatened with the rack, revealed Norfolk's part in the process. He also vilified the Queen of Scots far beyond the questions in hand as a serial husband-killer who, if she had married Norfolk, would have similarly brought his life to a premature end. The Bishop's interrogator was stunned by the torrent of allegations; to Cecil he wrote, "Lord, what a people are these! What a Queen, and what an ambassador."[65]

---

* Elizabeth had to sign a warrant herself to allow, if necessary, two of Norfolk's servants to be tortured in the Tower. The usual procedure was to try the threat of the rack, and if that did not loosen the tongue of the prisoner then the full horror of the rack was to be used. She wrote: "if they shall not seem to you to confess plainly their knowledge, then we warrant you to cause them both, or either of them, to be brought to the rack, and first to move them with fear thereof to deal plainly in their answers. And if that shall not move them, then you shall cause them to be put to the rack and to fe[el] the taste thereof until they deal more plainly, or until you shall think meet." (*Collected Works*, 127.)

It was not Mary as his future wife who ended Norfolk's life with violence, but Elizabeth. With Norfolk found guilty of treason, the English Queen was put under enormous pressure from Parliament to sign his death warrant. She hesitated, she signed, she changed her mind four times in all, on one occasion she revoked the death sentence at two o'clock in the morning of the day projected for his execution. She could not bear to have the blood of such near kin on her hands.

Elizabeth was passionately exhorted by her Commons to arraign Mary for treason and thereby stop at source any more murderous plots. Tempers were frayed, voices raised and tears flowed, so strongly did they feel about the dangers Mary continued to pose. Realising that she had to give some concession to her loyal Commons, Elizabeth agreed to Norfolk's execution as the lesser of two evils. He went to the block with dignity on 2 June 1572, admitting his transgressions and asking forgiveness from his queen. To Elizabeth he had written, "The Lord knoweth that I myself know no more than I have been charged withall, nor much of that, although I humbly beseche God and your Majesty to forgive me, I knewe a greate deale too muche . . . For certayn it is, that these practyses of rebellions and invasions, were not brutes [rumours] without full intention. God, of his mercifull goodnesse, I hope, will disclose all things that may be dangerous to your excellent Majesty: and then I hope your highnes shall perceave that Norfolk was not such a traytor, as he hath, not without his own desertes, given great occasion of suspycion." News of his death sent Mary "into a passion of sickness,"[66] and she took to her bed with grief.

Shrewsbury was charged by Elizabeth to tell the Queen of Scots of the discovery of the plot and her part in it. He had to explain too that he was ordered to reduce her attendants to sixteen and temporarily restrict her movements and communications with the outside world. Mary, confronted with evidence of her own incriminating letters, her own writing even, and the confessions of her ambassador and messenger, not only denied everything but was self-righteous in her defiance. "I had of my own free will placed myself in the hands of the Queen his mistress," she told Shrewsbury, "relying upon her promises and friendship; that since she has detained me forcibly, if she suspects that I desire my liberty, I cannot help it. Nevertheless I am a free princess, and in that am not responsible to her or any other."[67]

Mary was courageous and clever in her response. She knew that legitimacy mattered to Elizabeth, and that it was necessary to the English Queen that actions were seen to be lawful. In a speech to her Commons some fourteen years later explaining why she would not comply with their urgent plea that she execute Mary, she elaborated on this prin-

ciple: "we Princes, I tell you, are set on stages in the sight and view of all the world duly observed. The eyes of many behold our actions; a spot is soon spied in our garments; a blemish quickly noted in our doings. It behooveth us therefore to be careful that our proceedings be just and honourable."[68] Mary also knew that, much more than any of her ministers and much more than Mary herself, Elizabeth was an idealistic monarchist who considered her to have a sacred authority which no mortal could put aside.

With the discovery of the Ridolphi plot there was a heightening of tension in Elizabeth's government. It was significant that even cool-headed, rational Cecil, now Lord Burghley, considered his country to be in a perilous position in relation to its neighbours. Weak, ill-equipped and vulnerable as it still was, he knew England was incapable of withstanding an onslaught from an alliance of the Catholic states. That such a concerted action was expected brought fear to Elizabeth's supporters and some frisson of excitement to Mary's. Rumours of other plots, possible traitors and potential routes of invasion were everywhere. The ports were watched, guards around the Queen increased and the militia placed in a state of alert.

Such nervous anxiety proved to be unmerited. Catherine de Medici, Queen Mother of France, long ago had given up the pretence of warmth and concern for her onetime daughter-in-law. She and her son, Charles IX, required that a woman who had been once Queen of France should be shown all due respect, but they were not about to risk war in order to rescue her from captivity. The news of the Ridolphi plot, however, and Mary's eagerness to ally herself with Spanish might, marked the end of even a pretence of anything more than mere verbal support for her from the French monarchy. Catherine de Medici had a revealing interview with Walsingham in the aftermath of the plot's discovery:

Catherine began, "[Mary] is alied to the King and to me, and brought up here . . . [but] she seketh an other way to ruinate hir self, to hurt hir freends, to deserve no pitie nor favour, and sorie we must be for hir. And if she be so dangerous (as yt aperith) we can not nor dare not require liberty for hir, which is so perillous to the Queene my sister's [Elizabeth's] State."[69] She continued that if, through Elizabeth's mercy, Mary's life should be spared, then Catherine and the King would trouble the English Queen no further.

On a personal level, the Ridolphi plot marked the end of any sisterly solidarity that might have existed between the two queens. Elizabeth was forced to accept that Mary was prepared to have her assassinated in order to gain her own freedom and subsequently the English crown. She had long realised that here in the heart of her kingdom was a charismatic

presence who seemed to have a fatal attraction for everyone who fell within her circle of influence. Mary, for her part, had recognised that Elizabeth may have longed to be rid of her but would not return her to Scotland where her Protestant lords were implacably set against her. Nor would she leave her free to go to France and there re-energise old alliances injurious to England.

Mary's next letter to Elizabeth, written from Sheffield Castle on 29 October 1571, acknowledged the irreparable deterioration in their relationship: "Madam, the extreme severity with which by your orders I am used, so convinces me, to my great regret, of the misfortune which I have, with many others, not only of being in your disfavour, but, which is worse, esteemed by you as an enemy instead of a friend, as a stranger instead of a close relation—even the more detested that it does not permit the exercise of Christian charity between parties so nearly related by blood and propinquity."[70] Her impervious self-righteousness made her very difficult to deal with. She emotively reminded Elizabeth in every letter of their close blood ties, the sanctity of their mutual queenship, the poignancy of her position as a lone woman, captive and away from friends, family and home. Her position was tragic, close to Elizabeth's own experiences, and affectingly expressed. But the implicit message was always self-justifying, sometimes pious and superior, yet fundamentally accusatory. Impossible as her situation was, Mary still operated on the principle she had demonstrated so strikingly during the Huntly rebellion a decade earlier—attack was the best defence.

Elizabeth wrote far fewer letters in reply to her distressed cousin. As she explained, often there was no answer she could give that would placate her. However, writing on 1 February 1572, she was moved to remonstrate against Mary's previous letter which, she objected, was full of "uncomely, passionate, and vindictive speeches." Elizabeth warned her, "to qualify your passions, and to consider that it is not the manner to obtain good things with evil speeches, nor benefits with injurious challenges, nor to get good to yourself with doing evil to another."[71] She then delegated all negotiations to the hapless Earl of Shrewsbury, who still remained as Mary's host–jailer.

In that phrase *to get good to yourself with doing evil to another*, Elizabeth was more obviously thinking of the plots against her own life. However, it was a phrase that could be applied to Mary's career so far, and the devastating effect she had on the men who were drawn to marry or assist her. Elizabeth did not like losing family members. Her cousin Lord Darnley, fleetingly Mary's husband and King of the Scots, had been murdered in confused and unhappy circumstances. Norfolk's treason lay

heavy on Elizabeth. When she wrote this letter he was still alive in the Tower, and she was under mounting pressure to have him executed. He was her leading nobleman, a suitor in the past for her hand and one of her inner circle. It made her wonder at the powers of persuasion the promise of Mary had exerted over this vain and susceptible man. Elizabeth had every reason to believe that her own life had hung in the balance, and still would, while her cousin's presence inspired schemes of rescue, and dreams of religious restoration and personal ambition. But there were other lives too. How many more men, important and close to Elizabeth perhaps, would become caught and ruined in that web of ambition and desire?

At the same time as she wrote her exasperated letter to Mary, Elizabeth commented to the French ambassador, "There seems to be something sublime in the words and bearing of the Queen of Scots that constrains even her enemies to speak well of her."[72] On the face of it, Elizabeth had all the advantages in the relationship between the two queens. Yet she was as much captive to the situation as was Mary herself, imprisoned by the insecurities of her own past and her deep-rooted respect, both philosophical and self-serving, for the divine elevation of them both as queens.

Elizabeth, in her actions and her letters, seemed intimidated at times by the reputation of her rival. Perhaps Mary's unimpeachable pedigree, her unquestionable legitimacy, was part of her power over her cousin. In this way she challenged Elizabeth's deepest vulnerabilities. Perhaps, too, Elizabeth was daunted by the mystery of Mary's almost sorcerous power of attraction, even on the briefest acquaintance. She had been wary of her personal charm from the beginning, "since her flying into our Realm,"[73] as she vividly put it in a letter to her ambassador in France. Why, even that most reliable and adamantine of men, her own Burghley, had attributed irresistible qualities to the Queen of Scots and feared the effect she would have on anyone, including those naturally averse, who fell into her toils: "she is able by hir great wytt, and hir sug[a]red eloquence, to wyn even such, as before they shall come to hir company, shall have a great mislykyng."[74]

Mary knew that magical powers of bewitchment were supposed to be hers. When she had first blazed over the English horizon, uninvited, as potentially inflammatory as a smouldering meteor, she had tried to allay her cousin's suspicions: "Alas! Do not as the serpent that stoppeth his heering, for I am no inchanter, but your suster and naturall cousyne . . . I am not of the nature of a basilisk, and lesse of the camelions, to turne you to my lykeness. And though I shuld be so dangerouse and curst as men:

yow ar sufficiently armeyd with constance, and with justice."[75] In the process, however, she just reinforced the uneasiness that here was a woman of supernatural power.

Elizabeth was armed with justice, but in her struggle with Mary this was to her disadvantage: how to act justly and yet safeguard herself and her country? Assailed by mysterious forces, by unknown plots and conspiracies against her life, Elizabeth recognised that her fate was inextricably linked with Mary's; that she too could not escape. "I am not free, but a captive," she wrote in some despair[76] during a long constraint that both queens, in their different ways, shared till death.

CHAPTER ELEVEN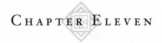

Singular Foes

I will appeal to the ever-living God, in whom onely
I acknowledge a Power and Dominion over us that are
Princes of equal Jurisdiction, Degree and Authority. And
upon him will I call, (with whom there will be no place
for Craft nor Fraud,) that in the Last day he will reward
us according to our Deserts one towards another.

LETTER FROM MARY TO ELIZABETH 1582

She wishes by way of invocation that God should
"retribute" to us at the time of His last Judgement
according to our deserts and demerits one towards
another, putting us also in mind that all disguisements
and counterfeit policies of this world shall then not
prevail . . . if that severe censure should take place it
would go much more hardly with her than we . . . can in
Christian charity wish for her.
For howsoever she is bold with men, who can judge but
of things outwardly, she ought to beware how she dallies
with God.

ANSWERING LETTER FROM ELIZABETH TO MARY 1583

The power of an island people, encircled by an unpredictable sea, is
forged in independence, self-reliance and insularity from continental influence. Inward looking, slower to change, an island race has an
enduring sense of identity and the confidence of knowing who they are,

where they have come from and where they are bound. Elizabeth's father, through desire for her mother and for herself, the unborn heir who should have been a boy, had ensured for his country a spiritual and ideological isolation too. Elizabeth's sister, Mary I, had attempted to rebuild the bridge with Europe and Catholicism, with catastrophic results. Elizabeth was herself quintessentially English and insular, an island queen who, despite her long life, her wide learning, linguistic skills and intellectual curiosity, never travelled beyond her immediate frontiers.

Yet within those limitations she claimed great strengths. She knew her people intimately, and was quick to remind them that she was like them and had been a subject too. She was proud that she was born of a domestic union and not from a dynastic alliance with a foreign power. Her claim that her blood was unsullied by foreign taint reinforced the chauvinism, superiority and suspicion shown towards foreigners that was beginning to characterise her people. Confident of their love and with her familial images as wife and parent, she promised them her care and loyalty to death, and was believed.

This comfortable fertile fortress, protected by an inhospitable sea, was safe even from incursion through her borders with Scotland now that the Protestant lords were well established there. The Scottish Queen's precipitate flight, however, and her continued unwelcome presence in the heart of Elizabeth's kingdom had breached the walls and once more thrown a bridge to Catholic Europe through which interest, influence and outright aggression could be channelled. Mary's nature was far from insular. She was not immediately identifiable as truly belonging anywhere. She had spent only seven years in her kingdom, always an exotic presence for whom her subjects initially felt a greater patriotic feeling than she could return. French was her natural language of choice and she never lost her accent. Her connections of family and religion extended from France to Spain and to the Pope himself, and her affections remained unwaveringly Francocentric, indelibly impressed with the charismatic family and the influences of a charmed youth.

As prisoner of the English Queen, Mary may have been deprived of personal and political power, but she was the symbol of something more powerful and more elusive than any individual could aspire to be. A born queen kept in captivity; a mother separated from her son; a Catholic martyr abused by heretic subjects and harassed by a godless queen; a French princess and Dowager Queen living in conditions far beneath her dignity; a beautiful, noble and ill-used woman in need of heroic rescue: these personae were already being woven into a Marian mythology of the Queen of Scots as sainted victim. She had become a magnetic pole for any dis-

senting opinion in Elizabeth's England and a focus of guilty shame for those sympathetic to her plight. Above all, she was a signal of hope for the Catholic population who dreamed of a counter-reformation, and a cause for every messianic hothead in need of a holy war.

The opposing mythology of Mary, forged by fearful English Protestants, was of a queen who had forfeited every divine right of monarchy through her immoral behaviour. In their over-heated rhetoric she was an adulteress and husband-slayer—worse, a regicide; a ruthless papist plotter intent on taking their own queen's life and subjecting their kingdom to a vengeful Catholicism. Through rumour, fear and alienation, Mary was easily transmuted into a mysterious, even diabolical, seductress whom men approached at their peril.

When the entrails of the Ridolphi plot were displayed to Elizabeth's councillors in 1572, the threat of a Catholic league against England, based on the legitimacy of Mary's claim to the throne, seemed imminent. The whole enterprise was sanctified by the papal bull excommunicating Elizabeth and denying her legitimacy as queen.

The relative tolerance of religious difference that marked the first decade of Elizabeth's reign was fractured not just by plots against her but by the instability of events in neighbouring countries. There was a growing religious extremism that disconcerted Elizabeth's secular political instinct for the non-committal and the inclusive. It was not just the conservative Catholic forces which were growing in confidence. The Puritan wing were also becoming more demanding, although posing less threat through their lack of powerful states as allies.

After the assassination of the Scottish regent Moray in 1570 by a Catholic Hamilton, the barely suppressed anarchy of Scottish politics once more gained the upper hand. Moray's eventual successor as regent, Darnley's father Lennox, was also killed by one of Mary's supporters in September 1571; as was the next regent, the anti-Mary Earl of Mar, just one year later, some said as a result of poison. The Spanish campaign against the Protestants in the Low Countries brought Huguenots streaming through the eastern ports of England seeking asylum, with tales of cruelty and suffering, and the threat of the imperial ambitions of this most implacably Catholic of states extending across the Channel too.

The religious wars in France had lasted almost a decade, periodically quiescent and then flaring into savage bloodletting and fanatical excess. A series of massacres of Protestants beginning on 24 August 1572, the feast of St. Bartholomew, convulsed the Protestant states with horrified disbelief. In the afterglow of a royal wedding feast, Catherine de Medici had initially intended a political act of assassination against certain Huguenot leaders, specifically Admiral Coligny, whose impressive char-

acter and powers of organisation were gaining unprecedented influence for the Huguenot party. The still mighty and ultra-Catholic Guise family had long vowed revenge for what they believed to be Coligny's implication in the murder of François Duc de Guise almost ten years before. They too were in on the plot, as was the Duc d'Anjou, soon to become Henri III. It was a plot to assassinate Coligny, but when he was merely wounded Catherine and her followers thought it too dangerous to leave his followers alive. What appeared to be a plan to kill the governing body of the Huguenot party turned into a bloodbath. The Parisian mob were encouraged to go on the rampage where every Protestant, and then anyone who crossed their paths, was destroyed in an orgy of killing.

This bloodlust lasted for days, sweeping across France and settling its bloodied fangs into other towns and districts until tens of thousands lay butchered in the streets and the fields. The emblem of St. Bartholomew was a knife, recalling his death by flaying: the massacre that was forever to bear his name was made notorious through its similar barbarous inhumanity. It was the most shocking episode in the French religious wars and was greeted with celebration by the new Pope Gregory XIII, who struck a commemorative medal, and Philip II of Spain, who congratulated the King and Catherine, his historic enemies, on a job well done. The militant faithful considered turning back the tide of European Protestantism as much an expression of God's will as Christianity's onslaught on the infidel Turk, and the sword therefore became a legitimate means of conservation and conversion. The papal medal on the reverse side depicted an angel with the cross in his left hand and a drawn sword in his right while before him lay the bodies of the slain, the inscription, *Ugonotorum Strages,* "the Massacre of the Huguenots," quite unambivalent in its meaning.

The news reached Elizabeth while she was hunting. Immediately the day's sport was abandoned and the court went into mourning. The predominant response was one of shock, puzzlement and fear. Elizabeth had only recently allowed her ministers to respond with some encouragement to the French King's latest offer of his youngest brother, the Duc d'Alençon,* as a possible husband for her. What appeared to be a policy of systematic destruction of the French Protestants filled her with outrage and alarm. All anyone could talk about at court was these latest

---

* Hercule became François Duc d'Alençon and then Duc d'Anjou, but is usually referred to as d'Alençon to differentiate him from his brother, the Duc d'Anjou who became Henri III in 1574. Monsieur was the more usual contemporary name for him, the name Elizabeth used when she didn't call him her nicknames of "frog" and "little fingers."

revelations of the perfidy of the French. Was this part of a greater Catholic plan which would spread to England's shores and sweep up the Queen of Scots as its heroine?

Mary's inheritance was both Stuart and Guise, and on all showings the courage, passion and charisma of her nature made her more her mother's daughter than her father's. It was wondered whether she would also prove herself as ruthlessly fanatic as her Guise uncles in the pursuit of her religion, in the willingness to destroy others. Certainly Mary was aware that her close blood ties and affective connection to this powerful family was considered suspicious. In a letter to the French ambassador she admitted, "they say that I love the house of Guise too much."[1] Elizabeth, however, was disinclined to use the horrors across the Channel as a way of reflecting more opprobrium on Mary. To the French ambassador who, soon after the massacre, asked her not to punish Mary further, she retorted: "The Queen of Scots has enough sins of her own to answer for, without ascribing to her those of other people."[2]

She was less understanding towards Mary's brother-in-law, Charles IX. Elizabeth wrote to him that even if this was punishment for rebels intent on relieving him of his life and his crown—an excuse frankly she doubted—it was "a terrible and dangerous example" to set by not taking these nobles for trial before executing them. She turned her outrage next to the reported treatment of the common people, "that women, children, maids, young infants and sucking babes, were at the same time murthered and cast into the river; and that liberty of execution was given to the vilest and basest sort of the popular [populus], without punishment or revenge of such cruelty done afterwards by law."[3] To his ambassador who delivered the King's version of events to her at court, Elizabeth interrupted the excuses with a thunderous expression, "even if everything had happened as the King said, and the conspirators had been rightly punished," she said sharply she would like to know "what blame was attributable to the women and children who were murdered."[4] The ambassador left soon afterwards.

Assassination had become a commonplace tool of policy among the European powers at this time. Yet it was striking how easy it was to gain close access to anyone in a position of power. The series of dead regents in Scotland was indication enough of how simple and unremarkable such a lawless act had become. Even in Elizabeth's court, full of rumours of individual plots against her, fearful of concerted actions by hostile states, access to her palaces and even her person seemed to be surprisingly relaxed. In one of the prayers composed while Mary was in captiv-

ity in her kingdom, Elizabeth expressed the ever-present awareness of uncertainty: "I see all things in this life subject to mutability, nothing to continue still at one stay . . . I hear ofttimes untimely death doth carry away the mightiest and greatest personages."[5]

Although Mary was at the mercy of Elizabeth and the English state, and vulnerable to some contrivance that appeared legal enough to justify her execution, closely confined as she was, she was much more protected from opportunist assassination than Elizabeth could ever be. The English Queen pursued her life at court and on regular progresses round the country, with immediate access to her nobles, her visitors and the people. There are fascinating travelogues of visiting foreign nobility who detail how they walked into any of the Queen's residences, inspected her living quarters, handled her plate and furnishing, gazed at portraits of her ancestors, turned up at church while she was at worship, joined the company around her and were presented to her, with very little barrier or protective protocol.

With so much turmoil abroad, with the Pope's call to action, and the Queen of Scots at home attracting support from disparate and dangerous factions, it was not surprising that Elizabeth's ministers and Commons should fear for her life. The Bishop of London wrote urgently to Cecil, "these evill tymes trouble all good men's heads, and make their heartes ake, fearing that this barbarous treacherie will not cease in Fraunce, but will reach over unto us . . . Hasten her Majestie homewards, her safe returne to London [from a royal progress] will comfort many hearts oppressed with feare."[6] During the Parliament of 1572, the members pleaded for the chance to try Mary for treason and thereby sentence her to death. Elizabeth, pressed by emotional speeches to safeguard herself and her country, would only agree reluctantly to the more modest suggestion that Mary be deprived of her right of succession. However, despite being passed by both houses, she unexpectedly backed away from ratifying the newly drafted bill.

Burghley was exasperated at her obduracy and apparent blindness to the danger: as long as Mary retained her claim on the English crown Elizabeth would not be safe from every kind of European or Catholic ambition against her. Anxieties grew to fever pitch when she fell ill with a pox that was immediately assumed to be a recurrence of the dreaded smallpox. No one was more fearful than Shrewsbury. If Elizabeth should die, Mary still remained the next in line to the throne. His position was perilous if in this sudden change of fortune his prisoner would become his sovereign, intent on revenge. After the execution of the Duke of Norfolk in early June 1572, Mary's bitterness against Elizabeth had been vitriolic. Shrewsbury had thought it wise to let Cecil know: "She still

continues great enmity, and gives no hope of other intent. It is too plain her heart is overhardened with deadly hate against the Queen's majesty—the more, therefore, her majesty's safety is to be thought upon."[7]

What faithful and literal-minded old Shrewsbury could not fathom, however, was the volatility of Mary's emotions. Living in the moment, thriving on sensation, Mary's expression of feeling was fundamentally intense but mutable; exuberance quickly followed despair, depression metamorphosed into action. Although, in her desperation to be free, she was an eager participant in any passing plot, she knew that her own life so easily could be forfeit in the chaotic process of a rescue attempt. Mary cannot have forgotten the pack frenzy of Riccio's murder and the danger to herself in the panicky aftermath.

Elizabeth too was capable of outbursts of uncontained emotion. The strain of living with Mary's presence, and the problems and dangers that she threatened sometimes got the better of her diplomatic cool. Introduced to Gondi, the French envoy, in the summer of 1578, "she told him loudly in the audience chamber that she knew very well he had come to disturb her country and to act in the favour of the worst woman in the world, whose head should have been cut off years ago." When Gondi reminded her that Mary was a sovereign queen and a kinswoman, Elizabeth angrily shot back at him, "that [Mary] should never be free as long as she lived, even though it cost her [Elizabeth] her realm and her liberty."[8]

After the Ridolphi enterprise, it was more than a decade before there were again significant conspiracies to rescue Mary or murder Elizabeth. Various plots of varying incompetence continued to come to light, thanks to Walsingham's efficient intelligence gathering, but none of them, until Throckmorton's involvement in 1583, caused any great consternation. Mary continued in her stately imprisonment, her household once more allowed to increase to royal proportions, and treated with increasing laxity until rumoured plots or threatening conditions abroad meant her activities were temporarily constrained. Her negotiations with Elizabeth turned to requests for more opportunities for outdoor recreation and expeditions to improve her health.

Her indoor leisure activities were still embroidering fine bed hangings and smaller pieces, their motifs charged with meaning, often in the company of the Countess of Shrewsbury. The gossip that animated these long hours of stitching was much enlivened by details of Elizabeth's last significant courtship that unexpectedly became a love affair. More than a decade after her amorous activities with Leicester had set the scandalmongers of Europe alight, Elizabeth's reputation remained

dubious, to her Catholic neighbours at least. Don John of Austria* had commented to his natural brother, Philip II, on the fleeting suggestion of a marriage between himself and the Queen of England: "I blush while I write this to think of accepting advances from a woman whose life and example furnish so much food for gossip."⁹

In fact, he was happier to consider marriage to Mary, admittedly a Catholic like himself, but a queen whose life gave more food for unfavourable talk than any queen living or dead. Elizabeth was vilified for being a heretic and, worse still, a woman and a monarch who had defied nature and God's law by refusing to marry. In choosing to rule alone, thriving in her heresy instead of being struck down for her sins, she challenged every principle, succeeding where all prejudice decreed she would fail. To the fanatical Catholic rulers of Europe, Elizabeth was an affront. Her unmarried state made her vulnerable to the judgements of others, but it also made her personally vulnerable to the promise of love.

The youngest French prince, François Duc d'Alençon, finally began his courtship of Elizabeth in earnest in the beginning of 1579. This youthful, over-excitable young man was described as "featherbrained" by Walsingham, who added dourly that this characteristic was true of most of the Prince's countrymen. Monsieur, as he was universally called, had added his support to the Huguenot struggle against the Spanish in the Low Countries. With his army in disarray, starving and beginning to desert, he faced an ignominious return to France. Instead he decided to try his fortune with Elizabeth. There were those in England who muttered cynically that he, like Aeneas, was seeking merely the easier option, with Elizabeth as the Dido he would betray. Already he had sent a series of extraordinary, passionately effusive letters, lauding her beauty and personal attractions to the skies and promising undying love, promising to die himself if deprived of her.

Elizabeth had embarked on this courtship, as she had on every other, as a diplomatic ruse, this time with the intent to make some kind of holding alliance with the French. The lowering presence of the Spanish, marauding the Protestant rebels in the Low Countries and just too close for comfort, was Elizabeth's real concern. Marriage negotiations were always a good way of disturbing an unfavourable status quo, unsettling the established power balance and delaying proceedings that might be injurious to her country. There were some alarming reports that the

---

* Don John was a dashing young prince who had become the hero of Europe since commanding the Christian fleet at Lepanto in 1571 in a historic victory against the previously indomitable Turkish fleet.

Spanish were building ships and fitting them out in Italy in such numbers that could only be explained by an enterprise against the English. This spectre of Spanish aggression loomed increasingly during the coming decade. The possibility, however faint, of an alliance between France and England menaced the Spanish in a way that English power alone could never achieve.

A major factor in the success of the Duc d'Alençon's courtship of the wily queen was a highly sophisticated courtier, Monsieur's best friend, Jehan de Simier. He travelled with an entourage of French courtiers to England in January 1579, with the express purpose of softening Elizabeth up before his master arrived in person. A series of extravagant entertainments were organised "with Tiltings performed at vast expense . . . to say nothing of other Courtly Sports and Pastimes, which are not so proper for an Historian to relate,"[10] so Camden, Elizabeth's earliest historian, related. The marriage had first been proposed when Elizabeth was thirty-eight and Alençon barely sixteen. From the start Elizabeth found the age difference embarrassing, saying she considered herself an old woman compared with this "beardless youth," a characteristic gleefully pointed out to her by the many detractors of the match. By early 1579, she was forty-five and Monsieur had become a man. Although Elizabeth would conduct other flirtations to flatter her vanity and beguile her loneliness, this would become her romantic swansong.

The impetus for this *coup de foudre* was Simier rather than his master. He was a man of forceful character with a capacity for Machiavellian ruthlessness.* Yet Simier was also a consummate courtier and practised in the ways of courtly love. He had an unexpectedly electrifying effect on the Virgin Queen. She was so taken with him that she insisted on seeing him daily, and simpered and posed and flirted so amorously that the whole court and the eagle-eyed ambassadors were agog. She also flagged her intimacy with him by awarding him a fond nickname, "monkey" or "ape," which punned in Latin on his name.

Simier seemed optimistic that his master's suit would be successful, "but will wait to say more till the curtain is drawn, the candle out, and Monsieur in bed." Whether he was sincere or merely diplomatic, he seemed almost as delighted with Elizabeth as she was with him. To Monsieur's commissioner in the Low Countries he wrote: "I swear to you that [Elizabeth] is the most virtuous and honourable princess in the world;

---

* Prior to his arrival in London, Simier had heard that while away, serving Alençon in his campaign in the Low Countries, his young wife had committed adultery with his younger brother. He sent his men ahead to kill this brother at the gate of his château, and his young wife died soon after, of poison, fear or grief, no one could say.

her wit is admirable, and there are so many other parts to remark in her that I should need much ink and paper to catalogue them. In conclusion I hold our master very fortunate if God will further this business."[11] Hopes were running high. The usually sedate French ambassador wrote to Catherine de Medici, Elizabeth's prospective mother-in-law: "This discourse rejuvenates the Queen; she has become more beautiful and bonny than she was fifteen years ago," adding optimistically, "Not a woman or a physician who knows her does not hold that there is no lady in the realm more fit for bearing children than she is."

It was juicy gossip like this that Mary Queen of Scots and the Countess of Shrewsbury shared over the embroidery. The women suggested a more commonplace reason for Elizabeth's rejuvenation—sex. According to the letter Mary wrote, detailing the most scandalous aspects of these conversations, she and the Countess had discussed Elizabeth's lascivious nature and how she had enjoyed sexual relations both with Simier and his master. It was not only the average Englishman, however, who was alarmed at Elizabeth's evident relish for this suit. The Spanish were busy working on undermining, through rumour and bribery, any support there may have been at Elizabeth's court.

Mary's interest in Elizabeth's potential marriage into the French royal family was not just for its entertainment value. She believed that such a match would substantially change her situation, hopefully for the better, and might even effect her release. She wrote to her long-time ally and ambassador, James Beaton, Archbishop of Glasgow, asking him to make overtures on her behalf to her youngest brother-in-law. Alençon had been only six years old when she had last seen him as she embarked for Scotland from France. The rackety life he had led subsequently, much of it at odds with his mother, Catherine de Medici, and his brother, now Henri III, meant Mary was uncertain of his religious or political allegiances, and concerned that he should be told of her own rights and complaints: "take care that no wrong be done to me, during his government, in the succession of this kingdom, demonstrating to him the right which I have to it." She then added the unrealistic gloss, "in the maintenance of which [right] I hope that the greatest and best part of England will hazard their lives."[12]

She was feeling hopeful again. To an optimist with an opportunistic nature, change was energising and if Elizabeth was to marry at last that would prove the greatest catalyst for change. Mary felt things were going her way and she was impatient to help them along: "in the state in which the affairs of this country are at present, and, as I again understand, those of Scotland are, it will be very easy to form great intrigues

and factions," she wrote to the Archbishop at this time, "and, in my opinion, I never have had so much opportunity and convenience for looking to the restoration of my affairs as now."[13] She followed the unpredictable romance of the English Queen and the French Prince, "my very dear frog" as Elizabeth fondly called him, with intense interest.

The English courtiers were just as interested but distinctly hostile: always suspicious of foreign men and their continental ways, they saw in Simier, "a most choyce Courtier, exquisitely skilled in love toyes, pleasant conceipts, and court-dalliances."[14] He had so bewitched their usually rational queen, so their rumours ran, that only by the use of "amorous potions and unlawfull arts" had he "crept into the Queenes mind and intised her to the love of [Monsieur]."[15]

Elizabeth's insecurity, her overweening vanity, her need for love, all were made more keen by the melancholy realisation that she was growing old. Her spies in France had relayed the cruel gossip which was circulating there and which she repeated indignantly to the French ambassador: "that Monsieur would do well to marry the old creature, who had for the last year an ulcer in her leg, which was not yet healed,* and could never be cured; and, under that pretext, they could send me a potion from France of such a nature that he would find himself a widower in the course of five or six months, and after that he could please himself by marrying the Queen of Scotland and remain the undisputed sovereign of united realms."[16]

It was particularly galling that this revealed Mary as her rival even here, popularly considered the more desirable match because she was a younger woman. Elizabeth's letters during this time emphasised her awareness of the passing of the years. To Monsieur she wrote "grant pardon to the poor old woman who honours you as much (I dare say) as any young wench whom you ever will find."[17] And this from an autocratic and impervious queen? Elizabeth proved to be far from fire-proof in the presence of Simier's skilful coquetry. His delicious flattery made her feel that she could defy time, that she still possessed youth and beauty, and that love and marriage might still be hers. His bold innuendo, the hints of Monsieur's persuasiveness between the sheets, reminded her of the longed-for consequences of desire.

The last time Elizabeth had allowed herself to imagine she could enjoy the pleasures of companionship, sexual fulfilment and marriage was in the fever of her love for Leicester. All the subsequent marriage negotiations had been business as usual for the Queen, of barely passing

---

* Apparently it was an ulcer just above her ankle which did not heal for seven years.

interest to the woman. Now, during this late courtship, Elizabeth for a while forgot her hard-learned lessons of self-protection and control. For a while she believed she could be as other women, pursue her love, share sexual pleasure, even give birth to the heir which would secure her beloved father's dynasty. She railed against her council members who increasingly opposed the match. Her cousin, Sir Francis Knollys, was emotionally reprimanded for blocking her last chance to fulfil her destiny as a woman: "It was a fine way" she said, "to show his attachment to her, who might desire, like others, to have children."[18]

The French were insisting on conditions that her council could not accept, that Alençon should be crowned immediately after marriage and have a large pension for life. They threatened to walk away from the marriage if these were not satisfied. Elizabeth's feelings were already deeply engaged. She had declared to her women of the bedchamber that she had determined to marry. She became "so melancholy since" her council's verdict, and felt diminished by the thought that Alençon was only interested in her for what advantages could be wrung from her and the country. To the French she wrote the timeless feminine plaint that she wanted to be valued for herself alone: "The mark that is shot at is our fortune and not our person," she complained.

This was a surprisingly romantic view of marriage, particularly a dynastic marriage, but it was upheld by her people's stated concern that her suitor was so much younger he might not love her for herself, instead using the marriage to advance his own interests. Elizabeth continued, with some defensiveness, that she could better understand the mercenary behaviour of the French if they were negotiating marriage with a princess who lacked beauty or intelligence, "But considering how otherwise, our fortune laid aside, it hath pleased God to bestow his gifts upon us in good measure, which we do ascribe to the giver, and not glory in as proceeding from ourselves (being no fit trumpet to set out our own praises) . . . we may in true course of modesty think ourself worthy of as great a prince as Monsieur."[19]

By the time Monsieur finally arrived, early one August morning and incognito, everyone's blood was up. Contrary to the usual deflation attendant on reality, Monsieur in person was even more delightful to the Queen than she had hoped. Elizabeth's fears about his ugliness and the scarring of his deeply poxed skin were erased by his exquisite gallantry, humour and the lively grace of his manner. To her cynical and disapproving courtiers, the Queen, simpering, fawning and showing off outrageously, was very close to making a complete fool of herself over this ridiculous Frenchman. In fact, Elizabeth's sensitivity about the age difference was given cruel credence by a report from Catherine de Medici,

admittedly a not impartial source, relayed in cipher by the Venetian ambassador in France to the signory just after this visit: "that Monsieur was somewhat embarrassed, when as a young man devoted to pleasure, he called to mind the advanced age and repulsive physical nature of the Queen [*le brutta qualità del corpo della Regina*], she being, in addition to her other ailments, half consumptive; . . . the lust to reign will contend with the lust of the flesh, and we shall see which of these two passions possesses the greater force."[20]

In the grip of unloosed feeling, Elizabeth's tautly strung self-control had unravelled in the skilful hands of the courtier-lover Simier. For a while she had forgotten her deep-rooted reservations, even her age, in the longing to be in love again. She wrote to Monsieur after his departure, exceeding the usual diplomatic utterance with rare abandon: "I confess there is no prince in the world to whom I would more willingly yield to be his, than to yourself, nor to whom I think myself more obliged, nor with whom I would pass the years of my life, both for your rare virtues and sweet nature."[21]

It would not be long, however, before reality asserted itself and duty called. Elizabeth's whole philosophy of monarchy was expressed by her in a letter to Simier: "how near it touches me that our people do not perceive in their Prince a negligence or a luke-warmedness for their well-being and safety; we were not born only for ourselves."[22] In fact the dour antagonism of her people for this match had worried her from the start. For a while her passions were so engaged that she managed to overlook this dark cloud threatening her hopes, but she was less able to ignore the disapproval and forebodings of her councillors. Her favourites were particularly put out. During the heat of the proxy courtship there were two attempts on Simier's life, with suggestions that at least one of them had been instigated by a murderously jealous Leicester. Elizabeth was outraged and mortified. This turned to white rage when Simier, in retaliation, revealed to Elizabeth something kept secret only from her—that Leicester had remarried the previous year. His bride was the widowed Countess of Essex, Francis Knollys's beautiful daughter, Lettice, a woman who had been her friend.

The resulting furore, the bitter accusations, the hang-dog Leicester, his rustication, Elizabeth's tears, all proved immense entertainment to Mary and Bess of Hardwick, plying their needles in Sheffield Castle. It proved another poignant reminder, however, to Elizabeth that *tempus fugit*, and even the companion of her youth, the love of her life, could betray her in love. A poem she wrote in the 1580s expressed eloquently the passing of youth and her melancholy acceptance of responsibility for what she had made of her life:

When I was fair and young, and favour graced me,
Of many I was sought their mistress for to be.
But I did scorn them all, and answered them therefore,
    "Go, go, seek some otherwhere,
    Importune me no more."

How many weeping eyes I made to pine with woe;
How many sighing hearts I have no skill to show.
Yet I the prouder grew, and answered them therefore,
    "Go, go, go seek some otherwhere,
    Importune me no more."

Then spake fair Venus' son, that proud victorious boy,
And said: "Fine dame, since that you be so coy,
I will so pluck your plumes that you shall say no more
    "Go, go, go seek some otherwhere,
    Importune me no more."

When he had spake those words, such charge grew in my breast
That neither night nor day since that, I could take any rest.
Then lo, I did repent that I had said before,
    "Go, go, go seek some otherwhere,
    Importune me no more."[23]

Elizabeth's frustrated love for Leicester may have been the inspiration for this poem. It may have been rather the regretful realisation that she could not pursue late passion and marry Monsieur. Then again the poem may have been more generally symbolic of change and loss, and the painful gaining of wisdom. Leicester was her enduring love, and although she was quick to anger and easily hurt, Elizabeth was always open to reason in the end. He had been a widower for eighteen years and the Queen was realistic. By then, both Leicester and she had accepted that their marriage could never be, not that this prevented Elizabeth from wanting him to be unconditionally hers, more devoted and loyal than any husband could ever be. Without much time in the wilderness, he was back in the centre of Elizabeth's emotional landscape, particularly as the passion for her "dear frog" faded to affectionate, if increasingly exasperated, friendship.

The unfortunate young man who apparently had discharged a firearm towards Simier, as he travelled with the Queen by barge up the river at Greenwich, protested his innocence of any evil intent and was released. Elizabeth had exercised a characteristic parental mercy,

according to Camden, for, "she was many times wont to say, *That she could believe nothing of her people, which Parents would not believe of their children.*"[24] She had certainly proved that she had the strengths and insecurities of a lone parent in her unwillingness to do anything that her children might veto.

Loyal as she was to her people, however, Elizabeth was capable of acts of savage retribution when threatened, for instance, by the power of print to disseminate dissension and revolt. The writer and distributor of a tract published in September 1579 entitled, "The Discovery of a Gaping Gulph whereinto England is like to be swallowed by another French marriage . . . , " were sentenced immediately to have their right hands hacked off. The offending work expressed in intemperate language what most of her populace believed to be the case—that the Valois princes were sly papists and worthless reprobates, that Elizabeth was too old for Alençon and he could not love her, that she anyway was past childbearing. In short, he was a rat who should not have been allowed even to look on their Queen.

Patriotic it may have been, but Elizabeth was still trying valiantly to reconcile her personal desires with her duties as monarch, and could not allow this powerful popular view the added force of widespread publication. By her brutal and precipitate action against the perpetrators, she acknowledged the growing power of print, which brought rapid and effective communication direct to the people, supplementing the official message of state or church. Elizabeth's subjects attending the public mutilation of these good burghers greeted the sentence with sullen silence and shock.

The Queen knew that her fantasy of love could not long survive. As she withdrew further from the courtship, she wrote to her French ambassador: "My mortal [foe can] no ways wish me a greater loss than England's hate; neither should death be less welcome unto me than such mishap betide me . . . Shall it ever be found true that Queen Elizabeth hath solemnized the perpetual harm of England under the glorious title of marriage with Francis, heir of France? No, no, it shall never be."[25]

Mary's growing realisation that Elizabeth's French marriage, like all her previous proposals, would wither unripened on the bough meant that she once more looked to Spain for her deliverance. Her thoughts were increasingly focussed on her son, James VI, who in the summer of 1580 was fourteen and already exhibiting an independent intelligence and capacity to rule. Morton was still regent, although not for long, and Mary showed a continuing maternal solicitude for James as well as a

political interest in what he might be able to do to effect her freedom, once he was free to rule himself. When she heard he was ill with some kind of digestive complaint her insistent letter to the Archbishop of Glasgow was eloquent of her "excessive sorrow and uneasiness." Having suffered from a similar complaint when she was young she recalled that wearing ivory close to her stomach had helped and urged that, in a ritual to safeguard his health, his weight in virgin wax be sent to the church of "nostre Dame de Cléry"* and a novena be said there. She asked also that a mass be sung daily for a year at the same church, and thirteen *trezains* [a base metal coin] be distributed to the first thirteen poor people who arrived on each successive day.[26]

While Elizabeth made much of her relationship as mother to her people, Mary was a real mother with a real son. She had been separated from this boy from the time he was barely one, when her disastrous marriage to Bothwell ended with her subsequent flight from Scotland. She had attempted through letters and gifts to maintain some sort of motherly contact, to keep his memories and affection for her alive and to influence his religious ideas. She feared but did not know fully that he had been brought up with the belief that his mother was closer to a jezebel than a madonna, responsible for the murder of his father and obstinate in her adherence to popery, which to the extreme Calvinists who surrounded him was close to witchcraft in its reliance on symbols, ritual and mystery.

He cannot have been so thoroughly shielded, however, from the influence of his mother's sympathisers. Certainly James seemed particularly proud of his glamorous Guise inheritance, writing to the Duc de Guise, when he was seventeen, to declare he was greatly encouraged "to imitate the virtues of our ancestors of the house of Lorraine, who have so borne themselves that their name shall be honoured to all eternity." It is likely some of his adulatory information came as a result of the flatteries from such Francophile sophisticates as the first favourite of many in his reign, his cousin Esmé Stuart.† He and another attractive youth, the

---

* The thirteenth-century church in the diocese of Orléans, a favourite place of worship and pilgrimage for the Valois kings. Orléans was an important city for Mary. It was here she had nursed her first husband, François II, to his death in 1560. It was also the setting for one of the great stories of French feminine heroism when at the battle of Orléans in 1429, Joan of Arc saved France from England. There is no reason to doubt that Mary was affected herself by the stories of this singular woman's heroic martyrdom and her subsequent immortality in the sentimental history of her country.

† Esmé Stuart, Duke of Lennox (1542?–83), cousin of James VI and some thought successor to his throne should he die childless. Handsome, charming, an adroit and plausible schemer, on his arrival in Scotland in 1579 he was immediately irresistible to the

Master of Gray, had just made the young King's acquaintance. James ended his paean of praise by noting that his worthiest attributes came from this ancestry, "from which I descend through my mother."[27]

When James finally had the choice, however, he did not wish to share his governance of Scotland with his glamorous but discredited mother, preferring instead to make his alliance with Elizabeth, thereby safeguarding his prospects of succeeding to the English throne. The Master of Gray, originally Mary's friend, had been sent to negotiate with Elizabeth in what Mary believed was a tripartite alliance, involving both her son and herself. In fact, the young Gray was keener to exclude Mary and court Elizabeth on behalf of James, in whom Scottish power now resided. He sent back a message to Elizabeth that James's affection was "such to your Majesty as though he were your natural son." To his own natural mother, James wrote without any of the filial love Mary had hoped would survive their separation: "as she was held captive in a remote place, [he had no choice but that] of declining to associate her with himself in the sovereignty of Scotland, or to treat her otherwise than as Queen-Mother."[28]

This complete loss of her son in every sense, physical, emotional and spiritual, was a devastating blow to Mary. She had to relinquish one of her dearest held illusions, that an instinctive filial love for her would survive everything. James lacked even a memory of his mother and this, combined with an ambition as fierce as her own to inherit the throne of England, meant ultimately he would reject her for Elizabeth. Mary unleashed on Elizabeth a pitiful rant of misery and revenge against the son she claimed to love more than anyone in the world. "Without him I am, and shall be of right, as long as I live, his Queen and Sovereign . . . but without me, he is too insignificant to think of soaring." She refused to be a Queen Mother "for I do not acknowledge one; failing our association, there is no King of Scotland, nor any Queen but me."[29]

As James's real mother, she had given birth to him at risk of her own life, and produced a son and heir of her own blood and dynasty. Now she was to lose him to the pretended mother, his godmother Elizabeth, the woman she had sought as a mother, a sister, a close blood relation for herself. Mary had been denied every intimacy for which she had begged and bullied. Even her rightful place as Elizabeth's successor had never

---

young, fatherless King. Ambition made him convert to Protestantism. After the execution of the regent Morton in 1581, his influence over James was at its zenith and he was rewarded with his dukedom. In 1582 he clandestinely agreed to command an army, raised by Philip II, to invade England. Philip's procrastination meant this came to naught, but controversy over Lennox's true religious affiliation meant he was forced to leave Scotland and return to France, where he died.

been acknowledged formally. Her precious son, however, in betraying her would gain the prizes she had desired always.

While captive, Mary's only means of affecting events was through letters, either official or coded, clandestine, contraband. Her letters to Elizabeth were in French, numerous, heartfelt and repetitive in their plaints. She was a clever and emotionally manipulative writer who managed very different tones of voice to different recipients. A typical letter to Elizabeth combined pathos and seduction with hidden menace, but never once was she close to accepting responsibility for any of the ill-fortune that had befallen her, or for the plots against Elizabeth in which she starred. In early May 1580 she wrote:

> *Madam, my good sister,—I have written to you several times during the last year, to lay before your consideration the unworthy and rigorous treatment which I have received in this captivity, notwithstanding the evidence which I have made a point of giving you, on all occasions, of my entire and sincere affection for you . . . I am constrained to beg and entreat you, as I humbly do, by my liberation out of this prison, to relieve yourself from the charge which I am to you, and from the continual suspicions, mistrusts, and prejudices with which [my enemies surrounding you] daily trouble you against me . . . Think that you can have me, out of prison, more your own, binding my heart to you by so signal a courtesy, than by confining my body within four walls.*

Mary then added an insight into her own sense of inviolable queenship and characteristic defiance, as candidly she explained, "compulsion not being the usual mode of gaining much from those of my rank and disposition, of which you may have some experience from the past." She reiterated her credentials as a sovereign queen, nearest relative to Elizabeth and "plus juste hérétière [most lawful heretrix]" and threatened she would soon die of her increasingly ill health. She ended with a request to be allowed to go to the baths at Buxton, which was granted, for three weeks at the end of July.[30]

Mary's imprisonment at this time was more of a house arrest with horse-riding and periodic therapeutic visits to the Buxton spa. Throughout she was treated with the full courtesy due to a queen, dining under her canopy of state and waited upon by servants of her own choosing. Although her mail had to pass through Shrewsbury's hands, there was a limited welcome to courtiers and visitors who requested access to the Queen. However, Walsingham's nose for traitorous activity had long been alert to the comings and goings of friends and correspondence

around the Queen of Scots. He arrested one of Mary's go-betweens, Jail-heur, but found nothing incriminating.

Her relief was palpable in her letter to Archbishop Beaton, written in code just a couple of weeks after her plaintive missive to Elizabeth. The change in tone was instructive; here was a woman who was decisive, business-like and ready for any adventure. She informed the Archbishop she would find someone to replace the exposed Jailheur to "obtain ser-vice in my more important and secret matters." One of these more important and secret matters was her request for help to Spain, the seri-ousness of which she wanted the Archbishop to underline by proposing "the removal of my son to Flanders or Spain, according as shall be agreeable to the King [Philip II]." Mary then went on to mention her letter to Elizabeth requesting her freedom. Should that fail, though, she promised her ambassador she was ready for any available plot or enter-prise: "I shall expose myself to the risk of such other invention as may present itself."[31]

The following year, Mary was writing to the Archbishop in similarly decisive vein: "I am earnestly exhorted to bring back my son to the faith, and to labour all at once for its restoration in this island, so as to engage in the cause all the Catholics in this country." She continued in sanguine vein, "Walsingham boasts of being acquainted with the plans of my cousin Monsieur de Guise for my deliverance, and also with the negoti-ations which have been entered into respecting it . . . offering likewise to prove that I have written to you in these very words,—'That I shall leave no stone unturned to escape from this imprisonment.' Consider from what quarter he could receive such information, and beware of it, I entreat you."[32]

Mary was in an impossible situation. Desperate to escape and reclaim her life and her crown, and even the crown of England too, she had to endure a long imprisonment from which hope of legitimate release had all but faded. Temperamentally she was not one to wait with patience for the tide, to resign herself to fate. She was a fighter who worked for freedom and paid whatever price. Secrecy, subversion and dreams of revenge gave her the necessary excitement and kept hope alive. Plotting was her lifeblood and games of risk saved her from insan-ity or chronic depression. Principal Secretary and arch spymaster Wal-singham recognised the recklessness implicit in the nature of such an adventuress. He knew that it was just a matter of time before he had Mary implicated up to her neck in a cast iron case of treason.

Only with overwhelming evidence did he, Cecil and the more radi-cal Protestants of Elizabeth's council hope to be able to rid themselves of the troublesome presence of the Queen of Scots. While she lived, they

believed she threatened the very core of Elizabeth's reign, the Protestant succession, the continuance of a peaceful Reformation, the safety of the realm. Religious wars had riven France and the Low Countries. Elizabeth's ministers feared civil war while Mary lived, but they knew well their own queen. Passionately attached to the concept of the inviolability of kings, she was repelled when it came to talk of their assassination. Desperate to keep faith with her people and not antagonise her Catholic neighbours, Elizabeth was determined that everything she did was seen to be legal. To destroy Mary, her ministers would need incontrovertible evidence.

Not only were Mary's hopes alive that some foreign power would come to spring her from jail into the welcoming, and militant, arms of the English Catholics, the English Catholics themselves were awakening to a new hope as their own faith enjoyed spiritual renewal. Although religious wars raged just across the Channel, Elizabeth had hoped initially that a policy of non-intrusive tolerance would ensure Catholicism conveniently withered in her realm through lack of nurture. In 1570 she had promised Catholics freedom from "inquisition or examination of their consciences in causes of religion"; as long as their religion was practised in private, and that outwardly they conformed and kept the law. Harried as she had been herself during her sister Mary's reign, this policy of freedom of conscience was close to her heart. She is reputed to have said to Philip II about his campaign against the Protestants in the Low Countries, "What does it matter to your Majesty if they go to the devil in their own way?"[33]

Elizabeth herself had never been driven by religious conviction and was more conservative certainly than the strongly Protestant Cecil, Leicester and Walsingham. But freedom of thought mattered to her and she pursued, until cornered, an evasive policy of laissez faire. The compromise and veiled hypocrisy she demanded of English Catholics who wished to maintain their faith, along with their liberty and wealth, were merely reflections of Elizabeth's own diplomatic style. She did not see why a certain pragmatic pretence should be rejected in favour of an awkward truth.

The papal bull of 1570 was the first alarm bell: taken literally, a true Catholic was exhorted to rid England of the heretic pretender to the throne, with the promise of heavenly reward. Bills proposed by the Parliament of 1571 to make every subject take Protestant communion were vetoed by the Queen, still insisting on freedom of conscience for all. However, a bill was passed which designated as high treason any attempt to convert an English subject into a subject of Rome, or even to be an English subject whose first allegiance was to Rome. It would take six

years, however, before a priest was prosecuted and executed for treason under this new act. More than a hundred would follow by the end of Elizabeth's reign.

While the papal bull breathed fire, the arrival of missionary priests, trained at the recently established Douai seminary in the Low Countries, gave heart to the Catholic faithful in England. They entered the country clandestinely and were greeted with great enthusiasm as they carried new blood into the cells of the disheartened resistance across England. Many of the priests were English exiles, hastily trained and ill-prepared for their missions. According to Camden, Elizabeth thought "these silly priests" were mostly innocent of "plotting the Destruction of their Countrey"[34] and were much more the instruments of their superiors' treasonous will.

A far from silly priest was the English Jesuit Edmund Campion. A brilliant scholar at Oxford, he had debated before the Queen during her historic visit to the university in 1566. She had been particularly impressed during the Natural History Disputation with his contribution to the proposal that the tides were caused by the moon's motion. Both Cecil and Leicester, who were present, offered to become his patrons. He had been a deacon in the Church of England in his twenties before converting to Catholicism and fleeing to Europe to train at Douai and then Prague. He arrived back in England in 1580 and was arrested, accused of plotting against Elizabeth to place Catholic Mary on her throne.

Even under torture Campion denied his motives were anything other than spiritual. He had written an apologia before embarking on his mission in which he denied any political intent: "I never had mind, and am strictly forbidden by our Father that sent me, to deal in any respect with matter of State of Police [policy] of this realm, as things which appertain not to my vocation, and from which I do gladly restrain and sequester my thoughts." But the Pope's bull, disputing Elizabeth's legitimacy, had made the spiritual political. Any support from these priests for the English Catholics would implicitly involve them in the treason of offering greater obedience to the Pope than to the Queen.

Elizabeth was sensitive to accusations of religious persecution and cruelty towards the missionary priests. Her government was careful to make the sophistical point that they questioned their suspects on political allegiances and steered clear of any spiritual matters. There was uneasiness too at reports of excessive cruelty being used to extract confessions (the Spanish ambassador had reported to Philip II that Campion had been viciously racked, even subjected to nails driven into the quick beneath each finger) and a declaration was published that

although Campion was put on the rack it was never so extreme that he was not "presently able to walk, and subscribe his Confession."[35] Under English law, torture was illegal but could be used by special dispensation, and, during these years of conspiracy and intrigue, it was one of the tools used frequently in the search for evidence.

The increasing influence of rebel priests and the upsurge of Catholic support meant that the Parliament of 1581 passed an act aimed at restricting aberrant behaviour. It became a dangerous and expensive world for English Catholics. Converts were subject to the charge of treason, as were the priests who converted them. The recusants who refused to attend church and accept the Protestant sacrament were liable to be fined twenty pounds a month, a sum to beggar even the wealthiest of families. Elizabeth had long resisted the pressures of her ministers to deal more decisively with her Catholic subjects and had consistently been more lenient in her attitude towards the confinement and punishment of Mary. Uneasy when having to conduct her rule in broad strokes of black and white, Elizabeth was much happier when lines were blurry and detail open to a variety of interpretations.

Suffering ever more savage reprisals against the priests and the laity who shielded them, the English Catholics were harassed, but their faith was spiritually invigorated. The executions, particularly of self-evidently courageous and principled men like Campion, fuelled a lively martyrology. However draconian their members of Parliament might wish to be in their measures against the Catholics, ordinary people were less willing to inform on or prosecute those neighbours who appeared to be otherwise peaceable, law-abiding citizens.

This revival of support energised Mary too. Temperamentally inclined to optimism and never short of confidence in her powers of attraction, she believed that there was a very significant body of dedicated English Catholics ready to take up arms for her cause. Mary sent the Spanish ambassador a remarkable message for Philip II: "[She] did not mean to leave where she is, except as Queen of England . . . her adherents and the Catholics were so numerous in the country that, if they rose, it would be easy even without assistance, but with the help of your Majesty it would soon be over, without any doubt."[36] With that she hoped to encourage armed Spanish intervention in the fates of herself and of Elizabeth.

Such naivety and over-confidence meant she gave her blessing to any schemes and intrigues that came her way, and would in the end even put her name to incriminating letters of intent. Just as the rise of Catholic solidarity in England gave Mary cause for hope, it also meant her position grew increasingly perilous. It would make it easier to impli-

cate her legally in the treasonous activity of others. Also as factions became polarised and fear took a grip there would be some prepared to assassinate Mary rather than risk losing English autonomy and their Protestant monarch.

In the final decade of Mary's life there came a variety of plots based on this papal plan. The spiritual imperative to restore to England the true faith and the rightful heir was stamped with the Pope's—and therefore, to the English Catholics, God's—imprimatur, while the force to effect this was expected to come with Philip II's army and the spontaneous uprising of Mary's newly invigorated supporters. Ever vigilant, Walsingham was full of foreboding but frustrated by the reluctance of his sovereign to act swiftly and harshly in protection of her self, her religion and her realm. It was to his advantage to prove the ubiquity and ruthlessness of the plotters, and persuade Elizabeth to stiffen her resolve against the Catholics and Mary herself, the focus of their hopes.

The discovery at the end of 1583 of what was to become known as the Throckmorton plot was further proof to Walsingham, Cecil and Leicester that the status quo between Mary and Elizabeth was too dangerous to leave undisturbed. For a while Elizabeth had appeared willing to accommodate again a plan put forward by Mary two years before. In return for her freedom and recognition of joint sovereignty with her son James of Scotland, Mary declared herself ready to relinquish her claim on the English throne while Elizabeth lived, denounce the papal bull of excommunication, safeguard the Protestant religion in Scotland, and proclaim an amnesty for all those who had wronged her in Scotland and England. Mary's willingness to accept such terms exhibited either a sincere desire for freedom at any cost or, as Walsingham warned, a lax approach to promises and treaties which could be modified or even ignored as occasion demanded. In the end it was James himself who declined the power sharing, and temporarily broke his mother's heart at his betrayal of her maternal illusions.

Mary's insistence during the revived negotiations in the summer of 1583 that she was a practitioner of "plain and upright dealing," desiring "nothing so much as her majesty's good favour," and "greatly wearied . . . of her long captivity. She is much decayed in health . . . ,"[37] sounded rather hollow when it was discovered that simultaneously she was keenly engaged in the workings of another plot. After six months' surveillance, Walsingham emerged with evidence of close involvement of the Duc de Guise, the Spanish King and the Queen of Scots, with Sir Francis Throckmorton as go-between, in an ambitious plan of invasion, rescue and assassination, the dream being to place Mary on Elizabeth's throne through force, and return the heretic isle to Catholicism.

In November 1583, Throckmorton was arrested and confessed under torture. Mary denied everything. She had long ago decided that it was far more noble to be persecuted for her faith than for the tawdry machinations of treason. The combative Spanish ambassador, Bernadino de Mendoza, was summarily expelled from the English court the following January. "Being a man of a violent and turbulent Spirit," he did not go quietly. He insulted Elizabeth by telling her ministers that as she was a woman he had expected nothing better than her rank ingratitude. He threatened that "as I had apparently failed to please her as a minister of peace she would in future force me to try to satisfy her in war."[38] So injured was his pride he wrote to Philip II that the only point of life now for him was to avenge the insolence of the English, "even though I have to walk barefooted to the other side of the world to beg for [God's commission to do it]."[39] From his vantage point in Paris, he laboured to promote the next great plot against Elizabeth but died just before the insolent English rout of the Spanish armada.

Not only was Mary once more implicated in treason, her own personal behaviour again was under attack. The Countess of Shrewsbury, a friend no longer, had taken damaging allegations to court about the leniency of her husband's wardship of the Queen of Scots, due to the fact, she claimed, that he was in love and had enjoyed sexual relations with her. Mary was incensed and quick to write to the French ambassador begging him to acquaint Elizabeth, her council, the French King and Catherine de Medici, as well as all the Guises, with her innocence of "anything in the world contrary or prejudicial to my honour."[40] A second, but this time secret, letter was also intercepted and decoded by Walsingham's agents: in this Mary requested that the ambassador should pass on a veiled threat to Leicester, intimating that if nothing was done to clear Mary's name from "this false and unhappy imposture"[41] then she would reveal certain information concerning his intimate behaviour with Elizabeth, as well as his personal ambitions. (He had a scheme to marry his son to Arabella Stuart, Mary's niece-in-law, the Countess of Shrewsbury's grand-daughter, and a claimant to the English throne.)

None of these revelations consoled Elizabeth. The Throckmorton plot brought together her two most powerful enemies, Spain and France—in the form of the Guises—in nightmare alliance. The fear of invasion by a superior force had haunted her reign. The Pope's support for a religious crusade against Protestantism had made the sacred political. In June 1584 the assassination by a Spanish agent of the Prince of Orange in the middle of his campaign in the Low Countries brought Elizabeth's own death closer. There were increasing rumours also of a great Spanish fleet in the making, with the fear that it meant some

aggressive intent against England. In the heart of her kingdom too was the canker of a captive Catholic queen whose presence focussed every form of dissent and wrung sympathy from even the most incorruptible of hearts.

Although officially Elizabeth did not give them much credence, the stories the Countess of Shrewsbury had to tell of Mary's seductive presence subverting one of the most solid and trusty of Englishmen merely reinforced the mythology of the Scottish Queen's supernatural powers of attraction. All scurrilous rumour around Mary also undermined Elizabeth's struggle to maintain her own reputation and probity against the malicious talk that her status and sex always had attracted. Her answer to Mary's distress over these allegations expressed how closely Elizabeth identified with the need to maintain the honour of all queens: "we can neither forget [Mary's] quality nor her proximity in blood. We have always had special care to suppress the licentiousness of this corrupt age in speaking evil of princes, whose credit and reputation ought to be held sacred."[42] She feared the disrespect of the people and the condescension of her fellow monarchs who were keen to denigrate the feminine inadequacies of every queen. These many precarious elements hung heavily on Elizabeth. She was conscious of her own vulnerability, her country's poverty and weaknesses, and frightened always of war.

The confused details of another possible plot to assassinate the Queen involving one of the members of her own Parliament, William Parry, were revealed hard on the heels of the Throckmorton plot. In an atmosphere where potential assassins lurked at every turn, Cecil produced a declaration in October 1584 aimed at protecting Elizabeth's life by removing the reward expected on her death—a Catholic queen on the English throne. The signatories to this document swore to defend the Queen and to pursue to death anyone who attempted any violence against her. Its clauses were broadened to disallow the succession of any person involved in an attempt on Elizabeth's life. This became known as the Bond of Association, and by the end of the autumn was enthusiastically signed by tens of thousands of loyal subjects up and down the land. Elizabeth was touched by the evidence of her people's love and loyalty, and thanked her Parliament, promising as much care for her people in return: "I am not unmindful of your Oath made in the Association manifesting your great goodwills and affections . . . done (I protest to God) before I heard of it or ever thought of such a matter, until a great number of hands with many obligations were showed me at Hampton Court, signed and subscribed with the names and seals of the greatest of this land. Which I do acknowledge as a perfect argument of your true hearts and great zeal for my safety, so shall my bond be stronger tied to greater care for your good."[43]

Although it did not name Mary, the Bond was aimed directly at anyone who might act against Elizabeth in order to place her rival or that rival's heirs on the throne. If it was made law, which Parliament attempted that November, in effect it would have become Mary's death warrant. Should any other plot to assassinate Elizabeth be uncovered with the objective of placing Mary on her throne, even if there was no evidence that she had any part in it, she could be found guilty by association and summarily executed. Elizabeth was unhappy with the extremity of the proposed act and insisted that guilt should be established first, by a minimum of twenty-four councillors and noblemen.

Careful also not to debar James, Elizabeth ensured the heirs of a guilty party were not prevented themselves from inheriting. Mary, writing to Cecil in January 1585 from Tutbury Castle, was so keen to impress him and Elizabeth with her trustworthiness she offered to put her signature to the Bond of Association to prove "before God and on her honour" she was not "one who would wish to attempt, support, or favour an act so wicked as an attempt against her person or her kingdom."[44] Within eighteen months she was deep in the final conspiracy of her life in which the murder of Elizabeth and the invasion of England by Spain were integral parts.

During this Parliament an act against the Catholic missionary priests was introduced which ordered any priests ordained abroad to leave England within forty days or be executed for treason. Scores of priests, some already condemned and imprisoned as traitors, were deported to France, where the militant Spanish ambassador Mendoza noted with delight that these English attempts to stem the flow only served to increase the fervour of the "seminarists [who] go over daily to England with glad hearts and wonderful firmness to win the crown of martyrdom."[45]

This general alarm meant Mary was moved from Sheffield Castle and finally out of the care of the Earl and Countess of Shrewsbury. Shrewsbury had discharged his onerous duty over a period of fifteen years, during which time his health and his fortune had been significantly depleted. On taking leave of Elizabeth the following year he kissed her hand and thanked her fervently for having "freed him from two devils, namely, the Queen of Scotland and his wife,"[46] the indomitable Bess of Hardwick.

Mary was moved, with great forward planning and in the company of a body of armed men, to Wingfield Manor, to be temporarily in the care of the kindly old diplomat Sir Ralph Sadler. Now in his late seventies, he had been Henry VIII's ambassador to Mary's mother, Mary of

Guise, when she was regent of Scotland. At that time he had been impressed both by her, and by the beauty and vigour of her tiny baby, Mary herself. Nearly forty-two years ago she had been unwrapped and undressed in the middle of winter to prove to the King of England's envoy that the baby he coveted in marriage for his son Edward was both healthy and perfect, and likely to survive. If Sadler was touched by her then, inevitably he would be putty in the hands of the now grown-up and tragic woman, the deposed queen.

In January 1585, despite protestations and delaying tactics, Mary was transferred once more to the grim stronghold of Tutbury Castle. On the way Sadler, Mary and their party had unexpectedly to stay the night in a lowly house, kept by "an ancient wydow, namid Mrs. Beaumont." Mary's charming manners and gift of empathy in her concern to put at ease this unimportant woman gave an insight into why her own female servants, particularly, remained so affectionate and loyal to her all their lives: "So sone as [Mary] knew who was her hostesse, after she had made a beck [nod] to the rest of the wemen standing next to the doore, she went to her and kissed her, and none other, sayeng that she was comme thither to trouble her, and that she was also a wydow, and therefore trusted that they shulde agree well inough together, having no husbands to trouble them."[47]

One of Sadler's favourite sports was hawking. Mary too was an enthusiast and long ago had surprised her French family when she first arrived in France, aged not yet six, by exhibiting precocious expertise as a falconer. When Sadler sent for his hawks and falconers to while away what was an unhappy situation as jailer, he could not resist Mary's blandishments, even when it got him into trouble. On the arrival of his birds, she had "ernestly intreated me that she might go abrode with me to see my hawkes flie, a passetyme indede which she hethe singular delite in." Sadler could not deny her and allowed Mary to accompany him three or four times, even though it meant riding on horseback some miles down the valley from the castle. Elizabeth was far from happy when she heard of this breach of security in his keeping of the Queen of Scots, alarmed at a possible escape or rescue attempt. Sadler explained that he was an unwilling jailer and anyway had never had less than forty armed men on horseback with them. Weary of life, he said, he desired nothing more than to relinquish this unsought charge, to return home to prepare himself for death and "the euerlasting quyetnes of the lif to com."[48]

His wish was to be granted, for his duties as Mary's keeper were handed over in April 1585 to Sir Amyas Paulet, a scrupulous Puritan and the least susceptible of men. Sadler had mildly complained to Elizabeth that it was impossible to keep track of all the correspondence and con-

versation that eddied about the Queen of Scots, so large was her household and the numbers of Scottish, English and French servants and courtiers who came and went almost without check. Paulet immediately imposed his more austere will. He pared down her household and closed off the channels of her private mail, even for a while to the French ambassador. The casual expeditions were also stopped. There were no more summer visits to Buxton baths and certainly no more days hawking miles down river from the castle gates. If Paulet was unimpressed by Mary, she was equally dismissive of him: "he is one of the most gruff and rebarbative [*un des plus bizzares et farouches*] of persons whom I have ever known; and, in a word, fitter for a jail of criminals than for the custody of one of my rank and birth."[49] She also felt that should Elizabeth die, Paulet would have little compunction in eliminating her, rather than countenance a Catholic successor to the English throne.

Mary fired off an indignant complaint to Elizabeth at these new restrictions. Even as she wrote, however, it occurred to her that her letters were barely read by the recipient as they were "so long and customarily tedious, according to the subject that is daily provided to me for them." Through the years the stream of letters from Mary to her cousin veered from professions of love to the pathos of the victimised, through queenly outrage to veiled menace and threats of foreign intervention. Elizabeth at first had been sympathetic, sometimes intimidated, even amazed, but after nearly two decades when neither the content nor context had much changed she had grown distant; as Mary perceptively feared "you yourself will not always give yourself leisure to read my letters." Mary was not a fool and as a natural charmer and entertainer she also regretted the paucity of her experiences now, the narrowed horizons so different from the glamour and promise of her youth. She ended the letter with her unique combination of apology, accusation and pathos: "I regret that my letters convey to you only continual complaints and grievances; but still more the so pregnant cause which I have, to which I beseech my God to send a termination in some shape or other."[50]

Elizabeth did not immediately read this letter, if in fact she ever did. Despite the heightened awareness of her vulnerability to assassination and the complete lack of protection from anyone wishing her ill, she was on one of her annual summer progresses, greeted by crowds who pressed close with offerings, any one of whom could have killed her. Elizabeth had never forgotten that she owed her crown not only to God but to her people, and she recognised the power of her presence and the necessity of pageant and display.

Leopold von Wedel was a young German adventurer from Pomerania of independent means who arrived in England in the summer of

1585. In his informative diary, he not only admired the beauty of the fair-skinned English women but was surprised at their forwardness and the fact that they participated so wholeheartedly in public events: "the womenfolk in England wish to be in at everything,"[51] was his half-admiring aside. He also noted how accessible the Queen was, despite the level of anxiety raised by the discovery of various plots and possible assassination attempts. He had already been shown around her palaces, with great informality, noting the wealth and luxury of the furnishings and jewel-studded objets d'art; the pearl encrusted bed hangings of the Queen's bed of state and the even larger pearls embroidered onto the pillows, being amongst the details which caught his eye.

Wedel was struck by Elizabeth's popular touch despite the overwhelming grandeur of the pageant of her public life. Having been to church at Hampton Court she walked between two rows of her "common people," who as she approached fell upon their knees. "The Queen's demeanour, however, was gracious and gentle and so was her speech, and from rich and poor she took petitions in a modest manner."[52] Her surprising patience and affection seemed to be reciprocated by the populace many times over. Elizabeth managed to combine personal familiarity with semi-divine spectacle, with herself at the centre of the show. On her arrival in London in early November, ready for the annual festivities on the seventeenth, the twenty-seventh anniversary of the day she was proclaimed Queen, the glamour of the procession on horseback was recorded vividly by Wedel:

> [Burghley and Walsingham] were followed by the Queen in a gold coach, open all round, but having above it a canopy embroidered with gold and pearls . . . The Queen sat alone in the carriage. She was dressed in white and cried to the people: "God save my people," to which the crowd responded with "God save Your Grace." This they repeated many times, falling on their knees. The Queen sitting all alone in her splendid coach appeared like a goddess such as painters are wont to depict. Behind the Queen's coach rode my Lord Lester, who is an Earl of princely blood.[53]

Remarkably, this procession, almost three decades after that first triumphant entry into London on her accession, was fundamentally unchanged. Her two closest advisors then, Cecil and Lord Robert, some thirty years later were her closest still. Despite the passage of eventful years, only Walsingham had been added to the intimate family circle around Elizabeth, and this continuity and enduring loyalty was one of

the keys to the stability and success of her reign. Wedel appeared as caught up in the general emotion of fealty and gratitude to Elizabeth. A young man overwhelmed by the palaces he had visited, the pageants and jousting tournaments, the feasts and the balls, it was not surprising that he should declare the English as "rich, wealthy, very ostentatious and pleasure-loving."[54]

Just as this starry-eyed tourist was preparing to return to Germany, life in England was growing more difficult and dangerous for both Mary and Elizabeth. The Protestant rebels in the Low Countries were in disarray since the assassination of the Prince of Orange and were petitioning desperately for more help from Elizabeth than just the money and munitions she had supplied during the previous decade. Fear of Spanish aggression meant there were many in England who considered that Spain, having reasserted its authority over the Low Countries, would turn its warlike energies at last on England. Bowing to the passionate advocacy of an ageing Leicester, determined on his chance of military command in the Protestant cause for which he had long campaigned, Elizabeth reluctantly allowed her favourite to go to the Low Countries in command of her forces, with the title of the Queen's Lieutenant General.

Accoutred with magnificence, and in the company of an impressive array of noblemen, the portly Earl arrived in Flushing to an ecstatic welcome. He had a fleet of one hundred ships to transport his entourage and was in charge of thousands of foot soldiers and cavalry. Camden recorded how Elizabeth's decision to come to the "Netherlanders" aid meant "all the Princes of Christendom admired at such manly Fortitude in a Woman, which durst, as it were, declare War against so puissant [powerful] a Monarch: insomuch as the King of Sweden said, 'That Queen Elizabeth had now taken the Diadem from her Head, and adventured it upon the doubtfull Chance of War.' "[55]

To distract the Spanish further, Elizabeth let loose again Sir Francis Drake and his band of venture capitalists to prey on the Spanish colonies, their treasure ships and trade routes. This overt piracy enraged the Spanish further as the looted treasures enriched not only Drake's own coffers and those of the grandees who lent their support to his expeditions, but Elizabeth herself. Mendoza writing to Philip II explained the outrageous deal: "[Drake] did not take precise orders from the Queen, except to plunder as much as he could, to enable her to sustain the war in Flanders."[56] Her unashamed encouragement of her rapacious adventurers extended even to ennobling them. This insult combined with every other English outrage against his proud and powerful nation and drove the chronically cautious Philip II closer to waging outright war on English soil.

Elizabeth was the princess he had once saved from the bitter wrath of her sister, his wife Mary I. Now a presumptuous and ungrateful queen, a heretic who encouraged heretics within his own territories, she was about to face the consequences of his slow deliberations. The greatest Catholic power intended putting a brake on this renegade state. His duty as the military arm of the Catholic church, and with great commercial interests at stake, gave Philip every reason to act decisively at last.

Elizabeth was outwardly defiant, although anxious not to be seen as aggrandising her own kingdom. To the Prince of Parma she wrote: "Do not suppose that I am seeking what belongs to others. God forbid. I seek only that which is mine own. But be sure that I will take good heed of the sword which threatens me with destruction, nor think that I am so craven-spirited as to endure a wrong, or to place myself at the mercy of my enemy."[57] She always found it hard, however, to be decisive and now, as the Swedish King remarked, venturing her diadem on the doubtful outcome of war, she struggled with the consequent danger and expense and the threat of worse to come. The drain on her resources was emotional too; she missed Leicester, whose prominence in the war meant he was now in greater peril of losing his life. Even more alarmingly, he was pursuing his own grandiose plans. When he accepted, against his queen's express wishes, the title of Supreme Governor of the Low Countries, offered by the grateful rebels, Elizabeth's nervous tension exploded: "How contemptuously we conceive ourself to have been used by you," she wrote to her old favourite. "We could never have imagined . . . that a man raised up by ourself and extraordinarily favoured by us above any other subject in this land, would have in so contemptible a sort broken our commandment, in a cause that so greatly toucheth us in honour."[58] Leicester's contrary ambitions made Elizabeth all the more desirous of extricating herself from this troublesome and ruinous enterprise.

Like all her furious rows with Leicester, this one was soon over and Elizabeth was friends with him again. After the storms of more than thirty years' closest companionship, her letter to him in the summer of 1586, while he was still in the Low Countries facing failure rather than the triumph he had expected, makes her ease and intimacy with him clearly apparent. She began without preamble, "Rob, I am afraid you will suppose by my wandering writings that a midsummer moon hath taken large possession of my brains this month, but you must needs take things as they come into my head, though order be left behind me." She then ended a letter largely concerned with administration with, "Now will I end, that do imagine I talk still with you, and therefore loathly say farewell, Ô Ô,* though ever I pray God bless you from all harm, and

save you from all foes with my million and legion of thanks for your pains and cares." She signed it "As you know, ever the same,† E.R."[59]

The stresses on Elizabeth of expansion, as she engaged in her first foreign war, were mirrored by the stresses of containment endured by Mary under the stern Puritan regime instituted by Amyas Paulet. Neither queen was happy in these unaccustomed roles and both intended to escape them, Elizabeth through an initially secret treaty with Spain and Mary through another unrealistic but deadly conspiracy.

Mary's fascination with coded messages, secrets, plots and lies was in large part an expression of a risk-taker's need for excitement when confinement and constraint had closed off more conventional adventures. It was also a kind of revenge. As a clever and insightful spymaster, Walsingham recognised the Scottish Queen's peculiarly reckless temperament and hunger for action. The day before Christmas 1585 she was moved from Tutbury to Chartley, a great moated manor in Staffordshire. When a limited channel of clandestine communication was again made available to her on Walsingham's orders, courtesy of the local brewer and a small wooden box, to conceal her letters, submerged in a keg of ale, he knew that Mary would be incapable of resisting any projected madcap scheme that came her way. Just one month later, having recovered after another collapse in her health, she was writing to the French ambassador, via the keg of ale, with enthusiastic plans for continuing her covert operations. Authoritatively suggesting he beware of spies and the bribery of his staff, Mary launched off into a discussion of methods of conveying secret messages, unaware that Walsingham and his agents were reading every word:

"The plan of writing in alum is very common, and may easily be suspected and discovered, and therefore do not make use of it except in a case of necessity; and if you should use it, write . . . between the lines of such new books [sent in], writing always on the fourth, eighth, twelfth, and sixteenth leaf . . . And cause green ribbons to be attached to all the books, which you have caused to be written on in this manner." She also suggested writing on "white taffeta, lawn, or suchlike delicate cloth," advising the ambassador to add an extra half yard to the bolt of cloth which had been inscribed so "this word 'a half' may inform me that within there is something secretly hidden." Another ingenious hiding place occurred to her; letters in cipher could replace the cork inner sole

---

* The cipher used by Elizabeth in her letters for "eyes," one of her pet names for Leicester.

† Elizabeth's motto, *semper eadem*, which had also been her mother's.

of the high-heeled slippers which seemed to be delivered frequently to her women and herself.[60]

With the protective fervour of the Bond of Association now made law, the legal framework was in place by the beginning of 1585 to convict Mary in the event of her being implicated, even passively, in a plot to overthrow Elizabeth and place herself on the English throne. All Elizabeth's advisors knew that in order to get rid of Mary once and for all they would have to present Elizabeth with overwhelming evidence of her perfidy. Mary was never one to be passively part of anything dangerous or exciting when she could be wholeheartedly complicit and in the centre of things. So it was only a matter of management and time before Walsingham's crafty surveillance would have her in his web.

December 1585 was a busy month. If the relationship of Elizabeth and Mary was seen as a marathon chess match, this marked the beginning of the endgame. Just as Leicester sailed as a knight in splendour for the Low Countries, Mary took up her residence in Chartley and Walsingham apprehended at Dover a dubious priest and envoy to Mary, one Gilbert Gifford. He was persuaded to join the opposition, to become a double agent now, intent on opening communications with the Scottish Queen. Walsingham's own queen was distracted by the movements of her unruly knight and not fully aware of the trap being set for Mary. With a motley crew of English refugees, religious fanatics, double agents and romantic young hotheads, a plan to rescue Mary was merged with a simultaneous plot to take Elizabeth. It was a two-pronged move on Elizabeth's life and throne which would leave Mary vulnerable to a devastating checkmate, masterminded by Walsingham.

The catalyst was a priest, John Ballard, who sought out a young Catholic gentleman, Anthony Babington, a passionate supporter of Mary since he was a boy and had first had contact with her when she was held at Wingfield, near his family estates. Now, barely twenty-five and with the zealotry and arrogance of youth, he was determined to play the hero and rescue Mary. There was a new generation of idealistic and romantic Catholic youth who knew little of Mary's previous history yet found the poignancy of her situation, her adherence to her faith, her long captivity by a heretic sovereign, affecting and arousing. The papal bull had sanctified if not encouraged the murder of Elizabeth and for young men wishing to serve their God and earn their spurs, the death of the bad queen and salvation of the good seemed to be a thrilling and righteous enterprise. When Ballard suggested that Spanish and French forces were ready and willing to invade, the plan became more grandiose and concrete.

Mary was liberated by her new channel for sending and receiving contraband messages and wrote in May to Mendoza, Philip II's ambassador in Paris. She was in despair at her son's continued Protestantism and desire to make his political alliances with Elizabeth rather than with herself, his own mother. The last shreds of hope were abandoned with the news that James had made formal his alliance with Elizabeth by accepting a pension of £4000* a year. Certainly wishing to elicit support from the Spanish, and possibly seeking revenge on her ungrateful son, whose desire to succeed to the English throne was as great as her own, Mary made this extraordinary offer. "I have resolved that, in case my son should not submit before my death to the Catholic religion . . . I will cede and make over, by will, to the King your master, my right to the succession to this (i.e. the English) crown, and beg him consequently to take me in future entirely under his protection, and also the affairs of this country . . . I again beg you most urgently that this should be kept secret, as if it becomes known it will cause the loss of my dowry in France, and bring about an entire breach with my son in Scotland, and my total ruin and destruction in England."[61]

Mary was right. This action risked all those calamities and yet she seemed compelled to seek the most perilous path along which to career, unconcerned with the consequences. Her dealings with the conspiracy that was brewing around her showed a recklessness so extreme it could be thought suicidal. Contemporaries, even, recognised a certain self-destructiveness in her obsessive plotting and collaboration with any hare-brained conspiracy that raced past her door. The writer and her contemporary, George Whetstone, suggested that in her conspiracy letters "there is nothing more manifest, than that her malice thirsteth to death of her own life."[62]

Mary was highly conscious of her effect on others and aware that what she did had ramifications far beyond England's parochial shores. She had a strong element of self-dramatisation in her nature and a desire for transfiguration. She had already written to Elizabeth in 1585 that she would welcome the opportunity to sacrifice her life for her faith: "I am perfectly ready, with the grace of God, to bow my neck beneath the axe, that my blood should be shed before all Christendom; and I should esteem it the greatest happiness to be the first to do so. I do not say this out of any vain glory, while the danger is remote."[63] Although impatient and inexperienced in the chicanery of political life, she was astute enough in her directives to her ambassadors. To Beaton she wrote in

* Roughly equivalent to £750,000 today.

code from Chartley that summer, "Endeavour by all means which you can to discover for certain the design of the King of Spain for revenging himself against this queen, and especially if it is for an enterprise in this country, or only thereby to counteract the attempt of the Earl of Leicester in Flanders, and of Drake upon the Indies; because upon that depends entirely the resolution which I and all the Catholics here have to take for our part."[64] If Philip's avenging armies were aimed at England's shores then she would take hope.

As what became known as the Babington plot took root and grew, the assassination of Elizabeth became a central necessity. Babington's inflated plans involved six assassins and a group of a hundred gentlemen ready simultaneously to release Mary from captivity. In July he wrote to the woman he hoped to make his future queen, explaining that he and his co-conspirators were ready for the coming invasion of Catholic power. Quite unaware of how insecure his letters were he stated boldly in his letter to Mary his treasonous intent: "For the despatch of the usurper [Elizabeth], from the obedience of whom we are by excommunication of her made free, there be six noble gentlemen, all my private friends, who for the zeal they bear to the Catholic cause and your Majesty's service will undertake the tragical execution."[65]

This was a gift to the patient Walsingham. Now he had to wait and see if Mary would incriminate herself in her reply. Mary's eventual answer was everything they could have hoped. In a long letter and with a matter-of-fact tone she accepted all the details of Babington's scheme, but added her own logistical concerns about the need for foreign aid and for substantial quantities of armed men and money. She asked him to assure his aforementioned gentlemen friends "of all that will be required from my part for the entire accomplishment of their good intentions." Declaring that even should the plan to rescue her fail and she end up in the Tower, she would pray that Babington and his followers continue with their enterprise "pour l'honneur de Dieu"; she would die happy "when I shall know that you are delivered from the miserable servitude in which you [as English Catholics] are held captive."[66] It was a letter inviting foreign invasion and the utter overthrow of Elizabeth and the Protestant religion. Walsingham had his queen.

He wished to delay just a little longer in the hopes of uncovering more of the conspirators but Elizabeth, who had just recently been acquainted with the conspiracy, was shocked "that so dreadfull a Storm hung over her head, on the one side from her own Subjects at Home, and on the other side from Strangers abroad."[67] She commanded Walsingham to act immediately to round up what plotters he could, "Lest

(as she said herself) by not heeding and preventing the Danger while she might, she should seem rather to tempt God, than to trust in God."[68] Babington's immediate fellowship of assassins were, like himself, very young, aged between twenty and twenty-five. On news of his apprehension on 14 August, the bells of London pealed out in triumph and celebratory bonfires lit his enforced journey back to the city.

While the conspirators were being arrested and interrogated, Mary was kept in ignorance of the dangerous turn in the tide of events. Her spirits were buoyant, and when Paulet suggested a day's stag hunting she agreed with alacrity. She was in such an optimistic frame of mind that, when a body of strangers on horseback galloped up over the horizon, for a moment she believed these were her young gentlemen conspirators come to rescue her and carry her away. Unexpectedly and terrifyingly, she was confronted instead by Elizabeth's commissioners with the brutal message that she was under arrest for treason.

Separated from her servants, Mary was conveyed to Tixall, a nearby manor. She was confused and distressed. She had been taken completely unawares and for a while was frightened that her life would be ended then and there. During her days of seclusion at Tixall it appears her thoughts became settled on her final plan. This was to be the last time that she was to express in public any fear or anxiety as to her fate. While she waited for news of how Elizabeth would proceed against her, Mary must have known that whatever happened next the tedium and stasis of her prolonged genteel captivity was at an end. Anything was preferable to a return to those leaden hours of inactivity and hopelessness.

In her absence from Chartley, Mary's belongings were searched and incriminating letters and a variety of coding alphabets were found, "about 60 Indexes or Tables of private Cyphers and Characters."[69] In the careful inventory of her possessions were mentioned miniature portraits of Elizabeth herself, Mary's son James and mother, Mary of Guise, her father James V and all the previous Scottish kings from whom she was descended, back to James II. Her dead Guise uncles who had had such a powerful influence on her life, the Duke, and the Cardinal of Lorraine, were also represented, as was the present Duc de Guise, inheritor of that line of which Mary and her son were so proud.

Most distressing for Elizabeth amongst the discoveries were letters from some of her own noblemen swearing loyalty to her rival. Camden noted that Elizabeth bore these revelations in silence, disguising her true feelings, "according to that Motto which she used, *Video & taceo*, that is, I see, but say nothing."[70] The nobles themselves, however, in ter-

ror made great play as to their fealty to Elizabeth and abhorrence of Mary's deeds. Disloyalty upset and disturbed Elizabeth, unpopularity frightened her. Her suppressed emotion was discharged explosively at the French ambassador, whom she had summoned to her presence. "Well, what do you think of your Queen of Scotland? With black ingratitude and treachery she tries to kill me who so often saved her life. Now I am certain of her evil intent, and it may be she will not have another opportunity to behave like this,"[71] she raged.

The country was in a state of alarm. Rumours such as "10,000 Frenchmen had landed and captured three villages" gathered potency with the telling; the sight of three ships near the Isle of Wight, and a haystack set alight by chance, meant all the warning beacons were torched to summon the country to arms. Lord Buckhurst, the local governor, found himself suddenly in charge of four to five thousand men, armed and ready to defend England from invasion. Mendoza reported to Philip with glee the extent of the country's fear and confusion; eye-witnesses, just arrived in Paris, "are never tired of recounting it with infinite laughter."[72]

Elizabeth's vengeance was first of all directed at the young conspirators. Torture had wrung full confessions from them and death was the only punishment, but Elizabeth was adamant that it should be as cruel a death as was judicially possible. The death of a traitor was terrible enough if enacted to the letter, when the victim would be half hanged and then disembowelled still alive and sentient. Most executioners waited until the prisoner was dead before proceeding with the savage sequel. On 20 September, Babington and six of his fellow conspirators were brought to the scaffold. With the immediacy of the eye-witness, Camden wrote that they were "hanged, cut down, their Privities cut off, their Bowels taken out before their Faces while they were alive, and their Bodies quartered, not without some note and touch of cruelty."[73] Elizabeth was reputedly taken aback at the cruelty, and sensitive to reports of the watching crowd's pity and sense of shock, she commuted the sentence for the next batch of prisoners. They were hanged until they were dead, "by the Queen's express Command" and then cut down and quartered.

But what to do with Mary herself? By the confessions of these men and the freely given evidence of her two secretaries who had transcribed their mistress's incriminating letters, her complicity in the plot was clear enough to all. A trial for treason, invoking the newly ratified act of association, seemed the next logical step. There was uneasiness even then, however, among some councillors about the means used to entrap the Queen of Scots; others were wary of the presumption of subjects sitting

in judgement on a divinely ordained monarch. But these were mere cavils. To the majority of Elizabeth's councillors this was not the time to quibble when such gross intentions had been revealed. They were not about to allow the Queen to evade her duty to safeguard herself, her people and her realm, by pleading some metaphysical nicety be respected. They were determined that this time the Queen of Scots must die. All they needed now was for Elizabeth to agree.

Elizabeth had long recognised how equivocation and indecisiveness had been both her weakness and her strength; now she could procrastinate no longer. Years before she had told a French ambassador: "I know that it is true I have the imperfection of being longer than necessary in coming to a conclusion in these deliberations—a fault that has caused me much injury in the past . . . it is true the world was made in six days, but it was by God, to whose power the infirmity of men is not to be compared."[74]

As Mary left Tixall to return fleetingly to Chartley, she was greeted by a crowd of beggars who knew of her reputation for largesse to the poor. Mary gave them a sad valediction: "Alas, good people, I have now nothing to give you. For I am as much a beggar as you are yourselves." She can have meant this only as a self-dramatising metaphor, for she was still a queen with her jewels and her dowry to protect her from beggary. But the distribution of alms to the poor was an important part of her sense of herself as merciful and endearing. When Paulet had forbidden this activity, she wrote to the French ambassador that without this contact with the people she feared that in the locality she would be "reputed and held as some savage and complete stranger."[75] To connect with others and have an effect was the driving force of her life.

Soon after, Mary wrote a letter to the Duc de Guise outlining her plan for this the final act. She had always denied any implication in the treasonous plots that had sprung around her throughout her captivity. She had decided that she would stand on her unimpeachable sovereignty and die freely now as a martyr for her faith. Mary appeared to wish to dignify her struggle with Elizabeth by making it a microcosm of the religious wars of Catholic against heretic which were raging over the Channel: "I have declared to them that for my part I am resolute to die for mine [my religion] as she declared that she would do for the Protestant [religion]," she explained. Having determined on this course of public martyrdom Mary feared most the secret assassin, robbing her death of its power and meaning. She confided to her Guise cousin, "I am expecting some poison or other such secret death," a thoroughly plausible fear at that time.

She continued her letter despite, she said, the pain she suffered from her swollen arm: "the heart will not fail me in the hope that One who made me to be born what I am will do me the mercy of making me die for His cause." Her abandonment of Scotland was complete with her request that her body be sent to Rheims to rest beside her mother and her heart be placed beside her first husband, François II. She ended the letter with an intimation that her death would be avenged by the Catholic princes. But even as Mary bade her cousin an affecting farewell she requested that he pass a message on to Mendoza, the Spanish ambassador in Paris, that meant her betrayal of Guise and French interests in favour of the Spanish. The message—that she would not abandon what she had promised to Mendoza's friends—could only refer to the promise she had made to will her rights to succession of the English throne to Philip II, should her son continue to refuse to convert to Catholicism. A draft of this document in her own handwriting was found in her papers after her death.

As Mary was moved to Fotheringhay Castle in Northamptonshire on 25 September 1586, the stage was set for the final act in the struggle between the two queens. They would deny the roles of cruel oppressor and villainess that each had written for the other and display instead the archetypal characters that each had chosen for herself, as heroic populist queen and Catholic martyr. Mary the bold adventurer and enchantress had her chance to draw on her inner reserves for a dramatic consummation of her life that would gain her immortality at least. Elizabeth, until then the great equivocator, now made up her mind at last and through action transcended royalty to become an iconic queen.

CHAPTER TWELVE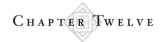

The Consequence of the Offence

Give me my robe, put on my crown; I have Immortal
longings in me.

ANTONY AND CLEOPATRA, ACT 5, SC.2

Elizabeth and Mary shared a grand sense of the dramatic. They were aware that their theatre was the world; everything they did was noticed and interpreted by a constituency much wider than their immediate kingdoms. They had the expectations of their ancestors upon them and the hindsight of history would judge them. Their public utterances rang with appreciation of their significance in the great drama of human affairs. Mary, addressing the commissioners sent to Fotheringhay in October, was exhorting Elizabeth. They were "to look to their Consciences, and to remember that the Theatre of the whole World is much wider than the Kingdom of England."[1] In that warning was her recognition that she was, above all, a European prince and a Catholic queen. She could look to her fellow Catholic princes to avenge her and to future generations to absolve her.

Elizabeth, addressing her Parliament in the following month, expressed her own awareness of the situation: "for we princes, I tell you, are set on stages in the sight and view of all the world duly observed. The eyes of many behold our actions."[2] Not only was personal privacy denied them, every public word and action was relayed, embellished or

interpreted, through the country and beyond to the capitals of European power.

Having protested with tears and anger at her impotence during the long years of her captivity, having complained volubly at every change of abode from castle to manor house and back again, Mary accepted the move to Fotheringhay without demur. With characteristic courage she had decided to embrace what she now recognised as the inevitability of death with the nobility of the righteous and the resolve of the martyr. In doing so she stage-managed her exit for maximum impact on history and the watchers of the world. Mary had shown already how well she rose to the most daunting physical challenges. Just as she had done when riding with her troops to battle, in taking control of her fate she became fearless herself, and awesome to others.

Elizabeth and Mary's last confrontation was a struggle for the moral high ground. Their reputations at stake, they sought now to justify their actions towards each other throughout their lives, with the eloquence of their own rhetoric and a canny use of propaganda. Both masters of their arts, they reduced to tears the members of Parliament and trial commissioners who heard their emotive submissions. Elizabeth was determined that Mary should admit her wrongdoing and ask for forgiveness, and she still clung to the possibility of saving her life and saving herself the agony of that capital decision, "a most grievous and irksome burden."[3]

One of Elizabeth's most famous letters, much copied and distributed in her lifetime to show Elizabeth's magnanimity and Mary's guilt, was to Sir Amyas Paulet, in the month Mary was conveyed to Fotheringhay, recommending his safe keeping of his royal prisoner:

Amyas, my most careful and faithful servant,

> *God reward thee treblefold in the double for thy most troublesome charge so well discharged. If you knew, my Amyas, how kindly besides dutifully my careful heart accepts your double labours and faithful actions, your wise orders and safe regards performed in so dangerous and crafty a charge, it would ease your troubles' travail and rejoice your heart . . .*
>
> *But let your wicked mistress know how with hearty sorrow her vile deserts compels these orders, and bid her from me ask God's forgiveness.*[4]

In her communications on the discovery of the Babington plot, Elizabeth intimated more than once that if only Mary would admit her guilt and show herself ready to make amends then she would be happy to pardon her. Mary herself knew this was the bargain. Even after being found

guilty, she wrote to Mendoza, the Spanish ambassador, suggesting that if she would only admit her guilt and ask for forgiveness her life might be saved: "I am threatened if I do not plead for pardon, but I reply that they have already condemned me to death."[5] Mary's stance was uncompromising; she wanted martyr not traitor to be the judgement of history.

For her part, Elizabeth conveyed a wistfulness that she and Mary had never met and been able to conduct their relationship unencumbered by the weighty matters of politics, religion and the balance of European powers. To her Parliament that November she memorably explained,

> I assure you, if the case stood between her and myself only, if it had pleased God to have made us both milkmaids with pails on our arms, so that the matter should have rested between us two; and that I knew she did and would seek my destruction still, yet could I not consent to her death . . . Yea, if I could perceive how I might be freed from the conspiracies and treasons of her favourers in this action—by your leaves she should not die.[6]

To Mary she sent a similar message via her councillors: "if the consequence of the offence reached no further then to ourself as a private person, wee protest before God we coulde have bene verie well contented to have freely remitted and pardoned the same."[7] If these sentiments were even half-sincere it was interesting to see that she considered how simple and less threatening their relationship would be if they had been merely private citizens. Elizabeth went on to explain that the fact they were queens and represented opposing religions and alliances abroad complicated the situation and increased the danger. The danger Mary represented emanated more from those adherents and interests that attached themselves to her cause. The need to execute her only became a pressing debate because the security of the realm, not just Elizabeth's life, was at risk.

To break this cycle of plots and threats of invasion, Elizabeth's ministers desperately argued for Mary to be tried, found guilty and executed for treason. With this intent, the thirty-six commissioners assembled at Fotheringhay by 12 October 1586, ready to proceed. They hoped to persuade Mary to attend the trial in person as her recognition of the proceedings would add an extra dimension of legality. Although it was decided she should be tried under the newly minted Act of Association, there were some doubts as to whether their country's laws could be applied to a foreign queen, particularly one who had sought asylum and then been constrained against her will.

Mary knew that by the terms of this new Act she was clearly guilty by association, at the very least. Her own defence was to stand on her sovereign power and immunity from the laws of an alien state. "It seemeth strange to me, that the Queen should command me as a Subject, to submit my self to a Trial. I am an absolute Queen, and will doe nothing which may be prejudicial either to Royal Majesty, or to other Princes of my place and rank, or my son. My Mind is not yet so far dejected, neither will I faint or sink under this my Calamity." She also made an affecting plaint by stressing how bereft she was of friend or counsel, deprived even of her personal papers: "The Laws and Statutes of England are to me altogether unknown, I am destitute of Counsellors, and who shall be my Peers I cannot tell. My Papers and Notes are taken from me, and no man dareth appear to be my Advocate." She continued to deny everything and would admit only one thing, "I have recommended my self and my condition unto foreign Princes."[8]

Elizabeth had been exasperated throughout the nineteen years of Mary's captivity by her obdurate refusal to accept responsibility or guilt for any of her actions or enterprises. In this perilous situation where she was about to authorise a trial of a fellow sovereign and foreign queen, watched by the world, she needed Mary to submit to her authority in some small way. Her reputation as a just queen required that Mary relinquish her haughty stance of injured innocence, her insistence that she was persecuted purely for her faith alone.

This was precisely what Mary intended to maintain. It was now clear that she would never freely admit any guilt or any conscious complicity in treasonous acts against Elizabeth. She was absolutely sure that the way to escape notoriety and claim immortality was to prove herself a martyr for her faith. Mary had to deflect the gaze from the wreckage of her reign and the ruination of her reputation through an act of nobility and courage. A heroic death went a long way towards reconciling a less than heroic life.

Elizabeth was not sympathetic to Mary's bid for transfiguration. On hearing that she was refusing the right of the English commissioners to try her, Elizabeth despatched an imperious broadside to Mary, post haste. This was in response to Mary's insistence that she be tried only by her peers, not by those inferior to her in status. Elizabeth was her only available peer but she insisted her councillors were there as her representatives. It was indicative of Elizabeth's ire that this letter carried no titles and no address, just a peremptory statement of fact and intent:

You have in various ways and manners attempted to take my life and bring my kingdom to destruction by bloodshed. I have never proceeded

harshly against you, but have, on the contrary, protected and main-
tained you like myself. These treasons will be proved to you and all
made manifest. Yet it is my will, that you answer the nobles and peers
of the kingdom as if I myself were present. I therefore require, charge,
and command you make answer for all I have been well informed of
your arrogance.

Yet even given the sharpness of the riposte, Elizabeth appeared still willing to pardon Mary if only she would bend her pride, submit to Elizabeth's authority and admit her guilt. Her valedictory sentence was
peremptory: "Act plainly without reserve, and you will sooner be able to
obtain favour of me." [9]

Mary continued to argue fluently and persuasively against the legality of the trial and, despite her protestations that she knew nothing of
English law, she showed herself more than capable of debating legalistic
points with the best of her interlocutors. When they threatened to proceed anyway against her, even in her absence, she gave a brave, defiant
answer, "That she was no Subject, and rather would she die a thousand
Deaths than acknowledge herself a Subject."[10] Her long years of
enforced inactivity had given her endless opportunities for rehearsing
the wrongs done to her; now at last with an attentive audience, Mary
could not resist running through her catalogue of woes. The commissioners eventually stopped her in mid flow and asked her to answer
plainly if she would attend the trial, yes or no. Her grasp of the weak
points of the prosecution against her was impressive. She declared:

> The Authority of their Commission was founded upon a late
> Law made to intrap her; That she could by no means away with
> the Queen's Laws, which she had good reason to suspect; That
> she still had a good Heart full of Courage, and would not dero-
> gate from her Progenitours the King's of Scotland, by owning
> herself a Subject to the Crown of England; for this was nothing
> else but openly to confess them to have been Rebels and Trai-
> tours. Yet she refused not to answer, provided she were not
> reduced to the Rank of a Subject. But she had rather utterly per-
> ish than to answer as a criminal person.[11]

Mary was lame and her physical suffering added a distinct pathos to her
appearance. This, together with her passionate self-righteousness,
affected the more chivalrous and soft-hearted of the councillors. Sir
Christopher Hatton, one of Elizabeth's privy councillors and prominent

in uncovering the Babington plot, was not so easily moved. He pointed out to the Scottish Queen the way she should best proceed: "appear to your Trial, and shew your Innocency; lest by avoiding Trial you draw upon yourself a Suspicion, and stain your Reputation with an eternal Blot of Aspersion." He added that should Mary clear herself "the Queen herself will be transported with joy, who affirmed unto me at my coming from her, that never any thing befell her that troubled her more, than that you should be charged with such Misdemeanours."[12]

Mary did agree to appear at her trial, despite suspecting that it would have no effect on the verdict. Her dramatic temperament led her to prefer to be centre stage in any arena. Mary had spent nineteen years out of power, away from the glitter and attention of court life. Through these long years she had felt abandoned by all governments, been refused consistently any interview with Elizabeth, barely offered acknowledgement of her requests, let alone a hearing to defend herself. She still maintained a strong sense of her importance and her ability to affect events. Now thirty-six of the most powerful men in England had assembled and here Mary had a stage and an opportunity to present herself and her case in public for the first time. Every word would be relayed with urgency to Elizabeth, who had held herself increasingly superior and aloof from Mary's plaints. Now all of them would have to pay attention.

Fotheringhay was the theatre for her final act of revenge and salvation. The only way to redeem her reputation and make sense of her life was to control the manner of its ending. She saw her death in these histrionic terms; writing to Mendoza she referred to the scaffold as "a stage whereupon I am to play the last act of the tragedy."[13] Now that her death was inevitable, she no longer sought Elizabeth's approval or pardon. The only world that Mary hoped to impress now was a Catholic one, the redemption she sought was spiritual and the immortality she craved was as a martyr for her faith. If she could manage that then she would not only establish her rightful place in history and the hearts of her supporters, she also would store up posthumous trouble for Elizabeth and her counsellors too.

On the morning of 15 October, Mary was led into the great chamber for the commencement of her trial. Because she had been secluded from London and the centres of power in the country, many of the nobility there assembled had never seen the Scottish Queen before. The lurid tales of her past history and her reputed supernatural charm had endowed her with a glamour and fascination. Even though now middle-aged, her height and demeanour meant she was still a compelling presence.

The stage was ready. Burghley had worked carefully on the symbolic detail of the setting. On a raised platform at the head of the room was placed the chair of state under a canopy of state. This was to represent the presence and authority of Elizabeth, Queen of England, and remained empty throughout. A smaller chair, placed further into the heart of the room, was designated for Mary Queen of Scots. The commissioners were seated on benches down either side of the long room. Mary objected to the inferior position of her chair. "I am a queen by right of birth and my place should be there under the dais [canopy of state],"[14] she is reputed to have said, pointing to the empty throne intended for the absent Queen of England.

The charges were read out against her, "that you have conspired the destruction of [the Person of the most Serene Queen Elizabeth] and the Realm of England, and the Subversion of Religion." Mary defended herself eloquently and emphatically, and admitted not one scintilla of evidence that could prove her guilt. The Babington letters were read out; she absolutely repudiated any suggestion that she had known him, let alone knowingly written him letters or received any from him. She demanded that she be shown the originals with her signature upon them.* Babington's confession she tossed back at her inquisitors: "If Babington or any other affirm it, I say plainly, They lie. Other mens Faults are not to be thrown upon me." Her "stout Courage" and forceful denials were punctuated with explosive bouts of weeping, one of which accompanied a statement of loyalty to Elizabeth: "I would never make Shipwreck of my Soul by conspiring the Destruction of my dearest Sister," she declared with feeling.[15]

The most damning evidence, however, was that given by her two secretaries Nau and Curle, whose confessions, recorded independently and not under torture, tallied with each other. They confirmed that the letters Walsingham had intercepted, deciphered and copied had been written on Mary's dictation. She even parried this damning evidence with cool composure: "As well the Majesty as the Safety of all Princes must fall to the Ground, if they depend upon the Writings and Testimonies of Secretaries . . . If they have written anything prejudicial to the Queen my Sister, they have written it altogether without my Knowledge, and let them bear the Punishment of their inconsiderate Boldness."[16]

In a letter the following month to the Spanish ambassador, Mendoza, who was complicit in the general detail of the Babington plot and

---

* Her prosecutors only had the copies made by Walsingham's secretary, Phelippes. In order not to arouse the suspicions of the writers and recipients, the letters were intercepted, deciphered, copied, and then resealed and sent on.

closely sympathetic to her, Mary wrote as if she accepted that her secretaries had spoken the truth: "Nau has confessed everything, Curle a great deal, following his example, and all is on my shoulders." [17]

In court she maintained her powerful, eloquent presence, insisting that her protestations be registered that she was a sovereign queen who did not recognise the authority of Elizabeth over her but came to the court voluntarily, "to vindicate herself from the horrible imputation that had been laid to her charge."[18] She continued to take the floor, undefended by anyone. Quite alone and having to act as her own counsel, she argued her case with passion. She was determined to promote the religious component of her arraignment which her prosecutors were equally adamant in denying: "[my religion] has been my sole consolation and hope under all my afflictions, and for its advancement I would cheerfully give my best blood, if so be I might, by my own death, procure relief for the suffering Catholics; but not even for their sakes would I purchase it at the price of the blood of others . . . It is, in sooth, more in accordance with my nature to pray with Esther than to play the part of Judith."*[19]

The trial was adjourned and the commissioners returned to London to meet again in the Star Chamber in Westminster on 25 October. Although they had not been asked to travel to Fotheringhay and give evidence before Mary, her secretaries here appeared in person to confirm their evidence about the letters. The commission, unanimously except for one vote,† pronounced Mary guilty of having "compassed and imagined within this Realm of England divers Matters tending to the Hurt, Death and Destruction of the Royal Person of our Sovereign Lady the Queen."[20]

When the councillors went to Elizabeth to give her the news, the French ambassador reported that she sank to her knees and remained in prayer for at least fifteen minutes. She asked God to "inspire her how to

---

* Esther interceded with Xerxes, the Persian King, to save the Jews, whereas Judith cut off the head of the Babylonian general Holofernes in order to save her people.

† Lord Edward Zouche (?1556–1625) was only twenty when he bravely and uniquely set himself apart from his fellow peers and sovereign in this sensational trial. In youth he considered himself feckless and his passion for creating gardens had apparently helped lose his patrimony. In old age he seems to have attained more conventional honours, including in 1620 being one of the first members of the New England council in Virginia. He was buried in a vault connected to his wine cellar, a fact which inspired this from his friend Ben Jonson: "Wherever I die, oh, here may I lie/Along by my good Lord Zouche/That when I am dry, to the tap I may hie/And so back again to my couch."

act for the greater glory of His name, the greater safety of her kingdom, the greater security of her person." Elizabeth in this prayer reiterated the fear she had at "putting to death a woman, a Sovereign Queen like herself, relation of all the great Princes of the world, and closely allied to herself by blood." Aware perhaps of her audience, she also shared with her maker how hard she found the decision, given that she herself was a woman, "and the most tender hearted on earth."[21]

Elizabeth may have been a little disingenuous, but she was not being melodramatic. Her fear was real on a personal, spiritual and political level. When the momentous news of the verdict reached the European courts there was talk of retaliation. Spain's long planned revenge for England's heresy, for her own fleet's piratical depredations on Spanish treasure ships and foreign colonies, for Elizabeth's intransigence, was prodded into life by the projected execution of Mary. In December 1586 a despatch from the Venetian ambassador in Spain reported in cipher, "the King [Philip II] and his Ministers are extremely anxious to avenge themselves on the Queen of England, but two considerations of great weight present themselves, the questions of how and when."[22] The Guises too were busy stoking French antagonism to Elizabeth for her treatment of their kinswoman. The general feeling abroad was that the English Queen would never be so rash as to allow the execution of the Queen of Scots to proceed, "there is no reason in the world why England should commit an act which would rouse all Christendom in wrath against her."[23]

With such threats from beyond her shores, Elizabeth's own anxiety and alarm was exacerbated by Mary's ecstatic embrace of her sentence: "so far was she from being dismayed thereat, that with a settled and steadfast Countenance, lifting up her Eyes and Hands towards Heaven, she gave Thanks to God for it." Even more disconcerting was Mary's sense of triumph when told by the commissioners that as long as she lived the reformed religion in England would never be secure. She greeted the news "with a more than wonted Alacrity, giving God Thanks, and rejoicing in her Heart, that she was taken to be an Instrument for the re-establishing of Religion in this Island."[24]

Greatly troubled as to what to do, Elizabeth faced a delegation from her Lords and Commons that November, most of whom were pleading that she execute Mary as soon as possible as the only way to re-establish security in the country. She wished to show her gratitude for their loyalty and her understanding of their fears. She explained that although infinitely grateful to God for every gift and mercy He had shown her, in keeping her safe from constant perils, the greatest miracle to her was her people's love: "as I came to the crown with the willing hearts of my sub-

jects, so do I now after twenty-eight years' reign perceive in you no diminution of goodwills, which if haply I should want, well might I breathe but never think I lived [without which I might as well be dead]."

She then addressed the pressing problem of Mary: "it is and has been my grievous thought that one not different in sex, of like estate, and my near kin, should fall into so great a crime . . . I secretly wrote her a letter upon the discovery of sundry treasons, that if she would confess them and privately acknowledge them by her letter to myself, she never should need be called for them into so public question." Acutely sensitive to Mary's charge that the Act under which she had been found guilty was made law expressly to entrap her, Elizabeth specifically denied this was the case. She declared it was more just to try Mary under this statute which allowed for judgement from a commission of the noblest in the land than to subject her to a common court of law and a jury of common men, which Elizabeth speciously claimed as "a proper course forsooth, to deal in that manner with one of her estate!"

Elizabeth was ever mindful of the need to prove herself as resolute as any king. She was aware of how Mary's transgressions fulfilled every expectation of female fallibility, reinforcing the suspicion that women could not rule. Well into the rhythm of her eloquence, Elizabeth explained how her experiences separated her from her cousin and made her worthy of her crown:

> I have had good experience and trial of this world: I know what it is to be a subject, what to be a sovereign; what to have good neighbours, and sometimes meet evil willers. I have found treason in trust, seen great benefits little regarded, and instead of gratefulness, courses of purpose to cross. These former remembrances, present feeling, and future expectation of evils, I say, have made me think an evil is much the better the less while it endureth, and so, them happiest that are soonest hence [in the face of evil the sooner one is dead the better] and taught me to bear with a better mind these treasons than is common to my sex—yea, with a better heart, perhaps, than is in some men.

Having proved her superiority, she ended her rhetorical flourish with the statement that brought the terrible possibility of her own death into the public mind, a mind now having to contemplate the execution of the Queen of Scots: "I would be loath to die so bloody a death [as assassination] so doubt I not but God would have given me grace to be prepared for such an event."[25]

The juxtaposition of her violent but innocent death with Mary's

emphasised on many levels their interconnectedness. Increasingly it seemed that one had to die for the other to live, but Elizabeth was determined to show too that even in dying, Mary's queenly courage could be matched by Elizabeth's nobility of spirit. By talking with equanimity of the greatest terror that her councillors faced, the murder of their sovereign, she assumed the mantle of the monarch she wanted to be. These great speeches of Elizabeth's were quickly published and distributed and there was a sense that she was addressing a wider public than solely these members of Parliament who had sought audience with her at Richmond Palace.

After the verdict Mary was divested of her canopy of state that had been symbolic of her status as queen throughout her captivity. In a letter to Beaton, she related how, since she had refused to admit her guilt and ask repentance of Elizabeth, the English Queen had ordered this dishonour, "to signify that I was a dead woman, deprived of the honours and dignity of a queen."[26] The following day Paulet offered to reinstate her canopy, explaining it was not Elizabeth but one of her council who had demanded its removal, but Mary refused. She had already replaced it with a crucifix. Mary's enigmatic motto "In my end is my beginning" had been embroidered on her cloth of state. Its removal symbolised the relinquishing of her temporal life as a queen in preparation for the eternal life as martyr and myth.

Mary explained to Mendoza her subsequent conversation with her jailers, who would be executioners, in which she argued for this new focus of her life:

> "It was a fine thing," they said, "for me to make myself out a saint and martyr; but I should be neither, as I was to die for plotting the murder and deposition of their Queen." I replied that, "I was not so presumptuous as to pretend to honours of saint and martyr; but although they had power over my body, by the divine permission, they had none over my soul, nor could they prevent me from hoping that, by the mercy of God who died for me, my blood and life would be accepted as offerings freely made by me for the maintenance of His church." [27]

Mary was determined on securing her spiritual reputation and personal salvation and her apparently serene self-satisfaction did not fail to irritate and disconcert Elizabeth. Just as she made much of her willingness to die for her faith, so Elizabeth was fond of declaring she would sacrifice her life for her people. At this time of danger averted and new perils to come her rhetoric was particularly resonant, bringing tears to the eyes of her

loyal audience of Parliamentary Lords and Commoners: "if by my death, other nations and kingdoms might truly say that this realm had attained an ever prosperous and flourishing estate, I would (I assure you) not desire to live, but gladly give my life to the end my death might procure you a better prince."[28] While Mary aimed for spiritual glory Elizabeth, always pragmatic and parental, sought more material insurance for her people. "I look beyond my lifetime to the welfare of my subjects and the security of my kingdom"[29] was her vision of a more practical immortality.

To condemn to death a fellow monarch and defenceless neighbouring queen made for all kinds of uneasiness and outrage both within her country and without. The ruling nobility in Scotland preferred their alliance with Elizabeth to any sentimental attachment for Mary. Although most were sanguine about the prospective execution of the Queen of Scots, the people were not. They had once called her a whore and threatened to burn her, but her transgressions had been lost to memory. Her suffering, her unjust treatment, her enforced exile from their land and long captivity in the inhospitable heart of Scotland's old enemy, was a source of raw emotion. She was born of the proud race descended from Robert the Bruce and had provided them with a good strong male heir to carry on that line. They were incensed at the idea that the English could claim a legal right to destroy her.

James VI, ambitious for himself, pragmatic and clever, was unmoved personally by his mother's plight. By this time he was twenty-one years old and had known her only through letters and by repute. The discovery of the Babington plot, he felt, justified keeping her in closer captivity, claiming dismissively "it was meet for her to meddle with nothing but prayer and serving of God."[30] Her sentencing to death made him take account, however, of the outrage of his people.

James sent the duplicitous Master of Gray* to Elizabeth to plead for mercy, pointing out all the arguments that already exercised her greatly: the damage to her reputation for justice and clemency; the solidarity of sex, status and blood between the queens, and concern for himself, for

---

* Patrick, Master of Gray (d. 1612), became another of James VI (and I)'s favourites, apparently invulnerable despite a lifetime of double-dealing, intrigue and betrayals. He was part of Mary Queen of Scots' inner circle while she was in France and a close colleague of the Duc de Guise, who rewarded him handsomely. He returned to Scotland, probably with Esmé Stuart in 1579; both were agents of the Duc de Guise. Gray betrayed Mary's secrets to James and then to Elizabeth, who always saw through him, despite his being thought the handsomest man of his time, with exquisite French manners and a brilliant wit. After Mary's execution he was tried and found guilty of treason on a number of charges. James saved his life, welcoming him back to court after only two years' exile, where Gray continued to intrigue and betray. He still managed, however, to die in his bed.

"what Straits and Hazzard of his Reputation among his own People he should be plunged, if any Violence be offered to his Mother." The factor which most worried Elizabeth—that of the setting of dangerous precedent—was hammered home rather too heartily in James's submission: "How strange and monstrous a thing it would be, to subject an absolute Prince to the Judgement of Subjects. How prodigious, if an absolute Prince should be made so dangerous a Precedent for the prophaning and vilifying her own and other Princes Diadems."[31] But while this public entreaty was not entirely welcome, Gray reputedly "buzzed into the Queen's ear that Saying, *Mortua non-mordet*, that is, A dead Woman biteth not."[32]

Elizabeth was besieged with advice and threats on all sides. She knew she had long ago lost her good relations with Philip II of Spain but this meant her amicable alliances with France and Scotland were crucial for the security of her realm. Her isolation, and the sense of loneliness in making this the most momentous decision of her life, ran through her speeches and letters of the time. Reliant as she was on her trusty Burghley, and affectionate Leicester, they did not appreciate her profound emotional attachment to the idea of the sacredness of kingship, the sense that the relationship with God, his king and their people was a mysterious and hierarchical compact. To violate that divine order was to profane it. Elizabeth was horrified that the responsibility fell to her alone. In turmoil herself, she had to respond to another emotional petition from her Parliament at the end of November. Her answering speech to them was full of the anguish and uncertainties of her position.

"Neither hath my care been so much bent how to prolong [my life], as how to preserve both, which I am right sorry is made so hard—yea, so impossible. I am not so void of judgement as not to see my own peril; nor yet so ignorant as not to know it were in nature a foolish course to cherish a sword to cut my own throat . . . But this I do consider: that many a man would put his life in danger for the safeguard of a king. I do not say that so will I, but I pray you think that I have thought upon it."[33] This illustrated perfectly Elizabeth's powerful sense of the inviolability of monarchy, that she should think it preferable to risk her own life than break that taboo. Trespassing on God's territory in order to punish an anointed queen who, by definition, was above mere mortal intervention, filled her with dread.

From France, King Henri III sent his ambassador Bellièvre to plead for leniency. Elizabeth, pained, could only reply: "It is impossible to save my own life if I preserve that of the Queen of Scots, but if you ambassadors can point out any means whereby I may do it, consistently with my own security, I shall be greatly obliged to you, never having shed so

many tears at the death of my father, of my brother King Edward, or my sister Mary, as I have done for this unfortunate affair."[34] Her official letter in January 1587 to Henri III, in response to his forceful arguments for clemency, revealed a more angry and imperious expression of her tension and fear: "My God! How could you be so unreasonable as to reproach the injured party, and to compass the death of an innocent one by allowing her to become the prey of a murderess? . . . that you should be angry at my saving my own life, seems to me the threat of an enemy, which I assure you, will never put me in fear, but is the shortest way to make me dispatch the cause of so much mischief."[35]

Mary, herself, at the centre of the storm, seemed beatifically calm while all around her were fearful and grieving. She had always shown great care for her immediate servants and this concern was made more urgent as she contemplated her fate. She wrote both to Elizabeth and the King of France asking them to consider their safety and welfare. Her last weeks were busy with administration and communication, with speeding letters to the courts of Europe, desirous as she was to protect her posthumous reputation.

So eager were Elizabeth's ministers to have some sort of confession from the Queen of Scots before she died that Walsingham asked Sir Amyas Paulet to engage Mary in conversation as often as possible. The dour and disapproving Paulet admitted he had avoided any but the minimum of talk with his royal charge, but dutifully hung around and offered a willing ear. His self-sacrifice proved fruitless. Mary was in complete control of the situation and although more than willing to talk to anyone as she whiled away the long hours, and still clearly full of the injustices done to her, she was not about to tell Paulet, of all people, her guilty secrets. He reported somewhat irascibly to Walsingham: "followinge your direction I have geven her full scope and tyme to say what she would, and yet at some tymes fyndinge no matter to come from her worthye of advertisement; I have departed from her as otherwyse she would never have left me; and I am deceaved yf my Lord of Buckhurst [who had just left] will not geve the same testimonye of her tediousness."[36]

In her reply to Parliament's pleadings, Elizabeth expressed the kernel of her character and governing style when she asked them to be content for the present with "this answer answerless . . . assuring yourselves that I am now and ever will be most careful to do that which will be best for your preservation. And be not too earnest to move me to do that which may tend to the loss of that which you are most desirous to keep."[37] Here she was in the role she had most naturally assumed for the first twenty-eight years of her reign, like Janus, ambivalent between past and future, seeing both sides, judicious, measured, sometimes risking

stasis in the quest for equilibrium. But she was about to be forced into a more active and decisive form of leadership, and the transition period was painful for her and those closest to her.

Under mounting pressure from her ministers to face up to her responsibilities, Elizabeth finally allowed Burghley to draw up the warrant for Mary's execution at the beginning of December. The proclamation was read out in public and bonfires lit all over London in celebration. William Davison, joint Secretary of State, however, was left with the task of obtaining Elizabeth's signature. They all remembered with foreboding the Queen's painful indecision over the Duke of Norfolk's execution fourteen years before.

Close to Christmas and in the middle of this fevered anxiety, Mary's valedictory letter to Elizabeth arrived. Calm, magnanimous, wishing to make her peace with everyone, she mentioned the debacle over her canopy of state and said she "praised God that such cruelty serving only to exercise malice and to afflict me after having condemned me to death has not come from you." But like all her subtle letters to Elizabeth, the sweetness carried a hidden barb: Mary prayed that God would pardon all those responsible for her death, and "I esteem myself happy that my death will precede the persecution which I foresee to threaten this Isle, where God is no longer truly feared and reverenced, but vanity and worldly policy rules and directs all." She then delivered the *coup de grâce:* "Do not accuse me of presumption if, on the eve of leaving this world and preparing myself for a better one, I remind you that one day you will have to answer for your charge, as well as those that are sent before, and that my blood and the misery of my country will be remembered." She signed herself with royal assertion, "Your sister and cousin, wrongfully a prisoner, *Marie, Royne.*"[38]

Anxiously her ministers watched Elizabeth's reactions. Tears sprung to her eyes, but otherwise she was calm. They feared anything that might soften her heart or encourage her natural equivocation. Leicester reported to Walsingham that the letter "hath wrought tears, but I trust shall do no further harm."[39] It was Mary who had the upper hand, her power gained through action and decision. Elizabeth struggled with contradictory advice and demands, and her innate fear of commitment. Although she "sate many times melancholick and mute" muttering to herself "*Aut fer, aut feri* [bear with her, or smite her]" and "*Ne feriare, feri* [Strike, lest thou be stricken],"[40] she had not yet exhibited the same terrible indecision shown before Norfolk's execution.

The only way that Elizabeth could be induced to permit Mary's exe-

cution was if she feared that the country was in peril. At the beginning of the new year of 1587 a variety of sinister rumours began to gain credence as they inflamed an already anxious people. There was a general expectation that the Scottish nobility were preparing for war with England in the event of the execution of Mary; at the beginning of February, the Mayor of Exeter wrote to Cecil about a hue and cry that swept the West Country to "make diligent search" for the Queen of Scots "who is fledd." Other broadcast cries told that the city of London "by the enemyes is set on fyre"[41] and men were exhorted to assemble in armour and in haste and readiness to defend the kingdom. There was even another confused half-plot to murder the Queen, said to involve the French ambassador, L'Aubespine. Independently, it seemed he had started a rumour specifically to cause alarm, that "the Queen of Scotland, disguised as a sailor, had fled from her palace" and had reached the sea, intent on reaching Brittany. All this made for a febrile atmosphere of threat and ever-present danger.

Elizabeth was not shielded from any of this hysterical alarm. Suddenly on the first day of February, she sent for the death warrant and signed it without fuss. Davison could hardly believe his good fortune. Then Elizabeth called him back. Frightened of taking sole responsibility for such a deed, she asked Davison to write to Paulet to ask him secretly to murder Mary and make it look as if she had died of natural causes. Although he could not salve her conscience and rescue her relationship with God, in this way he would protect his sovereign from the outside world. Elizabeth feared that personal defamation, loss of diplomatic alliances and even military aggression would follow any judicial execution. Davison was reluctant and, as he had surmised, Paulet was absolutely opposed. His principled rejection of the idea enraged Elizabeth. So much for the empty promises of the Bond of Association, she railed: in the absence of will and action, such bold declarations of loyalty from her subjects were useless hot air.

There was much anxious discussion amongst her closest ministers as to what exactly Elizabeth wished should be done with this now signed and sealed death warrant. She was utterly confused and confusing in her directives. Davison, inexperienced at dealing with his fearsome, exasperating Queen, went to Hatton for advice and together they sought out Cecil. A council meeting was called for 3 February and they all agreed that they would proceed without further consultation, it being "neither fit nor convenient to trouble her Majesty any further."[42] With the precious document in hand, they dispatched Beale, the Clerk of the Council and a stalwart Protestant, to speed to Fotheringhay. With him went two executioners, their axe hidden in a trunk. The same day, 4 February,

Elizabeth told a nervous Davison about a distressing dream she had had. She dreamt, she said, that Mary had been executed.

At Fotheringhay, Mary was told late on 7 February that she was to die the following morning. Shrewsbury was saddened by having to impart such news; he was her longest serving jailer and another who had not failed to warm to Mary's charms. Her servants protested at the brutal suddenness and lack of notice, but the lords had come with directives not to delay. Mary accepted her sentence with composure: "I did not think that the Queen my Sister would have consented to my Death, who am not subject to your Law and Jurisdiction: but seeing her Pleasure is so, Death shall be to me most welcome: neither is that soul worthy of the high and everlasting Joys above, whose Body cannot endure one Stroak of the Executioner." She took much satisfaction from the fact that the Earl of Kent burst out with, "Your Life will be the Death of our Religion, as contrariwise your Death will be the Life thereof."[43] This confirmed how significant they considered the threat of her faith and how important she was as a flame of that faith.

Back in London, it appeared that Elizabeth was still half hoping that Paulet could be induced to contrive some underhand way of getting rid of Mary. At Fotheringhay, Mary was in calm control of the situation. She spent her last hours in consoling her servants, dispensing her goods and any money left to her and remaking her will. She also wrote letters to Henri III and her almoner. To all the sorrowful faces around her she offered hope, by bidding them, "leave Mourning, and rather rejoyce that she was now to depart out of a world of Miseries."[44] The rest of the time she spent in prayer.

By eight o'clock on the morning of 8 February, the day designated for her execution, Mary had long been up. She had asked her women to dress her as if for a festival and, in response to the knock on the door, processed slowly in the company of her servants to the Great Hall where the scaffold had been erected. There would be many witnesses to the portentous events that followed, their accounts capturing vividly aspects of the gruesome drama. "Forth she came with State, Countenance and Presence majestically composed," Elizabeth's chronicler Camden recorded. The Scottish Queen was dressed in black with a floor-length veil of finest white linen falling from her hair. In her hands she carried her ivory crucifix, her rosary hung from her girdle.

At the entrance to the room she was prevented from bringing in her full retinue of servants. Sir James Melville, her long time friend, was in tears before her. In the consolation she offered him she bade him take

the news back to Scotland that she had died constant in her faith and "firm in my Fidelity and affection towards Scotland and France." She asked to be commended to her son, to have him reminded how greatly she had desired the unification of Scotland and England. Although her letters to Mendoza and the Pope still stood, offering her rights to the English throne to Philip II, should her own son obstinately continue Protestant, she requested that Melville assure James VI "that I have done nothing which may be prejudicial to the Kingdom of Scotland."[45]

By calling on her consanguinity with Elizabeth, her status as an anointed queen and their shared sensibilities as women and sisters in a masculine world, Mary managed to get the presiding lords to agree she could be accompanied by six of her servants. She had been keen they were present not just for their support but also to bear witness and relate the detail of the extraordinary events of that morning to the foreign courts in which her reputation mattered most to her.

Mary was led to a low platform with a chair, a stool and the scaffold block, all draped with black velvet. A huge log fire was blazing in an attempt to keep some of the February chill from the room. Once Beale had read out the warrant, the Dean of Peterborough began an oration, urging her to repent and accept the true faith. Mary interrupted him, requesting he should not "trouble himself, protesting that she was firmly fixed and resolved in the ancient Catholick Roman Religion, and for it was ready to shed her last Bloud." When he attempted to pray for her sins, she and her servants recited their own prayers in Latin. She then prayed in English for her Church, her son and Queen Elizabeth, "beseeching [God] to turn away his wrath from this Island."

As was customary, Mary then forgave the executioners for what they were about to do. She seemed in a hurry to proceed and her women helped her out of her outer garments, in order to bare her neck for the axe. Her petticoat of deepest red suddenly showed startling against the sombreness of their surroundings: the colour heavy with symbolism as the liturgical colour of martyrdom. Binding her eyes with a linen cloth, she lay her neck upon the block, repeating continually "*In manus tuas, Domine* [Into thy hands, O Lord]." The watching officials and Mary's servants recoiled to see the first blow of the axe miss her neck and slice into the side of her skull. The second blow severed her head. The emotion was palpable. A queen had been killed on the orders of a sister queen.

The Dean of Peterborough cried out "So let Queen Elizabeth's Enemies perish" while the witnesses wept. All kinds of eyewitness reports replayed the ceremonial agony of the event and the rapt nobility of the Queen. Rumours became entwined with fact, inevitably embellished in the telling of something more awesome and traumatic than

anything they would ever see again. The Queen of Scots' head was held up for all to see, her lips still moving for a further fifteen minutes, it was said, in silent prayer; the lustrous auburn curls fell away in the executioner's hand to reveal the dead Queen's own grey hair cropped close, transforming her from a beauty to an old woman in front of their eyes; one of her favourite pets, a Skye terrier, smuggled in under her skirts, emerged howling piteously and would not leave the severed head of his mistress: all these stories wracked the hearts of the Marian faithful and filled Elizabeth's supporters with an uneasy shame.

With faith and courage Mary had turned defeat and death into transcendent victory. The martyr was made. Amplified by the fraught publicity of her execution, the myth was born. The English councillors present on the day realised this too, for they insisted that every splash of blood was scrubbed away, every object and relic removed and destroyed. Her body, quickly wrapped in a cloth, was carried away and immediately embalmed. Her servants were kept confined in the castle and England's seaports were closed. The sense of threat that had inspired Mary's execution did not abate with her death.

As Mary's star shot heavenwards, Elizabeth's sank. Through personal insecurity and fear she failed to show the necessary princely virtue. Her behaviour following Mary's death was uncontrolled, dissembling and in certain aspects ignoble. The demons of her youth had returned to haunt her. But for Elizabeth too, Mary's death would mark a turning point in her life and reign.

Burghley was afraid at first to tell Elizabeth that the deed was done. When she learnt the truth she appeared little concerned. For Elizabeth, however, the night was always a time when fears seemed to multiply and loneliness went deep: it was at two o'clock in the morning that she had lost her nerve over the execution of the Duke of Norfolk and in a last-minute panic rescinded his death warrant. Now on the night of the momentous news of Mary's death a similar fear and panic gripped her. But this time it was too late. In the morning she sent for Sir Christopher Hatton and berated him for his part in what she saw as a shameful duplicity. She ranted and raved, she blamed everyone, and declared to the world that Mary's execution was something she had never intended. Someone had to pay for the grief and anxiety that engulfed her: peremptorily she sent Davison to the Tower. Despite her councillors' pleading on their knees for clemency, by the end of the month she was even threatening to have him summarily hanged.

Elizabeth's storms, frightening and destructive while they lasted,

usually blew over pretty fast. This one did not. Her grief and anger seemed to grow with the days. Her now elderly and gout-wracked Burghley was banished from her presence. He remained out of favour for months, enduring from her the kind of defamation, by "calling him traitor, false dissembler and wicked wretch," that such a loyal man found hard to bear. Aged sixty-six and in great pain, he was reduced to writing to Elizabeth pleading to be allowed even just to lie at her feet, in hope that "some drops of your mercy [might] quench my sorrowful panting heart." [46] For a while the Queen was beyond reason, neither eating nor sleeping, distracted with woe.

Elizabeth was particularly careful of her fame abroad and fearful of what France and Scotland might do to avenge the Queen of Scots' death. Within four days and in the throes of her passion, she wrote to James VI denying she had authorised the execution of his mother:

> *My dear Brother, I would you knew (though not felt) the extreme dolor that overwhelms my mind, for that miserable accident which (far contrary to my meaning) hath befallen . . . I beseech you that as God and many more know, how innocent I am in this case . . . I am not so base minded that fear of any living creature or Prince should make me afraid to do that were just; or done, to deny the same. I am not of so base a lineage, nor carry so vile a mind. Thus assuring yourself of me, that as I know this was deserved, yet if I had meant it I would never lay it on others' shoulders; no more will I not damnify myself that thought it not . . . for your part, think you have not in the world a more loving kinswoman, nor a more dear friend than myself; nor any that will watch more carefully to preserve you and your estate . . . Your most assured loving sister and cousin, Elizab. R.* [47]

Breathtakingly hypocritical as it may appear on the surface, this letter nevertheless expressed the depth of her ambivalent anguish. Despite her miserable protestations, she "had meant it" and had shamefully "laid it on others' shoulders," but it was also true that she had not meant it and the guilt cut deeply into her heart. The extremity of Elizabeth's emotion and the fact she remained overwrought for so long suggested there was something more troubling to her in the execution of Mary than the obvious tensions of safeguarding her reputation, balancing the Catholic powers, and squaring her conscience with God.

At first there were fears of Scottish revenge. The country was in uproar. Robert Carey was chosen by Elizabeth for the task, that no one else would perform, of delivering that letter to the King of Scots. Riding north he was stopped on the border and warned he would be murdered

if he proceeded further. James suggested he go to Berwick instead, for the King admitted that "given the fury [the people] were in . . . no power of his could warrant my life at that time."[48] Certainly on the streets of Edinburgh ferocious attacks on Elizabeth had spontaneously erupted. An example of the kind of libel being freely circulated was this simple and salty verse, attached with a hemp cord tied like a halter:

> To Jezebel, that English whore;
> Receive this Scottish chain
> As presages of her great malheur [misfortune]
> For murdering our queen.

Where the Edinburghers were louring and full of vengeance, the Londoners were in a merry mood, intent on the kind of noisy celebrations that exacerbated the outrage of the Scots and French. As Shrewsbury's son had ridden through the city with the news of Mary's death, "instantly all the bells were rung, guns discharged, fires lighted in all the streets, and feasting and banquets and every sign of joy."[49] This came from the report of the French ambassador who witnessed one of the street fires too close for comfort. When he refused some local revellers' request for wood for a bonfire, they retaliated by lighting a great bonfire against his own house door, which burned for two hours. But her own people's exuberance was not enough to lift Elizabeth's spirits.

The warlike rumours from Scotland, however, soon died down, and James VI seemed willing to return to business as usual. To save his own face with his people he demanded a scapegoat, *"necesse est unum mori pro populo."* That scapegoat was Davison, but he did not have to die: he was released from the Tower after the defeat of the Armada when Elizabeth had recovered her confidence and was no longer desperate to hang on to the allies she had.

Henri III of France also registered his protest forcefully and threatened the English ambassador with similar violence from the Paris mob should he venture from his house. He refused for some months to receive Walsingham as Elizabeth's envoy, come to explain the execution of the Queen of Scots. They put on an impressive show of mourning for their Dowager Queen, with her Guise family as prominent mourners, while angry crowds vowed vengeance on the "Jezebel" across the water. But the French too did not have the stomach for war. Philip II, however, was being exhorted even by his confessor to attack England, "to avenge the wrongs done to God and to the world by that woman, above all in the execution of the Queen of Scotland."[50]

While Mary lived, Elizabeth's isolation as a regnant queen in a world

of men was relieved; there was a sympathy between them and, until James's birth, they were among the closest blood relations that either had left in the world. Although temperamentally opposed and living their lives to different ideals, Mary had insisted on stressing this familial female relationship: mother, daughter, sister, cousin; in every one of her multitude of letters over the years she reminded Elizabeth of their blood connection. There was an attraction too in opposites, a fascination with those who lived out the unlived side of oneself. Mary had recklessly pursued her heart in a way Elizabeth would never contemplate and Elizabeth had assumed authority in government that had won the world's grudging respect. Elizabeth and Mary had offered to each other a different way of seeing, a point of identity and contrast. In their solitary queenship, the existence of the other, a cousin too, meant each was not entirely alone.

And yet Elizabeth, pressurised by the male world, had sacrificed Mary, a member of her royal and human family. Perhaps it was not too fanciful to think that Mary, representing carnal femininity and motherhood, a queen who had produced a male heir, reminded Elizabeth of her own mother, bloodily put to death in the same way, by the will of men, for giving birth not to that precious son, but to Elizabeth herself, the undervalued girl.

These months after Mary's death were the emotional crisis of Elizabeth's life. For twenty-eight years she had reigned, proud of the peace of a kingdom kept by a queen averse to bloodshed, shy of commitment and prevaricating in her dealings. She had now been forced to draw her sword, and in the blood sacrifice of her close relation, had been initiated into becoming a bolder sort of queen. In the struggle of these months she had to leave behind the woman of hesitation and equivocation, born of the insecurity and fear of her youth, and embrace a larger, more active vision of herself. Elizabeth faced the consequences of her actions.

The English Catholics had lost the focus for their hopes, their alternative queen. As the internal threats diminished, however, the long-feared shadow of Philip II stretched across the Channel. Within a year, all eyes would be turned outwards to a greater foe: for most of Mary's English supporters hatred of the Spanish was a more motivating force than antagonism to their Protestant Queen. Mary's death had meant Elizabeth would have to remove her frugal coat and don the panoply of war.

Elizabeth and England stood alone. In the spring of 1588, she was fifty-four but still full of vitality. She had her great ministers around her,

Burghley, Leicester and Walsingham, but they were ageing now, their health failing, although their prodigious work rate did not flag. To this great triumvirate was added Sir Christopher Hatton, her new Lord Chancellor. Her court had an injection of new blood too in the form of the next generation of favourites, Sir Walter Ralegh, Leicester's beautiful stepson the Earl of Essex, and Burghley's brilliant son Robert Cecil: all these helped maintain the sense of family connection and continuity around the increasingly solitary Queen.

There had been rumours for the past four years or more of the amassing of a great Spanish Armada. Ships were being built in every allied port, food stockpiled, munitions and items of clothing ordered tens of thousands at a time, and men recruited across the empire. There was a sense of danger looming like a storm cloud over England. The exchequer was chronically short of money and Elizabeth was desperate to conclude some sort of peace in the Low Countries with the Duke of Parma. Her fear of all-out war with Spain had made her weak and vacillating but even while she sued for peace, she was forced into action by the news that the fearsome Armada had set sail at last.

It was May and England was thrown into a frenzy of activity, preparing to repel a full-scale invasion. Bad weather and good fortune played their part and by the time the English and Spanish fleets met it was 20 July. Camden's description of that first sighting of the Spanish fleet in the Channel was vivid with the eyewitness's excitement and awe. The galleons "with lofty turrets like Castles" were spread out before them in a crescent, extending some seven miles, "sailing very slowly, though with full Sails, the Winds being as it were tired with carrying them, and the Ocean groaning under the weight of them." The Armada consisted of 130 ships, "the best furnished . . . of any that ever the ocean saw, and called by the arrogant name of Invincible."[51] During the following week there were various running battles up the Channel, with numerous acts of heroism and derring do, a great deal of noise from the ordnance, and not much loss of men or ships on either side. Then on 28 July, the Spanish fleet were anchored just outside Calais, and the English selected eight of their least seaworthy vessels as fireships, "besmeared with Wild-fire, Pitch and Rosin, and filled with Brimstone and other combustible matter," and sent them downwind at dead of night towards the unsuspecting Armada. The burning ships were reflected in the water, "the whole Sea glittering and shining with the Flame thereof" and so panicked the Spanish that their fleet scattered, pursued by the lighter, faster English ships. A sudden storm caught the great Spanish galleons as they fled north to try and reach Spain around Ireland and Scotland's shores.

The fear of Spanish aggression that had accompanied the first thirty

years of her reign was now confronted. In facing the spectre of invasion and defeat, Elizabeth rose magnificently to her new role as a warrior queen, no longer the ever-watchful, ambiguous Janus, but Athena, the goddess of wisdom and war. Cecil's son Robert was amazed at the reaction of this new Elizabeth to the news of the fleets' first engagement: "how great magnanimity* her Majesty shows, who is not a whit dismayed."[52]

Two major armies were assembled, one at St. James's to protect the Queen and the other at Tilbury, at the mouth of the Thames, to repel the first invaders. Leicester was in charge of these 22,000 men and 1000 horses, and invited Elizabeth to visit the camp and show herself to the troops. She accepted with alacrity and on horseback rode among them with a staff in her hand. Some said she wore a breastplate of steel, others suggested it was gold—that was how she appeared invincible to her cheering, adoring troops.

The speech she gave to her army, in the full expectation that the Armada would reform and threaten her island once more, became as famous as any in English:

> My loving people, I have been persuaded by some that are careful of my safety to take heed how I committed myself to armed multitudes, for fear of treachery. But I tell you that I would not desire to live to distrust my faithful and loving people. Let tyrants fear: I have so behaved myself that under God I have placed my chiefest strength and safeguard in the loyal hearts and goodwill of my subjects. Wherefore I am come among you at this time but for my recreation and pleasure, being resolved in the midst and heat of battle to live and die amongst you all, to lay down for my God and for my kingdom and for my people mine honour and my blood even in the dust. I know I have the body but of a weak and feeble woman, but I have the heart and stomach of a king and a king of England too—and take foul scorn that Parma or any other prince of Europe should dare to invade the borders of my realm. To the which rather than any dishonour shall grow by me, I myself will venter [venture] my royal blood.[53]

This marked the apogee of her reign. Elizabeth, in embracing action and sharing danger with her people, inspired the popular imagination

---

* In early modern English magnanimity, literally greatness of spirit, meant above all a noble courage. The concept goes back to Aristotle, and was seen as one of the most important virtues, seldom applied to anyone other than men.

with the vision of a goddess of war. The Armada had been sent by Philip to visit God's punishment on her for her religion, her support of Spain's enemies and her execution of a Catholic queen. In repelling the greatest military power in Europe, she had proved herself as great as any king, perhaps even to herself. The Pope, Sixtus V, on the eve of the Armada and hoping for victory, had renewed his Bull of excommunication, yet even he could not hide his admiration: "Just look how well she governs! She is only a woman, only mistress of half an island, and yet she makes herself feared by Spain, by France, by the Empire, by all." Elizabeth was elated by her country's unexpected victory, exhilarated by her own success. That same month, she wrote to Mary's son: "this tyrannical, proud and brainsick attempt . . . hath procured my greatest glory that meant my sorest wrack [direst destruction]."[54]

The relationship of Elizabeth and Mary continued even after Mary's death. In effect compassed by both of them, Mary's execution had allowed her to fulfil her spiritual aspirations. Courting the death sentence rather than begging for mercy, she ensured her transcendence into myth. For Elizabeth, the Armada, launched partly in Mary's name, provided the greatest challenge of her reign. Mary's death had demanded that Elizabeth rise to a greater authority and through that demonstrate her magnanimous power. In facing down Spain, she too was elevated to an idealised majesty.

But these moments of transformation marked the point when both queens became less recognisable in their individual characters, as they were overlaid increasingly with the projections of others: their natures distorted to support opposing narratives and adorn the romance of kings. But it is in their relationship with each other, as women, cousins and rivals, that their inward experiences were illuminated, in all their complex humanity. In their struggle as queens to overcome the expectation of failure in a male-dominated world, they chose quite different destinies. Their natural sympathy and solidarity evaporated as they became polarised in a lethal opposition where one of them had to die. Yet in death they achieved an extraordinary compromise that was impossible in life. Mary's ambition had been to inherit the throne of England and Elizabeth's to maintain independence, and the religion her father had established in order to legitimise her birth. Both wished for Scotland and England to be united under their rule. In Mary's son this ideal became reality. In the process both Mary's blood and Elizabeth's Church triumphed. Great Britain was born as a Protestant state under a Stuart king, James I.

Notes

CHAPTER ONE
The Fateful Step

1. *State Papers, Foreign*, I, 107.
2. *Elizabeth I: Collected Works*, 95.
3. *Italian Relations of England*, Sneyd, p. 20.
4. *Annals*, Hayward, 1.
5. *Carmen, Epithalamia tria Maria*, trans. Wrangham, 23.
6. *Images of a Queen*, Phillips, 15.
7. Ibid., 16.
8. *Burghley State Papers*, 71.
9. *Letters*, Labanoff I, 59.
10. *The History*, Camden, 10.
11. *Virgin Mother, Maiden Queen*, Hackett, 52.
12. *Dissing Elizabeth*, ed. Walker, 30.
13. *The Reign of Elizabeth*, Black, 15.
14. *Queen Elizabeth*, Mumby, 280.
15. *Fragmenta Regalia*, Naunton, 40.
16. *Annals*, 3.
17. Ibid., 2.
18. *Dictionary of National Biography*, 315.
19. Ibid., 315.
20. *Bible, Genesis* 3:16.
21. *The Peloponnesian War*, Thucydides, 2.45.
22. *Elizabeth I: Collected Works*, 70.
23. Ibid., 52.
24. *Calendar of State Papers Venetian*, Vol. 7, p. 167 (24 March 1560).
25. *The History*, Camden, 39.
26. *Annals*, Hayward, 6–7.
27. *The History*, Camden, 53.
28. *Annals*, Hayward, 10–11.
29. *State Papers, Venetian*, VII, 6.
30. *State Papers, Spanish*, I, 7.
31. Ibid., 19.
32. *Elizabeth I: Collected Works*, 58.
33. *State Papers, Venetian*, VII, 3.
34. Ibid., 11 (23 January 1559).

35. *The History*, Camden, 18.
36. *The Queen's Conjurer*, Woolley, 60.
37. *State Papers, Venetian*, VII, 3.
38. Ibid., 12.
39. Ibid., 17.
40. *Annals*, 16.
41. *State Papers, Venetian*, 12.
42. *Annals*, 16.
43. *Elizabeth I: Collected Works*, 53.
44. *Annals*, 6.
45. Ibid., 7.
46. *Acts and Monuments*, Fox, 223.
47. Ibid., 224.
48. Ibid., 239.
49. Ibid., 240.
50. *Annals*, 18.
51. *State Papers, Spanish*, I, 51.
52. *State Papers, Venetian*, VI, 17.
53. For a close discussion of what exactly happened at Elizabeth's coronation see *The Coronation of Queen Elizabeth*, ed. Reginald L. Poole, *English Historical Review*, Vol. XXII, Longmans, Green and Co., 1907, pp. 650–73.
54. *The Coronation of Queen Elizabeth*, ed. Poole, 670.
55. *State Papers, Spanish*, I, 37.
56. *State Papers, Spanish*, I, 25.
57. Labanoff, 59.
58. *Sadler's State Papers*, I, 379.
59. Ibid., 380.
60. *State Papers, Venetian*, VII, 17.
61. *State Papers, Spanish*, I, 17.
62. *Elizabeth and Mary*, Mumby, 229.
63. *Elizabeth I: Collected Works*, 59.
64. Ibid., 51.
65. *The History*, Camden, 39.

CHAPTER TWO
The Disappointment of Kings

1. *History and Chronicles of Scotland*, Lindsay of Pitscottie, I, 406.
2. *Leviticus*, xx, 21.
3. *State Papers, Venetian*, IV, 873.
4. *Anne Boleyn*, Sergeant, 52.
5. *Ballads from Manuscripts*, ed. Furnivall, 374; quoted in *Anne Boleyn*, Warnicke, 126.
6. *Anne Boleyn*, Warnicke, 166.
7. *Camden Miscellany*, XXX, vol. 39, 1990, Lancelot de Carles, 1536, in Introduction to "William Latymer's Chronickille of Anne Bulleyne," 37.
8. *Girlhood of Queen Elizabeth*, Mumby, 3.
9. Ibid., 4.
10. *State Papers, Henry VIII*, XIII, XI, p. 132.

11. *State Papers, Spanish*, IV, 40.
12. *State Papers, Henry VIII*, IX, 187.
13. *State Papers, Foreign*, I, 530.
14. *State Papers, Venetian*, V, 27.
15. *Nursing Mirror*, 27 December 1962, "The Death of Queen Catherine of Aragon," MacNalty, 275; *Henry VIII*, Scarisbrick, 334 note 3.
16. *State Papers, Spanish*, V, 19.
17. *Anne Boleyn*, Sergeant, 261.
18. Ibid., 27.
19. *State Papers, Spanish*, IV, 824.
20. *Anne Boleyn*, Sergeant, 272.
21. Ibid., 284.
22. *State Papers, Foreign*, I, 529.
23. Ibid., 527.
24. *Witchcraft in Tudor and Stuart England*, Macfarlane, 170.
25. *Dictionary of National Biography*, I, 1061.
26. *State Papers, Henry VIII*, XII, 339.
27. *Hamilton Papers*, I, 358.
28. *State Papers, Henry VIII*, XVII, 657.
29. *State Papers, Spanish*, VI, 189.
30. *Sadler's State Papers*, I, 88.
31. *The Youth of Queen Elizabeth*, Wiesener, I, 14.
32. *Sadler's State Papers*, I, 61.
33. Ibid., 228.
34. Ibid., 228.
35. Ibid., 250.
36. Ibid., 253.
37. Ibid., 289.
38. *State Papers*, Henry VIII, V, 355.
39. *Histoire d'un Capitaine Bourbonnais au XVIe siècle*, Jacques de la Brosse, 1485–1562, ses Missions en Ecosse, de la Brosse 320–1, cited in *Mary of Guise*, Marshall, 139.
40. *Hamilton Papers*, II, 325.
41. *Elizabeth I: Collected Works*, 5.
42. *Elizabeth I: The Word of a Prince*, 37.
43. *Elizabeth I: Collected Works*, 9.
44. Ibid., 97.
45. Ibid., 10.
46. Ibid., 15.

CHAPTER THREE
The Education of Princes

1. *Actes and Monuments*, Foxe, 116.
2. *The History*, Camden, 10.
3. *Annals*, Hayward, 46.
4. *Childhood of Queen Elizabeth*, Mumby, 29.
5. *The Six Wives of Henry VIII*, Fraser, 365.
6. *Burghley State Papers*, 96.

7. Ibid., 95.
8. Ibid., 102.
9. Ibid., 96.
10. Ibid., 99.
11. Ibid., 99.
12. Ibid., 96.
13. Ibid., 96.
14. *Elizabeth I: Collected Works*, 17–19.
15. *The Whole Works of Roger Ascham*, ed. Giles, I, 272–3.
16. *Elizabeth I: Collected Works*, 21.
17. *Burghley State Papers*, 62.
18. Ibid., 69.
19. Ibid., 69.
20. Ibid., 70.
21. Ibid., 70.
22. Ibid., 70.
23. Ibid., 71.
24. Ibid., 102.
25. Ibid., 89.
26. Ibid., 89.
27. Ibid., 70.
28. Ibid., 108.
29. Ibid., 108.
30. *Elizabeth I: Collected Works*, 32–34.
31. *Burghley State Papers*, 108.
32. *The Sayings of Queen Elizabeth*, Chamberlin, 3. This was taken from the often unreliable seventeenth-century biographer Leti.
33. *Hamilton Papers*, II, 9 August 1548.
34. *Balcarres Papers*, III, 132; *English Historical Review*, XXII, ed. Poole, 47.
35. *Balcarres Papers*, III, 122: *English Historical Review*, XXII, 49.
36. *Additions aux Mémoires de Castelnau*, I, Le Laborier'ere; *The Brood of False Lorraine*, Williams, I, 50.
37. *Balcarres Papers*, III, 19, *English Historical Review*, XXII, ed. Poole, 44.
38. *Lettres de Diane de Poitiers*, Guiffrey, 34–5; *English Historical Review*, XXII, ed. Poole, 49.
39. *Mary Queen of Scots*, Fleming, 19.
40. *Balcarres Papers*, II, *The Love Affairs of Mary Queen of Scots: A Political History*, Hume, Nash, 39.
41. *English Historical Review*, XXII, ed. Poole, 48.
42. *Balcarres Papers*, III, 130.
43. *The Love Affairs of Mary Queen of Scots: A Political History*, Hume, 41.
44. *La Premiere Jeunesse de Marie Stuart*, de Ruble, 181; quoted in *Mary Queen of Scots*, Fraser, 91.
45. *Lettres*, Labanoff, VII, 277.
46. *Queen in Three Kingdoms*, ed. Lynch, 39.
47. *Lives of the Queens of Scotland*, Strickland, III, 31.
48. *Lives of the Queens of Scotland*, Strickland, II, 136.
49. Labanoff, I, 9–10.
50. *The Love Affairs of Mary Queen of Scots: A Political History*, Hume, 46 note.
51. *Latin Themes of Mary Stuart Queen of Scots*, ed. Montaiglon, 34.

Index

A NOTE ON THE TYPE

This book was set in Janson, a typeface long thought to have been made by the Dutchman Anton Janson, who was a practicing typefounder in Leipzig during the years 1668–1687. However, it has been conclusively demonstrated that these types are actually the work of Nicholas Kis (1650–1702), a Hungarian, who most probably learned his trade from the master Dutch typefounder Dirk Voskens. The type is an excellent example of the influential and sturdy Dutch types that prevailed in England up to the time William Caslon (1692–1766) developed his own incomparable designs from them.

Composed by North Market Street Graphics,
Lancaster, Pennsylvania

Printed and bound by Berryville Graphics,
Berryville, Virginia

Designed by Soonyoung Kwon